Medical Humanities

This textbook brings the humanities *to* students in order to evoke the humanity *of* students. It helps to form individuals who take charge of their own minds, who are free from narrow and unreflective forms of thought, and who act compassionately in their public and professional worlds. Using concepts and methods of the humanities, the book addresses undergraduate and premed students, medical students, and students in other health professions, as well as physicians and other health care practitioners. It encourages them to consider the ethical and existential issues related to the experience of disease, care of the dying, health policy, religion and health, and medical technology. Case studies, images, questions for discussion, and role-playing exercises help readers engage in the practical, interpretive, and analytical aspects of the material, developing skills for critical thinking as well as compassionate care.

Thomas R. Cole is the McGovern Chair in Medical Humanities and Director of the McGovern Center for Humanities and Ethics at the University of Texas Medical School at Houston. Dr. Cole has published many articles and several books on the history of aging and humanistic gerontology. His *The Journey of Life: A Cultural History of Aging in America* (1992) was nominated for a Pulitzer Prize. His book, *No Color Is My Kind*, and accompanying film, *The Strange Demise of Jim Crow* (1997), were nominated for a National Humanities medal. His work has been featured in the *New York Times*; on National Public Radio, Voice of America, and PBS; and at the United Nations.

Nathan S. Carlin is Associate Professor at the McGovern Center for Humanities and Ethics and Director of the Medical Humanities and Ethics Certificate Program at the University of Texas Medical School at Houston. He has coauthored two previous books, *Living in Limbo: Life in the Midst of Uncertainty* (2010) and *100 Years of Happiness: Insights and Findings from the Experts* (2012). He has also published more than 100 journal articles, book chapters, and book reviews in about a dozen different journals.

Ronald A. Carson is Professor Emeritus at the Institute for the Medical Humanities, University of Texas Medical Branch at Galveston. He has received fellowships from the Institute on Human Values in Medicine, the Council for Philosophical Studies, and the National Endowment for the Humanities. He is an elected Fellow of the Hastings Center, a former president of the Society for Health and Human Values, and a recipient of that society's annual award. He has written many articles, chapters, and book reviews. He is coeditor of four books, including *Practicing the Medical Humanities: Engaging Physicians and Patients* (2003).

Medical Humanities
An Introduction

Thomas R. Cole
University of Texas Medical School at Houston

Nathan S. Carlin
University of Texas Medical School at Houston

Ronald A. Carson
University of Texas Medical Branch at Galveston

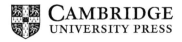
CAMBRIDGE
UNIVERSITY PRESS

CAMBRIDGE
UNIVERSITY PRESS

One Liberty Plaza, 20th Floor, New York, NY 10006, USA

Cambridge University Press is part of the University of Cambridge.

It furthers the University's mission by disseminating knowledge in the pursuit of education, learning, and research at the highest international levels of excellence.

www.cambridge.org
Information on this title: www.cambridge.org/9781107614178

© Thomas R. Cole, Nathan S. Carlin, and Ronald A. Carson 2015

First published 2015
4th printing 2017

Printed in the United Kingdom by Clays, St Ives plc

A catalog record for this publication is available from the British Library.

Library of Congress Cataloging in Publication Data
Cole, Thomas R., 1949– author.
Medical humanities : an introduction / Thomas R. Cole, University of Texas Medical School at Houston, Nathan S. Carlin, University of Texas Medical School at Houston, Ronald A. Carson, University of Texas Medical Branch at Galveston.
    pages   cm
Includes index.
1. Medical ethics.   2. Medicine and the humanities.   I. Carlin, Nathan, author.
II. Carson, Ronald A., 1940– author.   III. Title.
R724.C546   2015
174.2–dc23   2014020978

ISBN 978-1-107-01562-3 Hardback
ISBN 978-1-107-61417-8 Paperback

CONTENTS

FIGURES

PREFACE

This volume represents the first textbook in medical humanities. After decades of teaching in both medical and undergraduate schools, we wrote the book because there was still no single resource for interested students and faculty. While there are edited volumes in medical humanities, these books do not offer a coherent vision of or engagement with the field. We wrote this book to present such a vision and engagement.

We define medical humanities as *an inter- and multidisciplinary field that explores contexts, experiences, and critical and conceptual issues in medicine and health care, while supporting professional identity formation.* Our vision of the field is rooted in the humanistic educational ideal that aims to form individuals who take charge of their own minds, who are free from narrow and unreflective forms of thought, who are compassionate, and who act in the public or professional world. The book aims to stimulate and enhance both critical thinking and character development. We aim not only to bring the humanities *to* students but also to evoke the humanity *of* students.

The book is designed to serve as the backbone of courses in medical humanities, whether they are general introductory courses or more specialized courses (e.g., in literature, history, philosophy, religious studies, or social science). The chapters can be assigned sequentially or by section, or by the theme of a particular chapter (e.g., the history of medical technology, death and dying, just health care, or suffering and hope). The volume can be used with undergraduate students, graduate students, medical students, or other students in the health professions. It contains additional resources and materials that will engage advanced students and enable teachers to use the book in graduate courses.

The chapters are structured to maximize ease of comprehension and student interaction. All chapters open with an abstract and close with a summary. In addition, most chapters contain several distinctive elements: (1) a case study or primary source to engage students more actively in the practical, interpretive, or analytical aspects of the materials; (2) a visual image – a photograph, print, or painting – along with commentary, questions, and references for further exploration; (3) exercises for critical thinking and character formation, including questions for discussion, role playing, and suggested writing exercises; and (4) further resources, including suggested reading and viewing as well as lists of relevant journals and related organizations or groups.

Writing the book was a huge undertaking. It has grown out of many years of colleagueship and friendship, which has made the process more enjoyable (if such a thing can be said of writing a textbook) and has made possible consistency in perspective and authorship. Ronald A. Carson served as director of the Institute for the Medical Humanities at the University of Texas Medical Branch in Galveston and built it into a leading medical humanities research and teaching center from 1982 until 2005. Carson mentored Thomas R. Cole, who went to work at the Institute in 1982, where he founded the first graduate program in medical humanities and directed it for more than a decade. In 2004, Cole moved to Houston to found the McGovern Center for Humanities and Ethics at the University of Texas Health Science Center in Houston. There he began working with and mentoring Nathan S. Carlin, who went to work at the McGovern Center in 2009, where he serves as director of the Certificate Program in Humanities and Ethics and also administers a program in interprofessional ethics. Cole and Carson had wanted to write a textbook together for years. But writing a textbook is hard – and especially so for a field as diverse and vast as medical humanities – so they recruited Carlin (because he has somewhat of an architectural mind) to coauthor the book with them.

The book that you are holding took more than four years to produce. Perhaps a word about the process of writing this book is in order. Carlin proposed the original structure of the book, dividing it into four sections: history, literature, philosophy, and religion. This made intuitive sense to Cole and Carson, so the next step was to divide the writing assignments. Cole, a trained historian, wrote the history section. As a teacher of literature and medicine, Carson authored the literature section. And Carlin, a pastoral theologian, wrote the religion section. The philosophy section was divided among all three authors. With a few exceptions, this is how the writing assignments were determined. Cole also enlisted Benjamin Saxton to coauthor almost all of his chapters. Saxton, whose graduate training is in English, coauthored Chapters 1–6, 8, and 15. Carlin and Cole wrote the Introduction, and Cole wrote the Epilogue.

This book was a collaborative effort in every respect. For example, Carlin wrote the first draft of the book proposal and the introduction and then received feedback from Cole and Carson, revising accordingly. The rest of the book followed this basic process: an author would draft a chapter, then the others would critique it, and the author would make appropriate revisions. In the course of writing this book together, the authors engaged each other in numerous day-long meetings and conference calls, critiquing each other's work. At the last stage, Cole went through every chapter and made editorial suggestions to help unify the book. This collaborative process is what gives the book a more consistent voice than is possible in an edited volume. We should also note that we made every effort to remain faithful to various forms of academic discourse, meaning that sometimes the chapters vary – intentionally – in style. Finally, we should note another editorial decision to insert birth and death dates after the first mention of significant persons born before 1951.

There are many people to whom we are grateful, both personally and professionally, and many of these persons helped bring this book into being. We would like to thank Beatrice Rehl, Anastasia Graf, and Isabella Vitti at Cambridge University Press. Many colleagues provided extensive feedback, including Amir Cohen-Shalev, Jack Coulehan, Jason Glenn, Andrew Lustig, James Schafer, and Delese Wear – this book is much stronger for their feedback. Other colleagues also provided us with valuable feedback and/or insightful conversations along the way, including Andrew Achenbaum, Bryant Boutwell, Marcia Brennan, Howard Brody, Jai Gandhi, Brian Hurwitz, Tess Jones, Marc Kaminsky, Samuel Karff, Steven Linder, Rebecca Lunstroth, Laurence McCullough, Kate de Medeiros, William Metcalf Deutsch, Guy Micco, Kirsten Ostherr, Steven Smith, and Jeffrey Spike. Others provided other forms of help: Beatriz Varman served as a fact checker, Angela Polczynski looked up sources, and Shirley Pavlu helped with administrative responsibilities relating to the book's production.

We would also like to thank two research consultants in particular: Andrew Klein and William Howze. Klein helped with the team's early efforts to orient the project within the field of medical humanities and also contributed to the chapters' supplementary materials (e.g., case studies and abstracts). Howze, an art historian and video producer, selected the works of art that accompany each chapter and wrote the reflective essays embedded within the chapters. Howze previously collaborated with Cole to edit and produce the documentary *The Strange Demise of Jim Crow*. Many of the works come from the collections of the Museum of Fine Arts, Houston.

To secure images of works of art used in this book, a number of individuals were particularly helpful. For their generous assistance to select these works and to provide image files, we wish to thank Rebecca Dunham, Veronica Keyes, and Marti Stein. Several works are by Texas artists represented by Moody Gallery in Houston. For her enthusiastic support of this project, we wish to thank Betty Moody and her associates Lee Steffy and Adrian Page. Artist and teacher Gael Stack, also represented by Moody Gallery, offered thoughtful advice and heartfelt encouragement. For bringing to our attention the striking sculpture by Stephen De Staebler in front of the Moores Opera House at the University of Houston, we wish to thank Ted Estess, and for permission to reproduce it here, we are grateful to Michael Guidry and Jill Ringler. Without the patient assistance of rights managers at other museums, picture agencies, and similar organizations, it would not be possible to publish the range of images included in this book. In particular, we wish to thank Emma Aderud, Casey Anderson, John

Benicewicz, Capucine Boutee, Beth Braun, Natalie Costaras, Clive Coward, Joe Maloney, Emilie Le Mappian, Kay Menick, Katie Mishler, Maria Elena Murguia, Kathleen Mylen-Coulombe, Michael Slade, Alison Smith, Kajette Solomon, Alison Strum, and Judith Thomas.

We would like to thank the John P. McGovern Foundation for its continued support for the McGovern Center for Humanities and Ethics. And Cole would like to thank UTHealth, especially President Giuseppe Colasurdo, for a sabbatical during the 2013–2014 academic year.

Finally, a few dedications: Cole would like to dedicate this book to the memory of Christopher Lasch. Carlin would like to offer his dedication to Donald Capps. And Carson offers these words: "For Richard C. Reynolds and Melvyn H. Schreiber, to whom I owe a debt I cannot repay but herewith gratefully acknowledge."

Thomas R. Cole, Nathan S. Carlin, and Ronald A. Carson
January 2014
Houston, Texas

Introducing Medical Humanities

Of the physician's character, the chief quality is humanity, the sensibility of heart which makes us feel for the distress of our fellow-creatures.[1]

– John Gregory

INTRODUCTION

"I had undergone three heart surgeries in two years," Dr. Steven Hsi writes, "numerous tests, dozens of visits to doctors' offices, extended stays in hospitals and long recuperative periods at home."[2] He continues:

> I was 43 years old, a successful physician, married to a wonderful woman and blessed with two fine sons – all of it assaulted by a rare heart disease of such catastrophic power that it did more than threaten my life. It nearly destroyed my family.[3]

Dr. Hsi and his family coped well enough, he writes, but no one, especially none of his doctors, asked him what he felt to be the most important questions: "What has this disease done to your life? What has it done to your family? What has it done to your work? What has it done to your spirit?"[4] "Regardless of the considerable compassion and caring of many of them," Dr. Hsi concludes, "no one asked the questions that needed to be asked. I have come to believe this oversight was the single most grievous mistake my doctors made."[5] Existential questions – questions about the meaning of life and death – are essential to medicine. This book is designed to help you engage the most important questions.

During the last fifty years, health care professionals have struggled with dehumanizing tendencies created by the unprecedented success of modern medicine and the commercialization of the health care system – not enough time to see patients; technology that shifts attention to machines rather than patients; growing incentives to put profits above patients; a biomedical reductionism that attends to pain but not suffering and to disease but not illness; and institutional cultures that undermine the health of physicians, students, and others who work in academic health centers.[6] Progress in biomedicine has also generated a great deal of moral uncertainty and ethical conflict. Since the 1960s, the new fields of bioethics and medical humanities have grappled with problematic issues such as the protection of research subjects, the goals of health care, the definition of death, the rights of patients, the cessation of treatment, the meaning of illness, and the distribution of health care resources.[7] Most of these topics lie within the purview of bioethics, which emerged as a field alongside medical humanities and was perhaps indistinguishable from it at first. Indeed, medical humanities considers and addresses many of the ethical problems addressed by bioethics and in some ways overlaps with bioethics.[8] However, medical humanities tends to focus not on the practical resolution of ethical problems but on their cultural and historical contexts, emotional and existential dimensions, and literary and artistic representations.[9] Medical humanities is also closely linked to newer reforms in medical education that address the erosion of public trust and the impersonal quality of relationships between patients and health care professionals. These efforts focus on, for example, professionalism, the renewal of spirituality, relationship centered care, cultural competence, and narrative medicine.[10] Each of these fields or movements seeks to address the dehumanization of medicine – experiences such as Dr. Hsi's – in one way or another; medical humanities is the most intellectually comprehensive of them.

While we offer our own definition of and vision for medical humanities below, perhaps it is best to begin by defining not medical humanities but the humanities more broadly. What are the humanities? Why do they matter? And how did they come to be engaged with medicine and health care?

DEFINING THE HUMANITIES

What we now call the humanities first emerged during the fifth century BCE in ancient Greece, when teachers of rhetoric focused on preparing free men to participate in democratic deliberation, which required mastery of the arts of language rather than the art of war. Then, as now, success in the public realm required the capacity for rational argumentation and persuasion.

The word "humanities" derives from the Latin word *humanitas*. Originally, *humanitas* – in English "humanity" – meant humane feeling, which today could be known variously as sympathy, empathy, compassion, pity, concern, or caring. It was also understood as a kind of virtue inspired by knowledge or a quality of refinement achieved by intellectual accomplishment. *Humanitas* in this sense was similar to the Greek term *philanthropia*, that generous spirit toward others that ideally results from education in the liberal arts. In the fourteenth-century Italian Renaissance, Petrarch (1304–1374 CE) rediscovered the term *humanitas* from Cicero (104–43 BCE) and shaped it into the ideal of forming a person who combines humane feeling with liberal learning and action in the world.[11] This threefold ideal was built into the tradition of liberal education in the United States and reformulated by Lionel Trilling (1905–1975) as the "humanistic educational ideal"[12] in the 1970s, when it first came under severe criticism from postmodernist thinkers. The humanistic educational ideal can be seen in strong form today, for example, in the work of Martha Nussbaum (1947–).[13] For all its limitations, we support this ideal, which is wholistic, fluid, and individual. This bears repeating: humanistic education aims at forming a whole person who is compassionate, knowledgeable, and who acts in the world. It aims to educate the emotions as well as the intellect, to enhance compassion as well as critical thinking, and to encourage active engagement in public and/ or professional life.

Defining the humanities today is not a simple task. They can be defined by subject matter, disciplines, or methods, but no final definition is possible or perhaps even desirable. Defined by its subject matter, the humanities reflect on the fundamental question, "What does it mean to be human?" As the Rockefeller Commission on the Humanities put it in 1980: The humanities "reveal how people have tried to make moral, spiritual, and intellectual sense of a world in which irrationality, despair, loneliness, and death are as conspicuous as birth, friendship, hope, and reason. We learn how individuals or societies define the moral life and try to attain it, attempt to reconcile freedom and the responsibilities of citizenship, and express themselves artistically."[14] Defined by disciplines, the humanities range from languages, literature, history, and philosophy to religious studies, jurisprudence, and those aspects of the social sciences (in particular anthropology, sociology, and psychology) that emphasize interpreting, valuing, and self-knowing. Defined by their methods, the humanities have been delineated by Ronald S. Crane (1886–1967) as the cultivation of four essential "arts: language, analysis of ideas, literary and artistic criticism, and historiography."[15] Rather than mathematical proof or reproducible results (i.e., scientific ways of knowing), humanities scholarship and education are dedicated to understanding human experience through the disciplined development of insight, perspective, critical understanding, discernment, and creativity. Still it seems that disciplines, subject matter, and methods – whether taken separately or together – cannot adequately characterize the humanities because the humanities ultimately emphasize description, interpretation, explanation, and appreciation of the variety, uniqueness, complexity, originality, and unpredictability of human beings striving to know – and to change – themselves and their world.

Since the 1960s, a cascade of new intellectual movements and projects has broadened the scope of the humanities beyond its traditional boundaries to include what Cathy Davidson and David Goldberg call "interdisciplinary humanities"[16] (e.g., ethnic studies; age studies; gender studies; disability studies; cultural studies; media studies; science, technology, and information studies; and global studies). Medical humanities, and its emerging sibling health humanities, are among these interdisciplinary forms of study called into being by social needs and problems that cannot be adequately addressed within the boundaries set by traditional disciplines and/or methods.

THE ORIGINS OF MEDICAL HUMANITIES

Before the late nineteenth century, there were no great research universities or medical schools in the United States. Learned physicians were trained at European universities and were steeped in the classical tradition of humanistic education. Medical students in London, Edinburgh, Paris, Padua, and Vienna had to be well versed in Greek, Latin, and the classical liberal arts and were required to read the works of Galen (131–201) and Hippocrates (460–377 BCE), among other predecessors, in Latin. History – knowledge of and identification with medicine's vision of its past – was a central dimension of their professional identity and authority.[17]

Over the centuries, what we now call the humanities became more specialized and focused on pure scholarship, increasingly divorced from the life of feelings and of moral and public engagement. In the second half of the nineteenth century, this tendency toward pure scholarship was powerfully accelerated by German research universities, which emerged as the exemplar of specialized research in all areas of the arts and sciences. The dynamism and growth of knowledge embedded in the ethos of science replaced the preservation and transmission of tradition inherent in classically based education.

At the end of the nineteenth century, as more and more American medical students and physicians traveled to Germany to study in experimental laboratories and to learn about clinical specialties, biomedical science was rapidly displacing the old humanistic medicine as a source of identity and authority. When enthusiasts brought back the German model to new university medical schools in the United States, some began to advocate a new vision of medicine as an *exact* science. Yet when Johns Hopkins University Medical School (based on the German model) opened its doors in 1893, its most ardent advocates worried about excessive specialization, reductionistic thinking, commercialism, and moral drift. They worried, in other words, about the dehumanization of medicine. So it might be argued that medical humanities has its origin here, when men like William Osler (1849–1919) and John Shaw Billings (1838–1913) looked for a way of preventing science and business from taking the "soul" out of medicine. Indeed, Osler both embodied and articulated the holistic ideal of *humanitas* or humanistic education. For him, medicine was an art as well as a science; it was a calling rather than a business and required education of the heart as well as the head.

When neurosurgeon Harvey Cushing (1869–1939) spoke at the dedication of the first American professorship in the history of medicine at Johns Hopkins in 1929, he yearned for an idealized medical culture that was irrevocably lost: "Medicine has become so scattered and subdivided," he declared, "that there is a crying need for someone to lead it from the wilderness and bind it together."[18] Osler, Billings, Cushing, and others looked to history as the key to the revival of humane and morally centered medicine. This form of historically based medical humanism (which has its contemporary adherents[19]) had both strengths and weaknesses. On the one hand, its strength derived from its emphasis on cultivation – the learned education and identity formation of humane physicians. On the other hand, it was limited by a white, male, upper class exclusivity: there was no room for women, Jews, African Americans, or other minorities. In addition, the Oslerian "great man" version of medical history had no awareness of the multiple ways that the history of medicine can be told. Judged by the standards of contemporary scholarship, it was insufficiently critical and self-critical and was based as much on nostalgia as on the search for historical truth.

There is also a fascinating twist in the recent history of the humanities in general and the history of medical humanities in particular. At the same time that a historically minded medical humanism was developing in medical schools in response to the dehumanization of medicine, the humanities located in colleges and universities were distancing themselves from the tradition of Western humanism. Beginning in the 1960s, professional academics in the humanities largely severed their connection to the ancient tradition of *humanitas*. By and large, the mainstream professoriate distanced itself from ideals of individual cultivation and civic engagement. Indeed, some took the tradition of Western humanism itself to task, as they came to see the humanist tradition as the product of "dead white men" who had enjoyed privileged lives, ignored questions of power, and neglected issues of race, gender, and class (and, more recently, age and sexual orientation). They argued that the ideas, images, and concepts from the humanist tradition were little more than tools used to justify the domination of white European (and American) males over colonized populations, women, and people of color.[20]

Ironically, medical humanities in its current form began to take shape in the late 1960s and 1970s at precisely the time when university scholars in the humanities disciplines were distancing themselves from the term humanism and the curriculum of "great books" of the Western tradition.[21] The most prolific and influential proponent of medical humanism in this period was Edmund Pellegrino (1920–2013), a physician-reformer who chaired the Institute on Human Values in Medicine and later became president of Catholic University, and eventually served as chair of the President's Council on Bioethics.

In a paper delivered in 1976, Pellegrino noted that the term humanism had become slippery and difficult to define. Nevertheless, he pointed out, in some circles medical humanism had achieved the status of a "salvation theme," meant to absolve modern medicine of its "sins." The list of "sins" Pellegrino noted was a long but valuable specification of problems usually lumped together under the rubric of dehumanization: "overspecialization; technical; overprofessionalization; insensitivity to personal and sociocultural values; too narrow a construal of the doctor's role; too much science; not enough liberal arts; not enough behavioral science; too much economic incentive; a 'trade school' mentality; insensitivity to the poor and socially disadvantaged; overmedicalization of everyday life; inhumane treatment of medical students; overwork by house staff; deficiencies in verbal and nonverbal communication."[22] As a Roman Catholic, Pellegrino was mocking the salvific tendency among enthusiasts of medical humanism, and he articulated more modest goals: "Medical humanism is really a plea to look more closely at what medicine *should be*, and increasingly *seems not to be*. It encapsulates a pervasive ambivalence felt by even the most ardent devotees of modern medicine: Can we balance the promises of medical technology against the threats it poses to persons and societies? ... [Human beings] have always sensed that the more tools they forged and the more machines they built, the more they were forced to know, to love, and to serve these devices."[23] Pellegrino realized that the classical humanist training of Osler and his forbears was gone forever. So it was best, he thought, to abandon the attempt to make every physician "a Renaissance man." Instead, Pellegrino outlined three essential goals for the humanities in medicine (the term "medical humanities" did not come into widespread use until the 1980s and 1990s). First, the humanities would help clarify the ethical issues and values at stake in clinical decisions (through his efforts at the Institute on Human Values in Medicine, Pellegrino played a major role in establishing bioethics in the 1980s.) Second, the humanities would inculcate habits of critical self-examination. And third, the humanities would "confer those attitudes which distinguish the educated from the merely trained [professional]."[24] From Pellegrino's list and language of goals for the humanities in medicine, we can see that his vision contained much of the *humanitas* ideal (a personal integration of knowledge, compassion, and action in the world), expanded somewhat beyond the gentlemanly version of medical humanists in Osler's generation. What was new in Pellegrino's vision of humanistic education in medicine was his recognition of the need for scholarship and guidance from scholars trained in the disciplines of the humanities.

THE TERM "MEDICAL HUMANITIES": DEBATES AND PROBLEMS

The field of medical humanities can be conceptualized, theorized, defined, and debated indefinitely. We offer here a few of the major ways of thinking about the field as well as our own definition that will guide our presentation of and approach to the topics covered in this book.

A Field or Discipline?

Medical humanities, as noted, draws on many disciplines, including history, literature, philosophy, religion, anthropology, sociology, and other arts and sciences. One area of debate is whether medical humanities is a field or a discipline,[25] and whether it is multidisciplinary (i.e., uses various disciplines and approaches, *separately*, to examine a topic) or interdisciplinary (i.e., uses various disciplines and approaches that are *integrated* in some way to produce a new form of knowledge).[26] Our own position is that medical humanities is a field, not a discipline, and is both multidisciplinary and interdisciplinary. These distinctions and debates are important and helpful, but the key point is that medical humanities draws from many disciplines to examine issues related to the development and practice of medicine and health care. In this sense, it is similar to other fields such as religious studies or gender studies that utilize various disciplines and methods to study a subject such as religion or gender. What is different, however, is that medical humanities, unlike many other academic fields, has an essential practical component because all medical humanities knowledge carries implications for the care of patients, the professional development of students, the continuing education of residents and physicians, and/or the health of populations.[27]

The Problem of Exclusivity and Hierarchy

In the debate over the term medical humanities, one objection is that the term privileges doctors over other health professionals, such as nurses, dentists, and public health professionals. The term, it is argued, is hierarchical and patriarchal and reinforces certain undesirable qualities of cultures of medicine.[28] For this reason, some writers suggest the term "health humanities." This spirit of inclusivity and equality among the health professions, which we support, is reflected in journal titles such as *The Cambridge Quarterly of Healthcare Ethics* as opposed to the more restrictive and potentially hierarchical term *medical* ethics. In recent years, the British literary scholar and broadcaster Paul Crawford has championed the health humanities intellectually and organizationally.[29] And in 2014, Therese Jones, Delese Wear, and Lester D. Friedman (1945–) chose to title their comprehensive collection of essays *The Health Humanities Reader*.[30] While we support (and have ourselves published in the service of inclusivity and equality of the health professions[31]), we retain the term medical humanities. One reason is that the vast majority of scholarship in health humanities focuses on medicine. Another is a matter of scope; this is, in fact, a textbook in medical humanities, not health humanities. Although there is a good deal of material on public health and on nonallopathic forms of healing and care, this book is primarily about medicine. No book can be entirely comprehensive, and what we are introducing – medical humanities – might in fact someday become a subfield of health humanities. In taking this perspective, we will keep in mind this critique of power and hierarchy and will incorporate such critiques into various chapters.

The Tension between the Practical/Instrumental and the Intellectual/Critical

Within medical humanities, there is also an important tension between the instrumental justification for and the intellectual practice of the humanities – that is, the tension between using the humanities to produce more humane physicians and better patient care versus practicing the humanities to generate new knowledge, insight, and critical thinking. Anne Jones (1944–), in one of the first articulations and justifications of medical humanities, warned against the assumption that studying the humanities make students more humane: "This expectation makes me very uncomfortable," she wrote in 1987, because "[t]his expectation is a burden, not just for literature, for but for all of the humanities. We all hope that it will [make one more humane], but there have been too many examples to the contrary for me to believe in any guarantee."[32] In addition, some scholars oppose the very idea of an instrumental justification for the humanities in medicine and the health professions.[33] In arguing against a purely instrumental approach, Jones, Wear, and Friedman write in support of "the intellectual practice of the humanities, which enables and encourages fearless questioning of representations of caregivers and patients in all their varieties, challenges abuses of power and authority, and steadfastly refuses to accept the boundaries that science sets between biology and culture."[34] We believe that the tension between the practical/instrumental and the intellectual/critical forms of medical humanities is a necessary and healthy one that will continue to energize this field where the growth of knowledge fuels both cultivation and critique.

CONCEPTIONS AND GOALS OF MEDICAL HUMANITIES

In "Medicine and the Humanities – Theoretical and Methodological Issues," Raimo Puustinen, Mikael Leiman, and Anna Maria Viljanen note several conceptions of medical humanities that we find to be helpful. They point out that in the last half century, there has been a growing recognition in clinical medicine that, as they put it, "the biological approach alone cannot address the various human phenomena that physicians encounter in their everyday practice."[35] In other words (and as noted above), there has been a paradigm shift away from what might be called medical reductionism to medical holism, where patients are not reduced to diseases and bodies but rather are seen as whole persons in contexts and in relations. The chief theorists of this paradigm shift in clinical medicine cited by these authors are George Engel (1913–1999) and his biopsychosocial model of medicine,[36] Eric Cassell (1928–) and his conception of personhood,[37] and Edmund Pellegrino and David Thomasma (1939–2002) and their philosophy of medicine.[38] Another important and more recent author here is the physician Christina Pulchalski, who has developed a model of spiritual care.[39]

Puustinen, Leiman, and Vijanen further note that along with the movement from medical reductionism toward medical holism, students and reformers in medical education in the 1960s began to question the more or less exclusive biomedical curricula of medical schools. Over the next thirty years, in "response to this criticism, courses on social sciences and humanities were included in medical curricula at many of the medical facilities in the United States."[40] They continue:

> It was assumed that incorporating humanities as a part of medical training could bridge the gulf between science and human experience. The aim was to educate more humane physicians and to recapture the notion of medicine as a learned profession.[41]

While Puustinen, Leiman, and Vijanen do not elaborate on these three goals of medical humanities – bridging the gulf between science and human experience; educating more humane physicians; and recapturing the notion of medicine as a learned profession rather than vocational training – we offer some critical reflection on these goals and specify a fourth goal that is moral and political.

Medical Humanities as Bridge between Science and Experience

For most of the twentieth century, clinical medicine focused almost exclusively on biomedicine and discounted psychological and social information. Challenging pure biomedicine in 1980, Engel articulated a biopsychosocial model of medicine that legitimized this data and refined the ways of gathering and integrating it into patient care.[42] Clinical medicine, Engel insisted, is not only biomedical; it is also psychological and social. Health and illness, in other words, cannot be understood with lab results alone but only by attending to the patient's psychological experiences and social environments. Engel's biopsychosocial model of medicine is a medical humanities enterprise in that it attempts to bridge the gulf between science and experience. Likewise, in 1991, Cassell also attempted to legitimate non-biomedical forms of data – specifically, data related to suffering as distinguished from pain (bodies feel pain, Cassell argues, but persons suffer[43]). Both of these medical humanities approaches are clinically focused.[44] Additionally, efforts to bridge the gulf between science and experience have been greatly strengthened by the philosophical distinction between "disease" and "illness."[45] Disease – what happens to the body – is understood through science. Illness – what the person experiences – is understood through eliciting patient stories,[46] and by asking questions such as, "What has this heart disease done to your family?" Providing opportunities for conversations about such questions makes possible emotional and spiritual *healing*, whether or not physical *curing* (to use another important distinction) is possible.[47]

Other such approaches to bridging science and medicine, to name only a few, include reading stories about illness and pathographies,[48] watching films and theatrical representations of illness,[49] and viewing paintings and sculptures that represent the body in pain.[50] A related theoretical question to the relationship between science and experience is whether medical humanities ought to be regarded as integrating science and humanities in medical education, or, rather, whether humanities simply should be added to a largely scientific medical education.[51]

Medical Humanities as Educating More Humane Physicians

One reason that medical humanities gained footing in medical schools was that, until recently, medical educators and administrators more or less assumed that teaching ethics courses would result in bolstering ethical and professional behavior. When it became clear that this assumption was not necessarily correct, a new and broader emphasis on teaching professionalism emerged. Jack Coulehan (1943–) offers several reasons why. The first is that the widespread use of expensive technology in medicine often led to a conflation of self-interest and altruism. CT scans and MRIs, for example, are powerful tools, but their unnecessary use drives up the costs of health care and reveals a conflict between patients' needs and physicians' self-interest. Another reason is that patients were becoming less satisfied with what technology was actually offering (e.g., when end-of-life care only prolongs suffering). Patients also began to complain that specialists seemed more interested in looking at their diagnostic machines than in listening to them. A third reason, which is related to the first, involves the rise of commercialism in medicine, an observation that patients had about the shift in the larger culture of medicine. The development of for-profit hospitals, managed care organizations, and physician relationships with pharmaceutical and biotech companies created new and visible conflicts-of-interest. In American medicine's commercialized culture, it became clear that students needed to be taught and physicians needed to be reminded that they are professionals and that a profession is morally grounded in altruism and fiduciary responsibility.

We suggest that medical education needs to provide some guidance about what being a professional means in the new culture of medicine, that is, how to be compassionate and humane caregivers operating realistically under the modern pressures of medicine.[52] Medical humanities attempts to cultivate certain key virtues in and values of medicine, such as altruism, empathy, compassion, as well as certain qualities of mind by means of various reflective, interpretive, and reflexive practices.[53] Educating more humane physicians, we further suggest, also means that medical humanities attempts to provide guides, tools, and venues for self-care.[54]

Medical Humanities as Recovering a Learned Profession

In a 1974 *JAMA* article, Pellegrino, whose path-breaking work we have referred to above, wrote, "In the growing litany of criticism to which our profession is increasingly exposed, there is one that in many ways is more painful than all the rest. It is the assertion that physicians are no longer humanists and that medicine is no longer a learned profession."[55] He continued, "The assertion is painful because there is some truth in it."[56] Physicians during the twentieth century became much more technically competent, but, in many cases, this came at the cost of their interpersonal skills – the professionalism critique – and at the cost of their broader education in culture and the arts. According to Pellegrino, "Society has the right to require that physicians be competent, that they practice with consideration for the integrity of the person, and that *some* of them also be educated men [and women] who can place medicine in its proper relationship to culture and society."[57] Writing as a physician and for physicians and medical educators, Pellegrino suggested that medical humanities ought to be, at least in part, an intellectual pursuit in and of itself. We would reemphasize our point above, namely, that medical humanities scholars, many of whom are not physicians, should also pursue intellectual questions simply for their own sake as well as a means of promoting medicine as a learned profession.

Medical Humanities as Moral Critique and Political Aspiration

Worthy as it is, the goal of recovering medicine as a learned profession is fraught with social and political problems. It is one thing to argue that medical education should involve more than vocational training – that it should also include critical reflection, the growth of self-knowledge, and exposure to historical, literary, philosophical, and religious inquiry – but it is quite another to specify what those materials are and to avoid uncritically reproducing the tradition of white, male, European, and American privilege. This challenge is squarely embedded in our textbook, which is necessarily based on scholarship and primary materials produced largely in this tradition. We therefore present this introduction to medical humanities fully aware that we are limited by our own perspectives, expertise, and knowledge, and by linguistic skills limited to the languages of English and German. We invite readers and scholars to respond with their own perspectives, interests, and expertise.

   Be that as it may, becoming learned means becoming critical *and* self-critical. It means, for example, learning about the shadow side of medical progress and accomplishment. So in this book, on the one hand, we focus on medicine's scientific and technological accomplishments, its highest moral and professional norms, but, on the other hand, we focus on the unintended consequences of medical progress, on the human exploitation often involved in producing medical knowledge, and on biopolitics and the problems inherent in medical power.

Another way of putting this is to say that medical humanities involves moral critique and political aspiration – that is, medical humanities is not only a scholarly and educational pursuit but also a moral and political (though not monolithic or sectarian) enterprise as it aims at goals such as respect for individuals, protection of the vulnerable, tolerance of difference, care for those in need, equality of access, and the pursuit of justice and health in the broadest sense. As noted above, like gender studies (which developed in response to sexism) or humanistic gerontology (which developed in response to ageism), medical humanities grew up alongside and in association with the patient's rights movements in the 1960s and 1970s. It is concerned with questions of power and justice, broadly conceived. This conception of medical humanities attends to political and social structures as they pertain to medicine, as well as to how medical knowledge is used and produced, and whose interests it serves. In this sense, then, medical humanities engages in critical moral inquiry about medicine and it asks what justice requires.[58]

OUR DEFINITION

Having made some initial comments on the origins, goals, and conceptions of medical humanities, we offer here our own definition of the field and its implications for how the book is organized and presented. We define medical humanities as *an inter- and multidisciplinary field that explores contexts, experiences, and critical and conceptual issues in medicine and health care, while supporting professional identity formation.* Our definition, then, has four main components:

1. Context;
2. Experience;
3. Conceptual and critical analysis; and
4. Formation.

We do not suggest that every piece of scholarship in medical humanities attends to all four of these categories; a given piece may focus exclusively on, say, context. Still, these categories, taken together, enable us to make sense of various bodies of knowledge that constitute the field. A few words about each of these categories are in order.

Context

By exploring *context* we mean using various disciplines, such as history and anthropology, to understand the cultural and temporal dimensions of medicine. The questions explored can be economic, social, political, and cross-cultural in nature. How is, for example, medicine practiced under the National Health Service in the United Kingdom, and how does that differ from the social organization of health care in the United States? When was the Hippocratic Oath developed, and whose interests and purposes did it serve in ancient Greece? How did medieval Christianity affect European views of disease? What is Buddhism's view of suffering, and how does that affect Buddhists' ideas about health and disease? In what ways did modern medical education evolve in the United States and Europe, and what problems did it entail for student learning?

By exploring contexts, we also mean paying attention to issues of gender, race, class, age, and sexuality with regard to medicine, particularly to how knowledge is produced regarding these categories. What, for example, is the relationship between sexism and gynecology? In what ways do cultural assumptions about gender and sexuality literally shape human bodies, as in, for example, practices related to intersexed infants? How do the economics of the pharmaceutical industry affect the construction of mental illnesses? Medical humanities aims to contextualize medical practice, health care, and the experience of illness by exploring continuity and change over time and by offering contemporary descriptions and analyses across cultures and societies.

Experience

By exploring *experience* we mean using various disciplines, such as literature and psychology, to understand how it feels to be a patient, a doctor, or a community affected by an epidemic. These questions are usually local and personal in nature. What, for example, is it like to suffer lymphoma? What is it like to live with diabetes? What does a heart attack do to one's family life, one's work life, one's sex life, and one's faith life? What is it like to be a medical student? What is it like to be a woman in medical school? What does a nurse feel like when treated badly by a physician? What is it like to be an African American or a Muslim on the faculty of an American medical school? What is it like to be a white male in these contexts? What is it like to be dying? What is it like to recover from a given illness? Such experiences can also be social, communal, or global, such as living with the effects of climate change or dying during epidemics of the plague, the Spanish Flu, or HIV/AIDS.

The arts – short stories, poetry, novels, memoirs, sculptures, music, painting, film, theater, and other forms – can help us address these "experience-near" questions in concrete and particular ways. These questions often may have very little to do with decision making in medicine, but they are essential for educating the emotions and strengthening the capacity to care and the ability to empathize with those who suffer. Other disciplines and approaches, such as phenomenology and religious studies, also can shed light on the experiences of illness, medical education, doctoring, and other forms of health care. Medical humanities attempts to examine narratives of medicine and frameworks of meaning in whatever form they may take.

Conceptual and Critical Analysis

By *conceptual and critical analysis* we mean using various disciplines, but primarily philosophy, to define and to clarify ideas, terms, and issues related to medicine. This type of inquiry is often more abstract than scholarship related to context and experience, and asks questions such as: What is health? What is disease? Or what is the difference between disease and illness, or between healing and curing? This line of inquiry also asks teleological questions about medicine, such as: What are the goals of medicine? The tools of analytic philosophy can be of great value in clarifying the meaning of various words and concepts, and the tools of Continental philosophy, too, can be of great value in examining how medical concepts are related to structures of power and discipline. Medical humanities aims to examine various ways of knowing and participates in the conceptual analysis of medical knowledge.

Conceptualization in medical humanities is often intimately linked to critical analysis. In examining various concepts of disease, for example, we become aware that many newly named diseases (e.g., erectile dysfunction, alcoholism, or attention deficient hyperactivity disorder) can be understood as "normal" human experiences. In bioethics, learning about the principle of justice can lead one to question the fairness of the allocation of scarce health care resources in the United States or any other country. If one sees relief of suffering as the primary goal of medicine, it follows that procedures that briefly prolong life at the cost of suffering and financial expense will be called into question.

Formation

By *formation* we mean kinds of pedagogy, forms of scholarship, and ways of teaching and learning that cultivate self-awareness and commitment to the welfare of others. We see the dimension of what is now called "professional identity formation"[59] as a specific contemporary expression of the educational tradition of *humanitas* – which, as noted, aims at forming individuals who personally embody a combination of knowledge, compassion, and action in the public or professional world – in this case, medicine and health care. Medical humanities assumes that the practice of medicine is not, or should not be, merely technical. Physicians are not merely plumbers of the body; they are, or should be, caring and compassionate witnesses to the experiences of patients and their significant others and to their own experiences.

It should be noted that one reason for the emphasis on formation arises from recent concern about lack of empathy and professionalism in medicine. These concerns can be intimated by means of the following questions: Why is it that studies of the empathy of medical students show that their empathy *decreases* as they progress through medical school?[60] How can this be understood, and how can it be addressed? How can and do medical students cultivate a professional identity? In what ways can medical students, physicians, and others in health care cultivate strategies of resilience? How can medical students deal with the joys and sorrows of medicine, of witnessing a baby open her eyes for the first time or of witnessing an older man close his eyes for the last time?

It should also be noted that the language of formation derives from the context of theological education, where students are formed to be ministers in a particular religious tradition or denomination.[61] Formation in secular medical schools or for other students in medical humanities looks different – doctors are not pastors or priests. Nevertheless, their professional identity and personality depends in no small way on their emotional, moral, and spiritual (by "spiritual" we mean the dimension of the self which is linked to an individual's highest values or source of meaning) growth. We suggest that the educational materials that students engage should form them to aspire to become persons who attend to the suffering as well as the flourishing of patients and others.

THE LAYOUT OF THIS BOOK

Our book has four main sections: History and Medicine; Literature, the Arts, and Medicine; Philosophy and Medicine; and Religion and Medicine. While the issues and questions covered in this book reach across formal disciplinary boundaries, we decided to organize the book according to these four disciplinary categories rather than by a list of topics and problems. These ways of knowing help us focus on the topics at hand – what we want to know, what we need to know, and what is worth knowing – and they serve as rough guides for organizing contemporary scholarship on inherently interdisciplinary topics and for presenting it in a clear and compelling way. The book can, of course, be read in whatever sequence that readers, teachers, and students find useful.

We conceptualize bioethics as a part of the larger project of medical humanities, even as we realize that, under this conception, scholarship in bioethics constitutes the majority of work in medical humanities. Such topics include the ethics of abortion, end-of-life care, futility, organ transplantation, the allocation of resources, confidentiality, and capacity, to name only a few. Since there are many books and textbooks on bioethics, we have chosen to weave bioethics throughout the text and emphasize, instead, other topics in medical humanities.

This book, as noted, has four sections – a word about each. The History and Medicine section includes such essential topics as the doctor-patient relationship, the history of disease, the history of technology, the history of medical education, the health of populations, and the history of death and dying. The Literature, the Arts, and Medicine section draws heavily on major works, themes, and methods in the fields of literature and the arts. Attention is given to narrative medicine as well as film criticism and the visual arts. This section uses various genres to present, evoke, narrate, and interpret experiences such as suffering, healing, aging, dying, doctoring, and being a student. The Philosophy and Medicine section uses various tools and perspectives in philosophy to clarify definitions and goals of medicine. This section works with classic categories in philosophy – such as ontology, epistemology, and ethics – as they pertain to medicine. Topics include definitions of disease and of health, the goals of medicine and the role of technology, philosophy and bioethics, and medicine and power. The Religion and Medicine section draws on religious studies and theology to address existential and spiritual issues as well as practical and cultural issues in medicine. Topics include religion and health, religion and bioethics, the relationship between religious experience and the experience of illness, religious and cultural issues in patient care, and suffering and hope.

THE CENTRAL ARGUMENT OF THE BOOK

While the book is a textbook and its chief aim is to provide an overview of and introduction to medical humanities, we nevertheless do have a point of view. Put simply, it is this: Medical practice and medical education today are the victims of their own success. The very science and technology that have brought enormous advances in curing disease, relieving suffering, and extending longevity have also outstripped medicine's moral bearings and overwhelmed the human dimensions of caring and learning. Medical humanities attempts to restore the balance, to help re-humanize medicine. But (and this is one of the original contributions of this book) it is not just patients who suffer from the dehumanization of medicine. Under today's stressful conditions of practice, physicians, nurses, allied health professionals, biomedical scientists, and students all find themselves at risk for becoming alienated or separated from the ideals that drew them to health care in the first place. These conditions lead to high rates of burnout, depression, impairment, and even suicide. Hence the re-humanization of medicine involves enhancing, restoring, and attending to the humanity of students and caregivers as well as of patients.[62]

Medical Humanities: An Introduction addresses the dehumanization of medical education and practice in two ways: First, it focuses on the experiences of medical students and of physicians by using materials from memoir and social research to film and literature. Second, it actively involves students and encourages them to generate their own ideas and contributions. Each chapter, therefore, contains visual images, case studies, and exercises designed to engage students actively in their own intellectual, moral, emotional, and existential learning – that is, their own identity formation. We hope that the intellectual discipline involved in analyzing, interpreting, contextualizing, imagining, writing, and narrating will help strengthen students' capacities for self-understanding, caring, empathizing, attending to, and deliberating. As noted above, one aim of the book is to teach students the content of medical humanities in order to help them learn and develop habits of mind and heart – "professional identity formation" – demanded in today's highly scientific, technological, impersonal, and stressful world of health care. The other more traditional aim is simply to convey up-to-date knowledge about medical humanities. Both goals are appropriate for undergraduate students as well as students in professional schools and practicing physicians. And both goals will help students ask the most important questions, those Dr. Hsi wished his physicians would have asked.

EXERCISES FOR CRITICAL THINKING AND CHARACTER FORMATION

QUESTIONS FOR DISCUSSION

1. What interests you about medical humanities?
2. How would you define medical humanities?
3. What is the purpose of medical humanities?

4. What topics and ways of knowing would you like to pursue in medical humanities?

SUGGESTED WRITING EXERCISE

This exercise will take fifteen minutes. Write, without any concern for style or grammar, about when you first realized that you had a strong interest in medicine. If you decided that you would one day go to medical school, write about when you came to this decision and what you felt like. If you are unsure about a life in medicine, write about this uncertainty. What attracts you to medicine? What makes you ambivalent about medicine? If you do not plan on going to medical school, what interests you about medicine or about health care?

SUGGESTED VIEWING

The Doctor (1991)
Commentary: http://litmed.med.nyu.edu/Annotation?act
    ion=view&annid=10006

SUGGESTED LISTENING

Yale University Medical School Article on Music and
    Medicine, with Audio Links: http://yalemedicine.yale.
    edu/ym_ws98/music/music_01.html

FURTHER READING

Jerome Groopman, *How Doctors Think*
Sandeep Jauhar, *Intern*

Danielle Ofri, *What Doctors Feel*
Emily Transue, *On Call*

ADVANCED READING

Gary, Belkin. "Moving Beyond Bioethics: History and
   the Search for Medical Humanism." *Perspectives in
   Biology and Medicine* 47 (2004): 372–385.
Rafael, Campo. "The Medical Humanities, for Lack of a
   Better Term." *JAMA* 294 (2005): 1009–1011.
Ronald A. Carson, Chester R. Burns, and Thomas
   R. Cole, eds. *Practicing the Medical Humanities:
   Engaging Physicians and Patients.*

Francis, Peabody. "The Care of the Patient." *JAMA* 88
   (1927): 877–882.
Edmund D. Pellegrino. "Educating the Humanist
   Physician." *JAMA* 227 (1974): 1288–1294.
Johanna, Shapiro, Jack Coulehan, Delese Wear, and
   Martha Montello. "Medical Humanities and Their
   Discontents: Definitions, Critiques, and Implications."
   Academic Medicine 84 (2009): 192–198.

ONLINE RESOURCES

Bio-Ethics Bites
http://podcasts.ox.ac.uk/series/bio-ethics-bites
Blog Post by Johanna Shapiro, "Toward the Clinical
Humanities"
http://humanizingmedicine.org/toward-the-clinical-
humanities-how-literature-and-the-arts-can-help-shape-
humanism-and-professionalism-in-medical-education/
The Healing Muse
www.thehealingmuse.org

The International Health Humanities Network
www.healthhumanities.org
The New York Times: Well Blog
http://well.blogs.nytimes.com/
New York University School of Medicine – Literature,
Arts, and Medicine Database
http://litmed.med.nyu.edu/Main?action=new

JOURNALS

The Art of Medicine Section in *The Lancet*
Journal of Medical Humanities

Medical Humanities
Medical Humanities Review, 1982–2005

PART I
History and Medicine

PART OVERVIEW
History and Medicine

The history of medicine is the oldest discipline of medical humanities. Actually, medical history, whose origins lie in the late nineteenth century, long predates and helps us to understand medical humanities, which is barely forty years old. At the turn of the twentieth century, distinguished American male physicians and educators first turned to history as a means of humanizing medicine. Although there are now serious doubts, debates, and visions, and the field has grown more diverse, this mission in medical education has remained remarkably stable.[1] With the recent rise, however, of medical humanities and bioethics, and the professionalization of the field of the history of medicine, the influence of history in medical education has been overshadowed by ethics, literature, the social sciences, and to a growing extent, religion/religious studies and media studies. One counterbalancing trend has been public policy historians such as Susan Reverby (1946–), David (1937–) and Sheila Rothman (1939–), David Rosner (1947–), Gerald Markowitz (1944–), and Howard Markel who have been active in developing programs in history, ethics, and public health, housed outside of medical schools.[2] Another is the testimony of physicians whose lives and work have been shaped by their knowledge of history.[3] History is an exciting and essential way of understanding medicine and health care, which are never static but rather constantly changing and evolving.

History offers perspectives on our present moment. It is where we turn to understand where we have been, where we might be going, and why. It is a field that identifies the guiding values, social contexts, power relationships, and contested cultural meanings that have formed the world we live in. In this overview of part one, we look briefly at the history of the history of medicine in the United States; identify the field's major scholarly trends and some of its most prominent authors; and summarize the basic themes and topics contained in the following six chapters.

As we saw in the Introduction, John Shaw Billings (1838–1913) and William Osler (1849–1919) of the new Johns Hopkins Medical School were among the first to articulate concern about the human costs of the new scientific medicine that they championed and led. As early as the 1890s they saw that biomedicine by itself was incapable of producing well-rounded and humane physicians who practiced the art as well as the science of medicine. They worried that specialization, excessive commercialization, and scientific reductionism were leading to a cultural impoverishment and undermining medicine as a genuinely learned profession. Osler, who helped found the Johns Hopkins Hospital Historical Club in 1890, embodied the both the new science and the classical humanist tradition in medicine and tried to harmonize them in his 1919 address, "The Old Humanities and the New Science." Osler was well versed in the ancient Greek and Latin authors, and he turned to history as a moral compass as he used medico-historical cases in his clinical instruction and pointed "to the great physicians of the past" in order to inspire and to exemplify professionalism. Osler called for veneration and engagement with the classical texts in science and medicine. He encouraged the formation of medical history clubs and also of personal book collections, library archives for rare book collections, and the cultivation of a literary humanism marked by gentlemanly honor and the assumption of moral wisdom.

The first professorship in the history of medicine in the United States was established at Johns Hopkins in 1929. At its dedication, the neurosurgeon Harvey Cushing (1869–1939) descried the scattered and divided nature of specialized medicine. Cushing envisioned medical history and historical libraries as a means of unifying and inspiring all elements of "our great profession."[4] William Welch (1850–1934), the first dean of the medical school and proponent of experimental and laboratory medicine, claimed that history of medicine was "the one subject of humanistic study properly falling within the scope of medical teaching."[5] Abraham Flexner (1866–1959), the prominent reformer of medical education, also worried about the loss of cultural values and saw medical history as a counterweight. By 1937, almost three-fourths of U.S. medical schools offered instruction in the history of medicine. It was a style of history taught by men who were not trained in history, focusing on classic medical texts, great male physicians, and the cultivation of humane clinical care.

In the 1930s and 40s, physician-historians such as Henry Sigerist (1891–1957),[6] Erwin Ackerknecht (1906–1988),[7] and George Rosen (1910–1977)[8] were among the first to write serious and scholarly histories of medicine, initiating a new brand of medical history focusing on the social rather than the individual dimensions of medicine. Rather than engaging the classics, cultivating gentlemanly learning and the individual doctor-patient relationship, these historians focused on public health, health care systems, and the social forces affecting health. As John Harley Warner explains, "Sigerist grew impatient with American physicians who cultivated a romanticized image of the doctor rather than assuming responsibility for bringing the fruits of scientific medicine to the entire population."[9] A contemporary physician-historian in this tradition who writes on issues of public health is Howard Markel.[10]

By the 1960s and 70s, amidst a larger cultural critique of medical power and authority, history again emerged as an antidote to the dehumanization of medicine. This time, the Oslerian style of medical humanism was itself a historical tradition, now reiterated by physicians such as Edmund Pellegrino (1920–2013). While Pellegrino critiqued the term "humanism" for its vagueness, he acknowledged that it still carried enough appeal to help attract support for the teaching of human values and the art of medicine.[11] History was now only one of several disciplines engaged in this scholarly and educational work. In the 1980s, the terms "medical humanities" and "bioethics" appeared in academic medical journals. And non-physician scholars specializing in literature, philosophy, and the social sciences as well as history were hired onto medical faculties.

In this context, a new generation, trained as social historians and not as physicians, wrote from a perspective that was sharply critical of the health care system, the authority of physicians, and the biomedical establishment. Pioneered by Susan Reverby and David Rosner,[12] the new social history of medicine established itself within traditional history departments and in medical schools with its quest to move, "beyond the great doctors" and beyond the great books of medicine to explore issues of power, race, class, and sex in the delivery of health care.

Recently, dually trained physician-historians such as Joel Howell, Kenneth Ludmerer (1947–), Howard Markel, and Robert Martinsen (1947–2013), have followed in the footsteps of Sigerist, Rosen, and Ackerknecht. However, the broader shift in the field has been a growing awareness of the need for collaboration between physicians and historians. As Howard Kushner puts it, "If a history of medicine uninformed by biomedical knowledge is untenable, then medical research uninformed by historical context is incomplete."[13] The following chapters provide readers with information about major historical developments in six topic areas:

- The doctor-patient relationship;
- Disease;
- Medical education;
- Medical technology;
- The health of populations; and
- Death and dying.

The information provided under these rubrics is "true" – that is, it is based on facts that historians have established and agreed upon. Empirical facts, however, always stand in need of interpretation. For example, we know roughly when the Hippocratic Oath was written and what its stated values are. But what are we to make of this? Do we emphasize that the Oath is the source of many of the essential professional values of medicine? Do we acknowledge that it is unclear whether most ancient physicians read or even knew about the Oath? Do we emphasize that it was taken by a small number of men who entered into a closed, almost familial guild? To take another example, we know that the invention of the stethoscope in 1817 marked a powerful diagnostic advance by making heart sounds more audible and precise. But it also had the effect of putting an instrument between the physician and the patient, which initiated a pattern whereby technological advances tended to undermine the personal relationship between doctor and patient. And for a final example, take the discoveries of bacteriology in the late nineteenth century, when physicians and scientists first discovered the microorganisms that are the causal agents of infectious diseases such as tuberculosis and cholera. Do we emphasize the accomplishments of the great men who established scientific laboratories and made these discoveries? Or do we emphasize that these diseases flourished in crowded urban conditions of poor hygiene, sanitation, and nutrition and could sometimes be prevented or controlled with improved diet and public health measures? In making interpretive choices, we have been mindful of various perspectives.

Condensing such a vast field of scholarship is a daunting task. Omissions or mistakes are inevitable, and we apologize in advance for both. In addition to choosing the six topics listed above, we have limited our coverage primarily to western Europe and the United States. In general, each topic is organized according to the following periods: antiquity, medieval, early modern, Enlightenment, modern medicine, and contemporary medicine. Our chapters are necessarily based on syntheses of what other historians have written.

Very few contemporary scholars have attempted to write about the history of medicine as a whole. One exception is Roy Porter's (1946–2002) monumental *The Greatest Benefit to Mankind.*[14] Another is Jacalyn Duffin's (1950–) *History of Medicine: Second edition*, which she refers to as scandalously short.[15] The work of Charles Rosenberg[16] (1936–) is so extensive and ranges across so many topics that Rosenberg might almost be considered to have covered the history of American medicine as a whole. Other comprehensive works are written by multiple scholars: for example, Mark Jackson's edited volume, *The Oxford Handbook of the History of Medicine.*[17] By and large, we have relied on seminal figures who have written on the topics of interest to us: e.g., Robert Baker (1937–) and Laurence McCullough's (1947–) edited *Cambridge World History of Medical Ethics*;[18] Gunther Risse[19] (1932–) and Charles Rosenberg[20] on the history of the hospital; Ellen More (1946–) on women in medicine;[21] Thomas Bonner[22] (1923–2003) and Kenneth Ludmerer on medical education;[23] Stanley Reiser (1938–) on medical technology;[24] John Harley Warner on therapeutics;[25] Paul Starr (1949–) on the rise of corporate medicine;[26] David Rothman on the recent history of bioethics;[27] William O'Neil[28] (1917–) and J. N. Hays[29] (1938–) on epidemic disease; Dorothy Porter on public health;[30] and Phillippe Ariès[31] (1914–1984) and Emily Abel[32] (1942–) on death and dying.

In attempting to make sense of historical developments in medicine, we have struck a balance between two primary interpretive frameworks: history as appreciation of scientific and technological progress; and history as a critique of self-interest, power, inequality, and the social determinants of health. Both frameworks support the educational goals of cultivating a humanistic sensibility and developing critical thinking. We encourage readers to challenge our interpretations and develop new ones as a means of actively engaging in the production of historical knowledge.

1 The Doctor-Patient Relationship

One of the essential qualities of the clinician is interest in humanity, for the secret of care of the patient is in caring for the patient.

Francis Weld Peabody[1]

ABSTRACT

This chapter explores the history of the doctor-patient relationship in the West. Beginning with a discussion of how this relationship was conceived in antiquity, it examines how the Hippocratic ideal became associated with the Christian duty to care for the sick and needy; how the beliefs of antiquity were questioned by Renaissance physicians who wanted to "see for themselves"; how professional ethics based on virtue arose in the eighteenth century in response to increased competition between practitioners; and how the modern ideal of the doctor-patient relationship based on a personal connection, careful physical examination, and trust arose in the late nineteenth century. Then, with a focus on recent cultural and structural challenges to this modern model, it considers how we might reconstruct the doctor-patient relationship to address recent challenges, such as patients' skepticism about doctors' genuine concern for them as people and doctors' concern with patients' lack of compliance and growing challenges to their authority.

INTRODUCTION

There has, of course, never been a single or monolithic "doctor-patient" relationship. Relationships between doctors and patients – even as they have changed over time – have always varied depending on the social class, race, and gender of both patients and doctors. From antiquity to contemporary medicine, relations between doctors and patients have also been affected by religious authority and belief, by competition in the health care marketplace, and by science and technology.

In light of contemporary concerns about the goals of medicine and quality of care, we focus here on ideals, particularly on the moral norms and ethical frameworks that have guided the doctor-patient relationship. From the medical morality of the Hippocratic tradition to the bioethics revolution of the 1970s, medicine has been characterized by the desire for healing and caring. In the second half of the nineteenth century, this desire took a modern form: the widely shared ideal of a strong, personal, trusting relationship between patient and doctor. Since the 1960s, the modern model of the doctor-patient relationship has been culturally challenged and structurally weakened, creating discontent for both patients and doctors. In the midst of health care reform and escalating costs in the United States, the reconstruction of the doctor-patient relationship remains a work in progress.

DOCTORS IN ANTIQUITY

Historical knowledge of Greek medicine begins with the appearance of ancient texts written by doctors who first supported themselves with fees earned in Athens during the time of Plato (427–347 BCE). There were no schools, no licenses, and no state recognition or monopoly. Instead, doctors plied their trade in the marketplace alongside exorcists, bonesetters, priests, gymnasts, and others competing for attention and income. Medicine however, *was* a male monopoly, and doctors were educated through a loose apprenticeship in which a student became a virtual member of his teacher's family.

Hippocrates (c. 460–377 BCE) stands at the pinnacle of ancient Greek medicine. In his view, medical knowledge should be grounded in observation, experience, and reason rather than in supernatural explanations of health and disease. The central notion in the Hippocratic Corpus – a collection of about sixty diverse texts that were actually written by others – is that health is equilibrium and disease is disequilibrium. Achieving health, then, meant restoring balance within the body and between the body and the environment. In spite of its secular outlook, Hippocratic medicine lived comfortably in the world of the Greek gods – including Aesclepius, the god whose rituals of healing are discussed in the next chapter.

The ancients clearly understood the healing power of the doctor-patient relationship. "Where there is love of man, there is also love of the art [of medicine]," noted one Hippocratic text: "Some patients [achieve] … their health simply through contentment with the goodness of the physician."[2] Hippocratic medicine also stressed that the doctor should always act in the best interests of the patient – what contemporary bioethics now calls the principle of beneficence[3] – and that the "good" patient should honor the physician and always follow his instructions. Modern notions of patient choice or autonomy would have made no sense inside the paternalistic world of the Hippocratics. Nor was there any awareness that the interests and values of the doctor and patient might diverge, since both wanted the same thing – recovery and cure.

However, not all doctor-patient relationships were equivalent. In ancient Athens, the medical treatment of slaves was quick and tyrannical; the purpose of care was to get them back to work. According to one Hippocratic text, some citizens could not be trusted to follow a physician's instructions and, thus, should be given an "emetic or a purge or cautery or the knife."[4] Free and rich patients were given time and attention – but not always the truth. Rather than offering their honest opinion, physicians were instructed to "promise to cure what is curable and to cure what is incurable."[5]

The Hippocratic Oath, perhaps the most famous text in the history of medicine, articulates moral values that continue to guide medicine and health care today. Some of the Oath's stipulations – the prohibition of drugs for abortion or suicide, for instance – remain controversial. Others – the prohibition of surgery and the promise of care for the teacher and his family – have been relegated to the dustbin of history. Despite its endurance and fame, the Hippocratic Oath emerged in a culture profoundly different from our own – a culture that accepted slavery and the subordination of women with no moral qualms. We still do not know who wrote the Oath, whether Hippocrates himself ever saw it, or whether most ancient physicians agreed with it, lived by it, or even knew about it.[6] Nevertheless, the Hippocratic Oath remains the historical lodestar for medicine's basic professional values.

CASE STUDY: THE HIPPOCRATIC OATH

The Hippocratic Oath, perhaps the most famous text in the history of medicine, articulates moral values that continue to guide medicine and health care today. The Oath discusses the privacy and confidentiality of patients, the primacy of patients' welfare, and a prohibition of sexual contact with or exploitation of patients.

"I swear by Apollo the physician, and Asclepius, and Hygieia and Panacea and all the gods and goddesses as my witnesses, that, according to my ability and judgment, I will keep this Oath and this contract:

To hold him who taught me this art equally dear to me as my parents, to be a partner in life with him, and to fulfill his needs when required; to look upon his offspring as equals to my own siblings, and to teach them this art, if they shall wish to learn it, without fee or contract; and that by the set rules, lectures, and every other mode of instruction, I will impart a knowledge of the art to my own sons, and those of my teachers, and to students bound by this contract and having sworn this Oath to the law of medicine, but to no others.

I will use those dietary regimens which will benefit my patients according to my greatest ability and judgment, and I will do no harm or injustice to them.

I will not give a lethal drug to anyone if I am asked, nor will I advise such a plan; and similarly I will not give a woman a pessary to cause an abortion.

In purity and according to divine law will I carry out my life and my art.

I will not use the knife, even upon those suffering from stones, but I will leave this to those who are trained in this craft.

Into whatever homes I go, I will enter them for the benefit of the sick, avoiding any voluntary act of impropriety or corruption, including the seduction of women or men, whether they are free men or slaves.

Whatever I see or hear in the lives of my patients, whether in connection with my professional practice or not, which ought not to be spoken of outside, I will keep secret, as considering all such things to be private.

So long as I maintain this Oath faithfully and without corruption, may it be granted to me to partake of life fully and the practice of my art, gaining the respect of all men for all time. However, should I transgress this Oath and violate it, may the opposite be my fate."[7]

1. What values are embedded in the Oath?
2. Which values remain important today?
3. Which values are controversial? Which do you accept or reject – and why?
4. What aspects of the Oath are no longer relevant to clinical practice today?

In the Rom[an era], Galen (c.1[3]0–201 CE) [adopted] and revised the Hippocratic legacy [laying the foundations of] a learned medicine that would flourish for m[...] [...] [attributed] to Galen reveal a vast erudition [...] ranging from discussions of bloodletting to [...] the soul. Like Hippocrates, [...] believed the [...] best interest of the patient. [...] conceal the truth from his p[atient]. Not[ing] how even the best physicians har[med] patients with their treatm[ent], Galen coined the maxim "Above all do [no] harm" and elevated it to a [...]

[handwritten annotation: women excluded from elite medicine — extension of love into medicine —]

MEDIEVAL RELIGIOUS NORMS: THE RESPONSIBILITY AND AUTHORITY OF DOCTORS

B[y the] fifth century, when Christianity was official[ly] sanctioned by the Roman E[mpire, the tradition of Hippocratic] medicine – which had previously been intertwined with the cult of the healing god Aesclepius – was adapted into a monotheistic framework. In church-dominated medieval communities, salvation of the soul took precedence over the health of the body. Yet, although the priest was elevated over the doctor, religion and medicine enjoyed a relatively peaceful coexistence.[9] The New Testament was in no way hostile to secular healing: According to the Gospels, Jesus performed some thirty-five miracles and his disciple, Luke, was called "the doctor."[10] The church fathers thus adopted Hippocratic ideals even as they transformed the classical virtues of compassion and philanthropy into the ethical obligations of Christian physicians.[11]

Perhaps the most important medical legacy of early Christianity is the extension of love – *agape* – into a communal obligation to care for the sick and the needy. The priority of caring over curing transformed (at least in theory) the social position of those with certain diseases (e.g., leprosy and mental illness) from stigmatized, outcast sinners into vulnerable souls in need of help and attention. This ethos also resulted in church-sponsored institutions – the first hospitals – that served the poor, the needy, and the sick.

Medical practitioners in the Middle Ages fell into two basic groups: tradespeople and clerical (or elite) practitioners. Tradespeople sold drugs and their services like any other trade. They solicited patients on the streets or worked in monasteries, municipalities, or royal households, and received cash, clothing, gifts, or an annuity for their services. Clerical practitioners were paid by the church or by powerful patrons to dispense healing just as they dispensed the sacraments – as a charitable duty. Practitioners, then, came from various walks of life and were engaged in many forms of work. Medieval England, for example, was filled with brewers who practiced surgery, abbots who delivered babies, friars who penned medical books, and even a chancellor of the exchequer who doctored the king.[12]

Because they were excluded from the university and the clergy, women could not practice elite medicine. They were, however, allowed to function in the "middling" levels of society where, like other tradeswomen, they could practice without interference from the church. Female midwives presided over childbirth along with neighbors and relatives who supported the mother. Other female healers learned their craft from a male member of their family. The Benedictine mystic Hildegaard of Bingen (1098–1179) was a rarity who, in her position as abbess of Rupertsberg, practiced medicine and wrote medical texts.[13]

MEDICINE AND THE RENAISSANCE

During the fourteenth century, a cultural and intellectual rebirth spread across Europe. Beginning in Italian cities, especially Florence, writers and philosophers celebrated the classical traditions of Greek and Roman culture. This revival of the arts and of humanistic learning aimed to purify European culture by returning to its origins. Humanist scholars provided new Greek translations of classical medical texts, corrected Arabic and medieval Latin errors, and made more texts available to more readers – a process facilitated by the invention of the printing press around 1440. The humanist scholar Desiderius Erasmus (1466–1536), for example, introduced a new edition of Galen's work. Although personally skeptical of doctors, Erasmus and other humanists promoted medical learning that was rooted not only in classical texts but also in the physical body and the material world.

In translating Greek, Roman, and biblical texts into the vernacular, Erasmus, Martin Luther (1483–1546), and others did more than merely recover texts from the classical tradition. They also insisted that any literate person could read and interpret for themselves. The same impulse toward individually validated knowledge can be seen in the term *autopsy* (seeing for oneself), which privileges observation over authority in the search for truth. As laypeople took this message to heart, self-diagnosis and self-therapy grew popular in Renaissance culture. Word of a successful healer spread quickly through a personal network of kin, friends, and neighbors. People who called on physicians were also quite ready to switch to alternative healers – or to trust their own judgment – if the official treatment did not work. "I have been aggravated by a bad disease for about three years," one Italian woman said in 1698. "I sought treatment from several people, including a certain Anna, later decided to stay away from her, and I went instead to the barber in San Mamol.... Thereafter I have treated myself."[14]

Seeing for oneself applied to scientific knowledge as well as medical treatment and self-care. Galenic or Hippocratic texts – both of which had taken on a dogmatic authority – were no longer immune from critique. Through careful observation and dissection, for example, Andreas Vesalius (1514–1564) demonstrated that Galen's anatomical findings were taken from animal dissections – especially apes – rather than from human bodies. By relying on these dissections, Galen had, in Vesalius's opinion, committed anatomical errors in his descriptions of muscles, bones, and internal organs.[15]

Historical change is never linear, however, and there is no single march toward truth. In spite of Vesalius's findings, Galenism was so entrenched that some scholars refused to accept the possibility that their great master could be wrong: one declared that, if there was an error in Galen's texts, then the fault lay with the corpse and not with Galen.[16]

THE ENLIGHTENMENT AND THE ORIGINS OF MODERN MEDICAL ETHICS

Ironically, the birth of modern medical ethics in eighteenth-century Britain resulted not from pure idealism but from intense competition between practitioners.[17] Those who were sick had many reasons to doubt both the competence and the ethics of British medical practitioners. Medical colleges often sold degrees to anyone willing to pay. Without medical societies or licensing boards, people simply declared themselves "regular" physicians. Unrestrained by contemporary notions of informed consent or autonomy, professors and students used indigent and working-class patients as mere props for teaching or for scientific experiments. Infirmary professors commonly advanced their careers and doctors pursued their economic self-interest at the expense of patients' welfare.[18]

In response, the medical faculty at the University of Edinburgh formulated a new ideal for the well-educated physician: caring for what would later be called "the whole person." John Gregory (1724–1773) transformed professional ethics from an older ethos based on gentlemanly honor to a modern medical ethics based on virtue. Gregory and his Edinburgh colleagues also stressed that scientific practice was a moral obligation. Between 1731 and 1867, all medical students signed a revised version of the Hippocratic Oath, which required physicians to:

> … practice physic *cautiously, chastely and honourably,* and faithfully to procure all things conducive to the health of the bodies of the sick, and lastly, never, without great cause, to divulge anything that ought to be concealed, which may be heard or seen during professional attendance. To this oath let the Deity be my witness.[19]

Gregory's medical lectures, which were rapidly translated into Spanish, French, Italian, and German, also shaped English physician Thomas Percival's (1740–1804) *Medical Ethics* (1803), which marked the first time that term appeared in the English language. Percival worked at the Manchester Infirmary where he developed a code of conduct to reduce conflict between warring physicians. His writings revolutionized medical morality and anticipated the framework for modern Anglo-American professional ethics – in particular, the view that the physician is obligated to respect the *"feelings and emotions"* of patients, including the choice to refuse treatment.[20]

In 1847, the year in which it was founded, the American Medical Association adopted a Code of Ethics based largely on Percival's writings. The AMA Code was a mixture of self-interest and altruism. Members agreed not to advertise, sell, or prescribe secret remedies and not to consult with "irregular" physicians – defined as persons whose practice was based on dogma rather than genuine medical knowledge. The Code also obligated physicians to treat patients with attention, steadiness, humanity, delicacy, and equality. Physicians were enjoined to practice confidentiality and were prohibited from performing abortions. They were not to abandon dying patients, and – in a new moral norm – patients were not to abandon their physicians without giving "reasons for so doing." Finally, members were obligated to care "cheerfully and freely" for indigent patients and, in times of epidemic disease, work to relieve suffering – even at risk to their own lives.[21]

Historians have shown that the ideals of the AMA Code of Ethics were sometimes honored in principle rather than in practice, which helps explain the popularity of alternative medicine, home remedies, and the large market for patent medicines in the nineteenth century. (It is safe to assume that unethical practices would not have been prohibited if they were rare.) Nevertheless, these norms – amalgamated from the Hippocratic, Jewish, and Christian traditions as well as from Gregory, Percival, and nineteenth-century American medicine – provided essential professional and ethical standards for the doctor-patient relationship.

This framework remained intact until the 1970s when the bioethics revolution emphasized the ethical and legal rights of autonomous patients.[22]

TRIUMPHS AND TRIBULATIONS: THE MODERN DOCTOR-PATIENT RELATIONSHIP

Throughout most of the nineteenth century, sick people only sought help for serious problems such as coughing up blood, a bowel obstruction, broken bones, or disabling symptoms of trauma. By the later part of the century, patients went to physicians for a wider range of ailments with less severe symptoms: colds, bruises, cuts, or skin problems. White, affluent urban dwellers – especially women and their children – increasingly submitted to the care and authority of white male physicians.[23] Since a doctor's livelihood depended on fees paid for his services he was under pressure to satisfy the desires and expectations of patients – not always an easy task among the well-to-do. As George Bernard Shaw (1856–1950) put it sardonically in *The Doctor's Dilemma* (1906): "The doctor who has to live by pleasing his patients in competition with everybody who has walked the hospitals, scraped through the examinations and bought a brass plate, soon finds himself prescribing water to teetotalers and brandy or champagne jelly to drunkards; beefsteaks and stout in one house, and 'uric acid free' vegetarian diet over the way."[24]

The practices of university-trained doctors gradually spread from well-to-do urban dwellers to other segments of the population.[25] Although many early twentieth-century patients visited doctors in their offices, house calls predominated. The "modern" doctor was above all a generalist, a family doctor. When a middle-class family member was sick, the doctor traveled to the patient's home on horseback, in a horse-drawn carriage, or by automobile. Relationships between doctors and patients were usually based in local communities and built up over many years. They were face to face, entailed a careful physical examination, and, at least ideally, based on trust. Patients did not expect to be cured, but they did expect to be cared for and comforted. Luke Fildes's (1843–1927) famous painting *The Doctor* (1891) offers an idealized image of the doctor that appeared at the end of the nineteenth century.[26] (See Figure 1.)

What state of mind does the doctor's pose convey? Consider the child's parents in the dark back corner. What does the mother's pose convey? Put your head down on your desk and clasp your hands as she has. Can you imagine what emotions she might be feeling?

Every work of visual art makes use of composition, lighting, and form to engage the viewer. For example, is it significant that an oil lamp throws light on the doctor's silk hat, frock coat, and wing collar while daylight illuminates the birdcage, the flowers on the windowsill, and

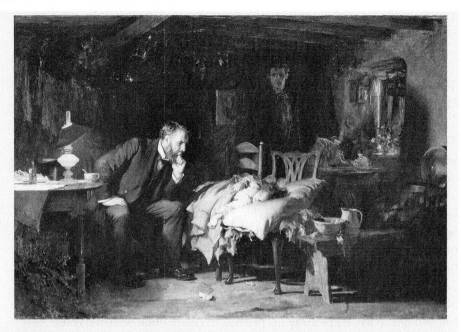

Figure 1. *The Doctor*, exhibited 1891, Sir Luke Fildes 1843–1927. Presented by Sir Henry Tate 1894. © Tate, London 2013.

the parents of the child patient? Notice the two chairs that the child is lying across. One is elegant with expressive curves and carving; the other is plain and common. What story do they tell? Why would the artist include them?

The Doctor, painted by the British artist Sir Luke Fildes, was exhibited by the Tate Gallery in 1891. Half a century later, in 1947, the American Medical Association used the painting in a misleading campaign against President Harry Truman's call for national health insurance. The AMA campaign literature claimed that "voluntary" health insurance would "Keep Politics Out of This Picture." Can you relate this 1940s debate to the opponents of the Affordable Care Act of 2010 who claimed that "Obamacare" would not let you choose your own doctor? Does *The Doctor* represent a typical doctor-patient encounter in the United States shortly after the Second World War?

The painting is now in the collection of the Tate Gallery, London. For more information visit: www.tate.org.uk. Look closely at the reproductions of works of art in this book and ask questions about them. Examine works of art wherever you encounter them.

What actually happened during these doctor-patient encounters? At its best, the most striking feature of this relationship, from the patient's perspective, was its familial quality. One elderly woman from Boston declared that, after seeing her physician throughout her adult life, "he was like a father to me."[27] Indeed, this man had been her parents' doctor, then her doctor as a child, and he continued to treat her into adulthood. In another woman's experience, doctors "came to the home with a little black bag and they sat by your bedside. And they knew your mother and father. They called them by their first name."[28] Such character-izations indicate the deep sense of kinship that – at its best – many patients felt with their doctors.

Physicians, too, left behind some interesting anecdotes.[29] In his *Horse and Buggy Doctor* (1938), American physician Arthur Hertzler (1870–1946) recalls one instance of old-fashioned surgical heroism. He had driven three hours to attend to a boy suffering from empyema (pus in the lungs):

> Grabbing a scalpel I made an incision in his chest with one stab – he was too near death to require an anesthetic. As the knife penetrated his chest, a stream of pus the size of a finger spurted out, striking me under the chin and drenching me. After placing a drain in the opening, I wrapped a blanket around my pus-soaked body and spent another three hours reaching home.[30]

This account offers a glimpse of the sometimes gruesome and imprecise nature of patient care. Hertzler himself admitted that "I can scarcely think of a single disease that doctors actually cured during those years ... [all that could be done was] to relieve suffering, set bones, sew up cuts and open boils on small boys."[31] Indeed, despite scientific and technological advances, doctors remained pow-erless against many lethal infectious diseases such as tuberculosis, diphtheria, meningitis, and scarlet fever until the 1940s and 1950s.

The major advances in clinical medicine occurred in rapidly changing urban hospitals, whose numbers grew from fewer than 200 in 1873 to almost 5,000 in 1923.[32] While a nineteenth-century physician could spend his entire career without stepping foot in a hospital, no physician after 1925 would graduate from medical school without substantial hospital training. Thanks to new methods of busi-ness administration, increasingly effective surgery, new techniques of antisepsis, scientific laboratories, trained nurses, and scientifically educated physicians, the hospital emerged as an essential institution in urban American life.[33] Surgeons, no longer relegated to a lower status by their traditional physician colleagues, now commanded their own separate operating rooms, performing procedures on as many as 50 percent of all hospital patients.[34] Hospitals, like orphanages and old-age homes, had traditionally been designed for long-term care of the poor and dependent. In contrast, the modern hospital increasingly treated paying patients who expected to leave the hospital in better shape than when they entered it.

Some doctors were able to move between the domestic world of nineteenth-century private practice and the rapidly growing medical realm of the twentieth century. Physician Richard Cabot (1868–1939), for instance, practiced both in his home office and in the Massachusetts General Hospital, where he advanced clinical hematology, medical education, and social work. Toward the end of his career, Cabot chaired the Department of Social Ethics at Harvard. He cham-pioned the role of hospital social workers long before it became common to understand patient care as a team effort.[35]

Despite its undeniable benefits, the "new" scientific medicine of testing and diagnostic precision stood in tension with the "old" medicine of compassion and care. Sir William Osler (1849–1919), who served as professor of medicine at Johns Hopkins University, may have overstated his case to make a point. "The good physician treats the disease," he wrote, "but the great physician treats the patient. . . . It is much more important to know what sort of patient has the disease than to know what sort of disease the patient has."[36] Harvard professor Francis W. Peabody (1881–1927) also warned that specialization and laboratory-based methods of diagnosis threatened the personal bond between doctor and patient. In prophetic comments, he noted that patients in advanced university hospitals were sometimes passed from one specialist to another, submitted to multiple tests, and treated for unimportant conditions. Tests and technology were no substitute for personal relationships, Peabody insisted. In his most memorable phrase, Peabody went to the core of the issue: "One of the essential qualities of the clinician is interest in humanity, for the secret of care of the patient is in caring for the patient."[37]

DOING BETTER AND FEELING WORSE

Peabody's fears were not fully realized until the second half of the twentieth century when a chronic dissatisfaction settled over both doctors and patients. Thanks to public health advances and improved dietary measures, medicine had dramatically reduced deaths from infectious disease and extended life for the masses. Yet even as doctors saved people who would have died only a generation earlier, an increasingly biomedical focus on disease threatened the care of the patient. People were "doing better and feeling worse."[38] As accelerated scientific innovations made their way into the offices of family doctors and onto the wards of a new generation of hospitals, observers worried that the personal and trusting clinical relationship was in jeopardy.[39] Patients felt skeptical about doctors' genuine concern for them as people, while doctors were troubled by patients' lack of compliance and growing challenges to their authority.

By the 1960s and 1970s, the modern ideal of the doctor-patient relationship was threatened by structural changes in medicine and shifting cultural values that challenged the authority of physicians. After World War II, with suburbanization and the increased mobility of the public, the medical profession was split increasingly into three distinct sectors of practice. First was the expanding group of doctors and trainees who, working in medical schools and hospitals, focused on research and training. Second were the office-based private practitioners who had moved to the suburbs in large numbers and whose standard of living rose dramatically. The third sector included doctors who occupied the lowest rung on medicine's ladder of prestige because they worked in rural areas, the inner city, or in state institutions.[40]

The growth of medical specialties in the United States also limited the availability of family doctors and primary care physicians, further reducing personal and lasting relationships between doctors and patients. This stood in marked contrast to Britain, where primary care doctors served as gatekeepers to specialists under the National Health Service. By the end of the twentieth century, primary care doctors in the United States rarely saw their own hospitalized patients, who were attended by new specialists known as "hospitalists." Under these conditions, patients and families could easily find themselves bewildered and without guidance from a physician who knew them or their relative as a whole person.

Perhaps the strongest force in the decline of the modern ideal of the doctor-patient relationship, however, was the corporate transformation of American medicine. Since the 1980s, the doctor as an independent professional and solo practitioner has given way to the doctor as an employee of hospitals, health maintenance organizations, group practices, and for-profit health care corporations.[41] In addition, the growth of private insurance payments, and the passage of Medicare and Medicaid in 1972 generated new sources of income and introduced another impersonal actor: the "third-party payer."

To be sure, medicine has always been a business as well as a profession. There has never been a "golden age" of the doctor-patient relationship. Nevertheless, until the 1980s, doctors had never been employees of large organizations dominated by bureaucratic authority and motivated by commercial gain. In addition, large pharmaceutical companies, device makers, and biotech companies also began hiring physicians as consultants and researchers – leading patients to suspect that some doctors were motivated by greed.[42]

In the first decades of the twenty-first century, such problems show no sign of abating. In fact, some observers believe that the strong, personal, trusting relationship between doctor and patient is no more. Of course, doctors still see patients, some in long-term primary care relationships. But physician encounters are often hurried, mediated by technology, paid for by third parties, and take place in impersonal hospitals, emergency rooms, or clinics.

Not surprisingly, physicians are often dissatisfied with their work. Studies in the new millennium showed alarming rates of burnout and depression. For decades, doctors had been hearing how important it is to treat "the whole person." Now it was becoming clear that there are two "whole persons" in the consulting room. Physicians too were suffering, a problem that attracted the attention of scholars in academic health centers.[43]

The doctor-patient relationship, then, is in trouble on both sides of the hyphen. To be sure, all is not lost. There is no shortage of sick and vulnerable patients who need access to health care and to the attention of competent physicians. And there is no shortage of altruistic and compassionate students and physicians committed to the relief of suffering and the cure of disease. Surveys reveal that most patients are actually satisfied with their doctors.[44]

In medical education, there are signs of renewed attention to the humane care of patients: courses and programs in medical humanities, bioethics, narrative medicine, spirituality in medicine, professionalism, and patient-centered care. Meanwhile, health care is now acknowledged as a collaborative enterprise. Doctors are not "captains of the ship" but leading members of a team that includes nurses, physician assistants, physical therapists, social workers, and a host of other health professionals. In fact, cultivating collaborative and respectful relationships with all members of the team may be the doctor's new secret to what Peabody called "the care of the patient."[45]

SUMMATION

This chapter explored the history of the doctor-patient relationship in the west. Beginning with a discussion of how this relationship was conceived in antiquity, it examined how the Hippocratic ideal became associated with the Christian duty to care for the sick and needy; how the beliefs of antiquity were questioned by Renaissance physicians who wanted to "see for themselves"; how a professional ethics based on virtue arose in response to increased competition between practitioners; and how the modern ideal of the doctor-patient relationship based on a personal connection, careful physical examination, and trust, arose in the late nineteenth century. Then, with a focus on recent cultural and structural challenges to this modern model, it considered how we might reconstruct the doctor-patient relationship to address recent challenges, such as patients' skepticism about doctors' genuine concern for them as people and doctors' worries about patients' lack of compliance and growing challenges to their authority. Overall, it emphasized that the doctor-patient relationship is always evolving, and that learning about its various historical configurations can help us understand the responsibilities and needs of physicians and their patients.

EXERCISES FOR CRITICAL THINKING AND CHARACTER FORMATION

QUESTIONS FOR DISCUSSION

1. Think about your favorite doctor. What do you value about him or her?
2. What is your ideal doctor? Where does that ideal come from?
3. For Hippocrates, what was the proper attitude of a doctor toward his patients? How does his attitude anticipate (or depart from) current relationships between doctors and patients?
4. In today's world of health care, the medical market is filled with alternative and complementary healers, with nurse practitioners and physician assistants. How does that complicate your understanding of "the" doctor-patient relationship?

SUGGESTED WRITING EXERCISE

Think back to your last visit to the doctor's office and write, for five to ten minutes, about your interactions with the physician. How long did you have to wait before the meeting? Where did the meeting take place? Had you seen him or her before? What did you talk about during the examination?

SUGGESTED VIEWING/LISTENING

The Diving Bell and the Butterfly (2007)
ER (television series, 2004–2009)
Good Will Hunting (1997)

Saturday Night Live, "Theodoric of York" (season three, episode 18)

FURTHER READING

Honoré de Balzac, *The Country Doctor*
Geoffrey Chaucer, *The Canterbury Tales*
Anton Chekhov, "Ward Number 6"
Anne Fadiman, *The Spirit Catches You and You Fall Down: A Hmong Child, Her American Doctors, and the Collision of Two Cultures*

Arthur Hertzler, *The Horse and Buggy Doctor*
Dr. Seuss, *You're Only Old Once!*
Bernard Shaw, *The Doctor's Dilemma*
William Carlos Williams, "The Use of Force"

ADVANCED READING

Michael Balint, *The Doctor, His Patient, and the Illness*
Rita Charon, *Narrative Medicine: Honoring the Stories of Illness*
Jay Katz, *The Silent World of Doctor and Patient*
Dorothy Porter and Roy Porter, *Patient's Progress: Doctors and Doctoring in Eighteenth Cent...*

Edward Shorter, *Doctors and Their Patients: A Social History*
David Rothman, *Strangers at the Bedside*

ONLINE RESOURCE...

The American Academy of Family Pl... ...ge: http://www. www.aafp.org/online/en/home.html
The American College of Physicians: ... ...Providers and acponline.org/
The American Medical Association: h...
ama-assn.org/

[handwritten note:]

modern concerns of goals in medicine & quality care:

— IDEALS (moral norms & ethic frames)

— characterization (desire for healing & caring)

— ... challenged & ... eally

2 Constructing Disease

"When I use a word," Humpty Dumpty said, in rather a scornful tone, "it means just what I choose it to mean – neither more nor less."

– Lewis Carroll[1]

ABSTRACT

This chapter explores the history of theories and conceptions of disease, while also attending to the epidemiological and symbolic impact of key diseases such as leprosy, bubonic plague, and influenza. Beginning with a discussion of the Hippocratic (or humoral) theory of disease, it examines how this theory came to be challenged by Renaissance humanists and, by the nineteenth century, overturned by the germ theory of disease. Then it considers some of the challenges facing us in the twenty-first century, including public health measures, the genetic revolution, and the "medicalization" of society.

INTRODUCTION

Societies, like Humpty Dumpty, decide what words mean. They decide who deserves sympathy and blame, the social role of the sick person, and the meaning of physical and mental illness. So too is society broken down into constituent pieces that have distinct perspectives and needs: patients, physicians, religious institutions, government, third-party payers, and pharmaceutical companies. Diseases, in other words, are not so much discovered by physicians and scientists alone as they are constructed by various competing social groups.

This chapter focuses on both the history of theories and conceptions of disease and the unusual epidemiological and symbolic impact of certain diseases (e.g., leprosy, bubonic plague, influenza). The history of disease is marked by fantastic progress. It is a story ranging from humoral theory, miasmatism, and germ theory to contemporary understandings of chronic, autoimmune, and genetic diseases. The recent history of disease also brings with it hopes for dramatic new cures via genetically personalized medicine, stem cell therapies, and nanomedicine. However, the history of disease is also filled with stubborn and unexpected realities: the emergence of chronic disease, medically induced illness, and new infectious diseases.

Disturbingly, medical knowledge has often been gained from the bodies of subjugated and marginal populations that were considered outside the boundaries of the fully human. Finally, the history of disease has recently been characterized by what sociologists call "medicalization," the process by which human problems are turned into treatable diseases and brought under the purview of medicine. Medicalization reminds us that labeling some conditions as diseases is a public as well as a scientific matter that raises questions about the goals of medicine, social policy, and the costs of health care.

ANCIENT THEORIES OF DISEASE

In general, ancient cultures understood the human body in terms of its relation to the environment, the cosmos, and the gods who watched over them and had the power to determine sickness or health. Yet there was no absolute division between "natural" and "supernatural" understandings of disease. Ancient Chinese medicine, for instance, was largely secular and naturalistic.[2] Even as classical Chinese medicine sought out a harmony between the body, the environment, and the cosmos, most Chinese citizens believed that illness was caused by malevolent ghosts, ancestors, karma, and sin. In the Hebrew Bible, we see a similar combination of the sacred and the secular. God is the physician of his people, yet physicians – common in ancient Israel by the second century BCE – carried out their healing work as human agents of God's will.

Likewise, in Greece, from the fifth century BCE the cult of Aesclepius coexisted with Hippocratic medicine. Ancient Greeks generally believed that disease was brought about by divine visitation, which only an appeal to the gods or magic could cure. Sick persons appealed to Aesclepius, the Greek god of medicine who was understood to possess a mythical healing power. After performing ritual sacrifices and prayers in Aesclepian temples, the sick entered a dreamlike state in which they received instructions for easing their suffering – perhaps bathing, rest, or an attention to diet. The cult of Aesclepius stood for centuries as the principal pagan response to disease, even as Hippocrates (460–377 BCE) and his followers rejected supernatural explanations of disease.[3]

Speaking of what is today known as epilepsy and was then called the "sacred disease," for instance, one Hippocratic author declared: "I do not believe that ...

[it] is any more divine or sacred than any other disease.... It is my opinion that those who first called this disease 'sacred' were the sort of people we now call witch doctors.... These are exactly the people who pretend to be very pious and particularly wise. By invoking a divine element they were able to screen their own failure to give suitable treatment and so called this a 'sacred' malady to conceal their ignorance of its nature."[4]

The Hippocratic approach to medicine, or *humoral theory*, dominated European medical thought well into the nineteenth century. The humors – basic four distinct bodily fluids or substances – were thought to be responsible for a health, disease, and a person's temperament. For the Hippocratics, the world was in balance when its basic components corresponded properly to each other: the humors (yellow bile, blood, phlegm, black bile); the seasons (winter, spring, summer, fall); the elements (earth, air, fire, water); the phases of life (childhood, youth, adulthood, old age); qualities (cold, hot, dry, moist); and the temperaments (choleric, sanguine, phlegmatic, melancholy). The preponderance of any given humor was thought to be at the root of illness: too much phlegm resulted in winter colds, while bile caused summer diarrhea and vomiting. Disease was thus understood as a condition of imbalance rather than as a specific pathological entity. Humoral imbalance, however, was itself caused by factors such as an unhealthy environment, individual predisposition, and hygienic regimen.[5]

Does this print appear to be a puzzle to be solved – something like a riddle – or is it an explanatory lesson?

For most of us today, it's a puzzle. In 1574, when it appeared in a book published in Leipzig by the physician Leonhart Thurneisser zun Thurn (1531–1595/96), it was meant to be a lesson that showed how the four humors – blood, phlegm, yellow bile, and black bile – corresponded to astrology, represented by the symbols for constellations and planets, and how they, in turn, shaped the character of men and women.

In the sixteenth century, medical theory continued to hold to the Hippocratic notion that disease results from disequilibrium of the humors. Does the distribution of elements on the page appear balanced and harmonious? Would you say that balance supports and reinforces Thurneisser's lesson? His complex ideas are represented by an equally elaborate graphic system of text, symbols, geometry, and drawing. The frame of a print or painting creates a relationship among the elements, whether those elements are realistic, schematic, or abstract.

To decipher the symbols, search the web for images associated with both the four humors and astrology.

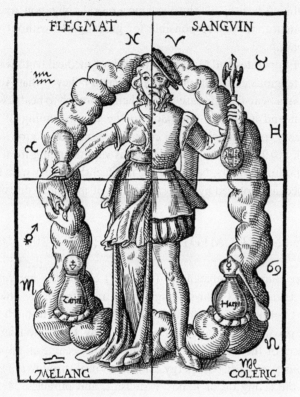

Figure 2. *The Four Humours,* from "Quinta Essentia" by Leonhart Thurneisser zun Thurn (1531–95/96) published in Leipzig, 1574 (engraving) (b/w photo), German School, (sixteenth century) /Private Collection / Archives Charmet/The Bridgeman Art Library.

Greek physicians focused their attention on patients with acute diseases that could kill quickly – those known today as pneumonia, mumps, malaria, and puerperal fever. The Hippocratic texts refer extensively to tuberculosis, one of the most destructive diseases in the ancient world, as *phthisis*, the Greek term for consumption.[6] Hippocrates theorized that consumption developed when external factors – climate, diet, exercise – combined with an individual's predisposition to the disease.[7] Chronic diseases – those that lasted longer than sixty days – were rarely mentioned, diagnosed, or treated.[8]

Roman physician Galen (129–210 CE) built on the Hippocratic corpus, which had evolved throughout the Hellenistic period (343–146 BCE). Galen believed, with Hippocrates, that the healer should restore a proper balance by treating one quality with its opposite. If the patient was too cold, he or she was treated by heating; if too dry, by dampening, and so on. For Galen, health extended beyond medical care to one's whole lifestyle, which included the proper balance of exercise, diet, sleep, environment, and daily routine. As a dietetic physician, Galen saw most disease as the consequence of a faulty regimen, and hence avoidable. A healthy life thus became a moral obligation, and a man with a healthy constitution was responsible for growing old without experiencing sickness or pain.[9]

For both Hippocrates and Galen, the pursuit of medical truth was not incompatible with religious explanation – in fact, Galen believed that Aesclepius had saved him from a near-fatal disease[10] – but their approach to health was grounded in empiricism and a holistic approach to the understanding of the cosmos. Humoral theory and Galenism also coexisted alongside a growing miasmatic theory, which attributed disease to poisonous vapors arising from swamplands and various polluted waters. Not until the nineteenth century were humoral and miasmatic theories replaced by the germ theory of infectious disease.

DISEASE IN THE MIDDLE AGES (400–1300 CE)

After Roman emperor Constantine (272–337) ended the persecution of the followers of Jesus in 313, Christianity played an increasingly powerful role in the healing, treatment, and understanding of disease. Although salvation of the soul was privileged over the health of the body, both physicians and clergy treated diseases of the body.[11] Indeed, medical care became an important act of Christian charity, as Christian clergy claimed to heal through the confession of sins, prayer, the laying on of hands, exorcisms, and miracles. Many Christian saints intervened on behalf of a sinful sufferer. Just as the ancient Greeks visited the Aesclepian temple in search of a cure for their ailments, so too did medieval wanderers visit holy shrines in Spain (St. James of Compostela) or England (St. Thomas a Becket in Canterbury).[12]

CASE STUDY: THEODORE OF SYKEON

The following passage showcases the miraculous healing power of Saint Theodore of Sykeon (c. 700 CE), a Byzantine saint who lived in Anatolia, the central region of modern Turkey. Theodore's biography records the saint's exploits of healing, which were typical of early Christian belief in medical miracles.

"The slave girl of a magnate had been possessed secretly by a demon for twenty-eight years so that she was always ill and did not know what caused the malady. Her master brought her to the saint praying that either by death or a restoration to health she might be liberated from her sickness. Saint Theodore took hold of her head and prayed that the cause of her illness might be made known and driven away. Immediately the demon in her was disturbed and tore her, shouting: "You are burning me, ironeater, spare me, strangler of demons, I adjure you by the God who gives you power against me." Theodore bade the demon be silent and told the girl to return in a week's time. On the following Wednesday she came and once more the demon in her became excited and abusive: "Oh this violence that I suffer from this harlot's child! Twenty-eight years I have possessed this girl and none of the saints found me out, and now this harlot's son has come and has made me manifest and handed me over to dread punishment. Cursed be the day on which you were born and the day that brought you here!" Theodore rebuked the demon with the sign of the Cross: "Even if I am the harlot's son, nevertheless to the glory of our Lord Jesus Christ the Son of God I bid you in his name leave the girl and never take possession of her again." The demon shouted in reply: "I do your bidding and go out of her, but after three days she will die." The saint answered: "Come forth and the will of the Lord be done. For a God-fearing man may not trust you, since your words are vain and false." The demon tore the girl, threw her down at the saint's feet and went out of her. And she, coming to herself, said: "It is through your holy prayers, father, that I have been healed, for I saw the demon coming out of my mouth like a foul crawling thing." Theodore prayed over her and dismissed her, bidding her remain in the church for seven days. And the word of the demon proved to be false, for after some days the girl and her master returned to the saint giving glory to God."[13]

1. How is Theodore able to heal the girl?
2. What religious beliefs are implied in the text?
3. What are some possible naturalistic explanations to the girl's illness? How do you think medieval practitioners would have responded to such diagnoses?

The disease that attracted the most attention during the medieval period, leprosy, offers a striking example of the way in which theology shaped social conceptions of disease. Known today as Hansen's disease after the scientist who first discovered the infectious microorganism *mycobacterium leprae* in 1874, leprosy causes a chronic, painful, and debilitating skin infection that can lead to the loss of fingers, toes, and facial features. Medieval authors thought that leprosy was the same disease referred to in Leviticus 13–14, which identifies a "repulsive scaly skin-disease" considered offensive to God.[14] Lepers therefore became stigmatized as unclean, nauseating, disgusting individuals. The association between leprosy and moral impurity was also consistent with the Galenic tradition that regarded health and morality as indivisible.

Leprosy suddenly disappeared from Europe around 1300 only to be replaced by a devastating epidemic. Bubonic plague, or the Black Death, rampaged through Asia before sweeping westward across the Middle East to North Africa and Europe. In the pandemic of 1347, Europe alone lost perhaps twenty million people – nearly a third of its population.[15] The onset of such a devastating disease demanded an explanation. Where did the Black Death come from? How did it afflict so many people in such a short period of time? What cures – if any – were possible?

Today, medical historians know that bubonic plague is a rodent disease in which a microorganism, *Yersinia pestis*, infects rodents (especially the rat). The "bubonic" form of plague strikes humans when infected fleas choose a human instead of another rodent host. When the flea bites its new host, the bacillus enters the bloodstream and leads to the characteristic swelling (bubo) in the neck, groin, or armpit. During the epidemic waves of the fourteenth century, some thought that the plague was a form of humoral imbalance resulting from "miasma" – the bad air or poisonous vapors found in unhealthy environments.[16] Others, sensing that the plague was contagious (spread from person to person) imposed quarantines that separated the poor, who lived in the most squalid conditions, from the rest of urban populations. Most medieval folk, however, believed that God had punished people for their evil ways.[17] This theological view was especially sobering since, unlike leprosy, which only affected specific individuals, the plague had afflicted all of Europe.

THE MEDICAL RENAISSANCE

In 1525, a new Greek translation of Galen's collected works led to renewed reverence, and even a slavish obedience, to the Galenic and Hippocratic tradition.[18] Yet the classical assumptions of humoralism that had dominated explanations of health and disease in the Western world did not escape unscathed from the Renaissance. Whereas some medical humanists restored texts to establish the authority of ancient Greek and Roman masters, others offered a "new science" in place of tradition.

The first significant challenge came from Swiss polymath Paracelsus (c. 1493–1542), who rejected both humoral theory and the elemental quartet of earth, wind, air, and fire. Instead, Paracelsus advocated a natural philosophy based on the chemical substances salt, mercury, and sulfur.[19] As a further departure from the Hippocratics, who believed that contraries cure, the Paracelsians insisted on cure by similitude. A poisonous disease, for instance, had to be cured by a like poison. Consequently, drugs compounded from mercury – arsenic, antimony, and others – were used as purges.

Neither "the ancients" nor "the moderns" had answers to the new diseases of sixteenth- and seventeenth-century Europe: typhus, many unidentified fevers, and especially syphilis. Known as "the pox" or "the great pox" to distinguish it from smallpox, syphilis spread throughout Europe in the early 1500s and behaved like a disease that no one had seen before. Although its origin is uncertain, most historians of medicine trace the appearance of syphilis in Europe to Columbus's exploration of the New World.[20] His arrival in Hispaniola

precipitated a disastrous epidemic among members of the indigenous population, reducing them from around one million to under 20,000 – a monumental,
tragic consequence of colonialism (see Chapter 6).[21] But the cultural transmission of disease also worked in reverse: According to the "Columbian theory of
syphilis," the Amerindians unwittingly transmitted syphilis to Columbus's crew
and, by extension, to Europe in the late 1400s.

Syphilis is now understood to be a sexually transmitted disease caused by the
spirochete organism *Treponema pallidum*, which was discovered in 1905.[22] The
disease made a great impression on early modern Europeans because of gruesome symptoms that include skin lesions, skeletal aches, and genital rashes. In
its final stage, syphilis damages several organ systems and may lead to dementia.
During the Renaissance, debates raged over what caused this terrible outbreak
and how to treat it. Galenic theory held that the pox was a humoral disorder,
with phlegm as the prime culprit; treatment, consequently, involved the expul-
sion of phlegm by spitting or sweating. Paracelsus, on the other hand, advocated
rubbing "Arabic ointment," or a type of mercuric sulfide, on the lesions.[23]

Syphilis was typical of the new plagues brought about by western exploration,
conquest, commerce, migration, and – most of all – the slave trade.[24] In addition
to the slave trade, syphilis was spread by international warfare, intercultural contact, unclean conditions, increased population density, and the ebb and flow of
refugees and peasants.[25] Because of its widespread impact, syphilis (along with
the bubonic plague) profoundly affected the way in which early moderns thought
about disease. Traditionally, Western medicine focused on diseased individuals
rather than on disease itself: The Hippocratics taught that disease (humoral
imbalance) resulted from congenital weaknesses, an unhealthy environment, or
sinful behavior. Any cures, consequently, involved restoring equilibrium or pla-
cating the gods. But from its first appearance, syphilis operated indiscriminately,
afflicting masses of people at the same time. This prompted a search for causes
of disease outside of the body, including a conception of disease as a distinct
external entity that might be spread from person to person.

THE SCIENTIFIC REVOLUTION AND THE ENLIGHTENMENT

These changes in medical thought were part of a seventeenth-century movement
conventionally known as the scientific revolution, which placed an emphasis on
empirical data and the power of human reason. Careful and repeated observation, not religious or medical dogma, would lead to new knowledge and permanent improvement of the human condition. The utopian philosopher-scientist
Francis Bacon (1561–1626) promised that empirical observation and systematic
investigation would transform society. "The improvements of medical practice,"

wrote Bacon, "which will become more efficacious with the progress of reason and of the social order, will mean the end of infectious and hereditary diseases and illnesses brought on by climate, food, or working conditions. It is reasonable to hope that all other disease may likewise disappear as their distant causes are discovered."[26]

In a direct challenge to Galenic medicine, English physician William Harvey (1578–1657) proved that the heart functioned as a muscular pump that pushed blood through a bodily circuit of veins and arteries in the body. In one test of his theory, Harvey cut open living animals that bled to death as their hearts forced blood out of their arteries. Rene Descartes (1596–1650), who attended one of these dramatic demonstrations, cited Harvey to support his own theory that animals and humans are essentially organic machines governed by the laws of mechanics. What separated humans from animals, in Descartes' view, was their faculty of speech and possession of an eternal soul.[27]

Two hundred years after Bacon, Enlightenment thinkers came to agree with him that health was a natural state to be attained and preserved – maybe even perfected. In the eighteenth century, philosophers such as Jean-Jacques Rousseau (1712–1778), John Locke (1632–1704), and Immanuel Kant (1724–1804) believed that God had created a benevolent universe that operated according to immutable "laws of nature," suggesting that scientists could discover the way these laws worked in the human body. Accordingly, the eighteenth century witnessed the emergence of new medical systems of classification and identification. Scottish physician William Cullen (1710–1790) developed a *nosology*, or disease classification, that treated diseases as real entities with their own distinctive signs.

New work in the study of diseased organs and tissues also transformed classifications of disease. Although a handful of physicians – especially Vesalius – had previously investigated signs of disease in the dead bodies of executed criminals, Giovanni Battista Morgnani (1660–1723) performed the first systematic investigations in modern pathological anatomy. Morgnani's monumental *On the Sites and Causes of Disease* (1761), based on 700 autopsies, demonstrated that visible traces of disease could be found in various organs.[28] By correlating symptoms of the living with these postmortem anatomical lesions, physicians were able to locate particular diseases in specific organs.

In spite of new knowledge and radical shifts in science and philosophy, therapeutic practice remained largely traditional. While the Galenic tradition was continuously refuted in theory, it was consistently upheld in practice. American physician and revolutionary Benjamin Rush (1745–1813), for example, remained faithful to the age-old therapy of bloodletting, which was thought to correct fevers, apoplexy, or headaches resulting from an excessive buildup of blood. For Rush, cure involved bleeding (venesection), blistering, purging, and vomiting. During the Philadelphia yellow fever epidemic in 1793, Rush's fidelity to "heroic medicine" – aggressive bloodletting, purging, vomiting, sweating, and blistering – killed as many of his patients as the disease itself.

THE BIRTH OF MODERN MEDICINE

As the leading medical theories of seventeenth and eighteenth centuries became more widely known, physicians began to think differently about disease and therapeutics. Diseases came to been seen less as systemic imbalances in the body's natural harmony and more as a set of distinctive signs and symptoms that could be analyzed, separated, and measured in isolation. The older "heroic" therapeutics gave way to an emphasis on diet and regimen along with the belief that, with time and rest, the body would heal itself.[29]

By the 1850s, the empirically determined "normal" began to replace the philosophically grounded "natural" as the paradigm of order and health. Physicians, in other words, measured health in terms of statistical norms rather than in terms of the patient's "natural" state of health.[30] Many of these principles of modern Western medicine emerged in the vast Parisian hospitals of Pitié-Salpêtrière and Bicêtre, where physicians and scientists studied – among other things – forms of mental illness (then divided into idiocy, dementia, melancholia, mania, and hysteria) and diseases of older people.[31]

The new science of biomedicine brought problems as well as benefits for clinical care. Following Morgnani's emphasis on anatomical lesions, Xavier Bichat (1771–1802) refined pathology by demonstrating that disease affected localized tissues rather than organs as a whole.[32] Once Bichat's tissue pathology established an ontologic foundation for observing and defining disease, a patient's experiences could be dismissed as secondary. If disease could be located in tissues or cells, there was no reason to attend to a patient's subjective description of symptoms. Bichat's contributions also paved the way for a new form of medicine – known as clinical or hospital medicine – that displaced the more individualistic, patient-centered medicine of the eighteenth century. A more limited way of seeing – philosopher Michel Foucault (1926–1984) has famously called it "the clinical gaze"[33] – eventually resulted in a focus on treatment of disease rather than care of patients.

Walter Benjamin (1892–1940) has suggested that every act of civilization is also an act of barbarism.[34] Unfortunately, the history of medicine provides evidence for this harsh generalization. New biomedical knowledge has often been obtained from observing, dissecting, or experimenting with bodies or persons considered less than fully human – the subjugated, enslaved, or marginalized populations housed in prisons, indigent hospitals, asylums, and mental hospitals.[35] Nineteenth-century medical schools resorted to grave robbing in order to garner enough bodies for research – particularly the graves of both free and enslaved African Americans. One American Southerner, for instance, endorsed a proposal that permitted local authorities to release bodies of executed blacks while also assuring the safety of white corpses: "The bodies of colored persons, whose execution is necessary to public security, may, we think, be with equity appropriated for the benefit of a science on which so many lives depend."[36]

The French focus on tissue pathology in the early nineteenth century set the stage for German study of cellular physiology and pathology in the second half of the nineteenth century. German polymath Rudolf Virchow (1821–1902), for example, urged his students to "think microscopically." He disagreed with the view that that cells originated from inorganic matter and, with his pronouncement *omnis cellula a cellula* – "every cell from a cell" – declared that each cell was created as a copy of a prior cell. For Virchow, pathology was a cellular affair: disease occurred when abnormal changes within one cell were transferred to other cells through division. Hence, biomedical science turned its gaze to increasingly smaller units: just as Morgnani had emphasized the organ and Bichat the tissue, Virchow highlighted the crucial role of cells in understanding disease.

The main idea of bacteriology or "germ theory" – that disease is caused by tiny infectious beings – was not entirely new in the nineteenth century. As early as 1546, Girolamo Fracastoro (1478–1553) declared that tiny seeds (*seminaria contagiosa*) carried disease. Using the newly invented microscope in the 1660s, British naturalist Robert Hooke (1635–1703) confirmed the presence of these infinitesimally small creatures and named them "cells." Today these microorganisms are known as single-celled bacteria or protozoa or their even smaller cousin: the virus.

French chemist Louis Pasteur (1822–1895) is usually considered the founder of the germ theory of disease. In 1878, Pasteur argued that microorganisms were responsible for disease, putrefaction, and fermentation. Once these organisms were known, he suggested, prevention would be possible by developing vaccines, a process pioneered a generation earlier by Edward Jenner (1749–1823).[37] To verify his findings, Pasteur presented a public display of anthrax injection to a group of cattle. His technique was to inject small quantities of microorganisms that had been made less virulent; the weakened organisms, as a result, triggered immunity without producing the symptoms of full-blown disease. The public demonstration proved not only the effectiveness of the vaccine – the vaccinated cattle survived while the others perished – but also Pasteur's savvy ability to popularize his ideas.

Robert Koch (1843–1910) stands alongside Pasteur as the cofounder of germ theory. In addition to establishing bacteriology as a scientific discipline, Koch discovered the bacteria that cause tuberculosis, cholera, and other diseases. These discoveries confirmed that individuals were often carriers of infectious diseases. They also established that these diseases took root and flourished in crowded urban conditions of poor hygiene, sanitation, and nutrition, thereby encouraging the development of new public health methods to protect urban populations from epidemics.[38]

Germ theory contributed to the gradual reorientation of public health toward the individual. People were increasingly seen as carriers of disease, and new methods were designed to prevent them from spreading infection. Like all new theories, germ theory was initially controversial. Authorities in London clung to the miasmatic theory of disease for years after Pasteur's and Koch's discoveries. Nevertheless, public health officials successfully prevented the spread of disease by isolating infected individuals – by quarantining, for example, sailors infected with cholera on ships. By the 1890s, most rank-and-file physicians supported germ theory. In the twenty years between 1880 and 1900, scientists identified an unprecedented number of bacteria, including those responsible for typhoid fever, leprosy, tuberculosis, cholera, diphtheria and tetanus, malaria, pneumonia, plague, botulism, dysentery, and syphilis.[39]

DISEASE IN THE TWENTIETH CENTURY

The discoveries of the bacteriological revolution did not quickly translate into effective treatments for patients. Robert Koch, for instance, rashly declared that he had found a treatment for tuberculosis, only to discover that his "tuberculin" was a failure.[40] From 1914–1918, a virus later known as Type A/H1N1 unleashed a devastating influenza epidemic that killed perhaps 50 million people around the world – far more than the combined number of soldiers killed during World War I and victims of the Black Plague.

Viruses are microorganisms that are even smaller than bacteria. They were later known to be the culprits in diseases such as smallpox, polio, measles, influenza, and AIDS. Viruses could not even be seen until the invention of the electron microscope in the 1930s and were not clearly understood until the 1950s. Although there is still no definitive treatment for viral diseases, vaccines for prevention were developed as far back as Edward Jenner's (1749–1823) vaccination for smallpox at the end of the eighteenth century. In the mid-twentieth century, Jonah Salk (1914–1985) and Albert Sabin (1906–1993) discovered vaccines for polio and various strains of influenza. Thanks to a worldwide effort, the World Health Organization declared in 1977 that smallpox had been eliminated from the earth.

The 1940s witnessed the first successful antibacterial medications: sulfa drugs and penicillin, which had been discovered by Scottish scientist Arthur Fleming (1881–1955) in 1928. Penicillin proved to be an effective cure for syphilis, certain forms of pneumonia, and strep throat, among other bacterial infections. The development of streptomycin led to a cure for tuberculosis. By the 1950s, drug companies were producing mass quantities of an expanding array of antibiotics that effectively treated patients who would have died from infectious disease just a few years earlier. Perhaps the most significant advance of Western medicine in the second half of the twentieth century was the ability to tame or eliminate infectious diseases through the application of preventive medicine, vaccination, and antibiotic drug treatment.

As in previous eras, these great strides in biomedical knowledge were shadowed by the exploitation of vulnerable and stigmatized populations. To test the effectiveness of penicillin between 1946 and 1948, for example, U.S. researchers in Guatemala used prostitutes to infect prison inmates, mentally ill persons, and Guatemalan soldiers with syphilis and other sexually transmitted diseases (STDs). To test antimalarial treatments during World War II, researchers from the University of Chicago working with the U.S. Army infected prisoners with malaria at the Stateville Penitentiary in Illinois.

After World War II, the Allied Forces held military tribunals in Nuremberg, Germany, where Nazi doctors were convicted of mass murder and criminal human experimentation. The 1947 Nuremberg Code articulated the major principles of ethically acceptable research with human beings: informed consent, absence of coercion, rigorously constructed scientific experimentation, and beneficence toward the research participants. Sadly, the Code did not significantly alter federally funded American experimentation with human subjects after the war. Researchers continued to rely on populations that could not fully exercise free and informed consent: prisoners, men enlisted in the army, the mentally ill, and indigent and minority populations. Perhaps the most well-known example of unethical human experimentation in the United States was the Tuskegee Study of syphilis in African American men in Macon County, Georgia, initiated during the 1930s by the U.S. Public Health Service. In order to study the "natural history of syphilis" researchers withheld penicillin from the men even though it was known to be effective against syphilis by the 1950s. The study was not halted until a reporter exposed the story in 1972.[41] Unethical research practices in the United States were not effectively constrained until the Belmont Report and the Federal Code of Regulations, which governed human experimentation beginning in the late 1970s.[42]

Ironically, progress in bacteriology and the antibiotic treatment of infectious disease in Western society gave rise to a new pattern of disease and mortality, usually known as the "epidemiologic transition."[43] Over the course of the twentieth century, mortality from infectious diseases (e.g., tuberculosis, malaria, typhoid, cholera, smallpox) declined substantially, causing the average age at death in the United States to increase from forty-one in 1900 to seventy-eight in 2006.[44] Meanwhile, the decline in deaths from infectious disease gave rise to an aging population, the growth of chronic disease, and increasing disability. Deaths due to chronic and degenerative diseases (primarily heart disease, cancer, stroke, chronic obstructive pulmonary disease) accounted for 76 percent of all deaths in the United States in 2002.

By the 1970s, many observers believed that infectious disease no longer posed a major threat in the developed world. Chronic diseases, accidents, homicides, smoking, and drinking had replaced infectious disease as primary causes of death. Some thought that deaths among younger people might be largely preventable. This perspective turned out to be sadly mistaken. It ignored mortality due to endemic and epidemic contagious diseases in Africa and Asia (poor and undeveloped countries have always suffered the heaviest burden of disease). And in an era of international air travel, new and recurring infectious diseases spread rapidly across the world. New viral hemorrhagic fevers, AIDS, and the return of previously contained diseases such as cholera, malaria, and syphilis were just a few of the diseases that posed serious threats to global health at the end of the twentieth century.[45]

THE GENETIC REVOLUTION AND MEDICALIZATION

Throughout the late twentieth- and early twenty-first centuries, scientists continued to plumb the infinitesimal depths of the human body. Genetics took Rudolph Virchow's insistence to "think microscopically" a step further, peering inside the cell nucleus in search of the secrets of heredity. In 1953, James Watson (1928–) and Francis Crick (1916–2004) revealed the structure of DNA, the molecule that transmits genetic material from one generation to another. Alterations or mutations of genes – which provide instructions for cellular growth and development – are now known to increase susceptibility to or cause more than 4,000 diseases.[46]

By 2003, thanks to the federally funded U.S. Human Genome Project, researchers had identified all 20,000–25,000 genes in human DNA. This information was stored in databases, allowing analysis and technology to transfer to the private sector for use in diagnosis, prevention, and treatment of genetic abnormalities involved in birth defects, mental retardation, autism, connective tissue disorders, and certain inherited forms of cancer or dementia.

At the end of the twentieth century, the rise of genetic medicine led to a good deal of hype and misinformation about the promises of gene therapy and molecular medicine. Contrary to popular understanding, most genes or genetic mutations create only a predisposition to disease. Epidemiologists and others have linked the prevalence of cancer to environmental pollution and chemicals found in food, plastics, and other household goods. A small percentage of inherited genes are known to cause disease alone – specifically BRCA 1 and BRCA 2, which lead to the development of breast cancer in 85 percent of women who carry them.

Great advances in understanding the genetic components of illness have not yet translated into any clear triumphs over cancer or other diseases. Nevertheless, the era of genetic engineering – transplanting healthy genes into sick persons or preventing illness by altering the genetic makeup of embryos – is rapidly approaching. Genetic engineering is replete with ethical and humanistic questions: Should we select embryos for desired traits or sexual selection? Should we alter or insert genes into fetuses to produce stronger athletes or "better children?"

It remains to be seen which of the dreams for cure and prevention will come to fruition and which of the nightmares about the manipulations of the human genome will become realities.[47]

In the second half of the twentieth century, while people were dying from chronic and infectious diseases whose definitions were unquestionably biomedical, an entirely new range of human problems were relabeled as disease. This process, which sociologists call "medicalization," transforms human problems into diseases or disorders and brings them under the jurisdiction of medical diagnosis and treatment.[48] Medicalization also turns certain normal life events or cultural deviances into disease. In the last forty years, for example, normal biological experiences such as menopause, infertility, childbirth, baldness, aging, and even death have been labeled as diseases. Certain conditions or behaviors considered deviant (e.g., alcoholism, drug addiction, homosexuality, and sexual abuse) were culturally reframed as "sickness" rather than "badness."

Medicalization lends credence to what might be called the "Humpty Dumpty" theory of disease. As Humpty Dumpty remarked in the epigraph to this chapter, words mean what societies *want* them to mean, and these meanings are open to contention and change. Homosexuality, for example, was defined as a medical pathology by the American Psychiatric Association in 1968 and then demedicalized in 1974 after strenuous debate and political pressure from the gay community.[49] Now-common maladies such as attention deficit/hyperactivity disorder (ADHD), anorexia and bulimia, chronic fatigue syndrome (CFS), post-traumatic stress disorder (PTSD), panic disorder, and premenstrual syndrome were not even named fifty years ago. As another example, the diagnosis of autism increased forty-fold in the first decade of the twenty-first century. This diagnosis did not represent an epidemic of autism – brought on, some say, by vaccination. Instead, it reflected the fact that public schools required a diagnosis of autism before they would authorize special services for children.[50]

Leaving aside the question of what constitutes a "real" medical condition, medicalization is part and parcel of the enormous expansion and transformation of medicine in the last half century. In 1950, for example, 4.5 percent of the U.S. gross national product was spent on health care. In 2006, this percentage had jumped to 16 percent. Even more strikingly, the number of physicians in the country nearly doubled during that period.[51] This dramatic expansion of medicine and health care, along with an insatiable public demand for health, created a vast increase in disease categories, diagnoses, and treatments.

When does medicalization become *over*medicalization? This question has no easy or obvious answer. As we have seen, throughout the history of medicine, societies decide what counts as illness. Decisions about what qualifies as disease today are made in an increasingly commercialized health care system. They are complex negotiations between various social actors and institutions, including scientists, governments and their reimbursement categories, pharmaceutical companies, private insurance companies, biotechnology companies, social movements, consumers, and patient advocacy groups.

The future history of disease will play out in the overlapping area between biological threats to human health and social decisions about what conditions are diagnosable and treatable. The implications for the ethics of health care, the economy, and the structure of society will be profound.

SUMMATION

This chapter explored the history of theories and conceptions of disease, while also attending to the epidemiological and symbolic impact of key diseases such as leprosy, bubonic plague, and influenza. Beginning with a discussion of the Hippocratic (or humoral) theory of disease, it examined how this theory came to be challenged by Renaissance humanists and, by the nineteenth century, overturned by the germ theory of disease. Then, with a focus on public health measures, the genetic revolution, and the "medicalization" of society, it considered some of the challenges facing us in the twenty-first century. Overall, this chapter pointed out that, throughout the history of medicine, societies have decided what counts as disease, and that this insight can help us to negotiate the increasingly complex network of social actors and institutions that influence how we think of health and illness.

EXERCISES FOR CRITICAL THINKING AND CHARACTER FORMATION

QUESTIONS FOR DISCUSSION

1. Have you or someone in your family ever had a serious disease? What was its impact?
2. Galen thought that disease was a consequence of a faulty regimen for maintaining health. What would he have thought of obesity?
3. Do you agree with Galen that maintaining health is a moral obligation? Why or why not?
4. Do you think aging is a disease?

SUGGESTED WRITING EXERCISE

Choose a television commercial that deals with questions of health in some way. Write for seven to ten minutes. Does the ad deal with things that concern you or your family? What do you notice about the relation between disease and society in the ad? What are some of its unspoken assumptions about health (and disease)?

SUGGESTED VIEWING

And the Band Played On (1993)
Contagion (2011)
Hysteria (2011)

The Libertine (2004)
Malaria: Fever Wars (2006)
Philadelphia (1993)

FURTHER READING

Daniel Defoe, *Journal of the Plague Year*
Siddhartha Mukherjee, *The Emperor of All Maladies: A Biography of Cancer*

Susan Sontag, *Illness as Metaphor*
John Updike, "From the Journal of a Leper," in *Problems and Other Stories*

ADVANCED READING

Peter Conrad, *The Medicalization of Society: On the Transformation of Human Conditions into Treatable Disorders*
Paul Farmer, *Infections and Inequalities: The Modern Plagues*
Mark Harrison, *Disease and the Modern World*

J. N. Hays, *The Burdens of Disease: Epidemics and Human Response in Western History*
Arno Karlen, *Man and Microbes: Diseases and Plagues in History and Modern Times*
Charles Rosenberg, *Framing Disease: Studies in Cultural History*
Sheldon Watts, *Disease and Medicine in World History*

ONLINE RESOURCES

American Public Health Association
http://www.apha.org/
Center for Disease Control

www.cdc.gov
Office of Disease Prevention
http://prevention.nih.gov

3

Educating Doctors

To study the phenomena of disease without books is to sail an uncharted sea, while to study books without patients is not to go to sea at all.

– William Osler[1]

ABSTRACT

This chapter explores the history of medical education in the west. Beginning with a discussion of how medical knowledge was established and transmitted in antiquity, it examines how many important medical texts were translated into Arabic in the Middle Ages; how scholars rediscovered and rethought these texts in the Renaissance; how medical education evolved during the eighteenth and nineteenth centuries to include new academic subjects such as physiology and chemistry; and how, by the middle of the twentieth century, medical education came to be associated with academic health centers. Then, with a focus on a 2010 Carnegie Foundation Report, it considers some of the challenges facing medical education in the twenty-first century.

INTRODUCTION

As all teachers and students know, education is a difficult business. Medical education is especially difficult because people's lives are at stake and because the acquisition of scientific and clinical knowledge is such a demanding process. The history of medical education is characterized by several pedagogical tensions. Do students learn best from texts and classroom lectures or from clinical apprenticeships and experience? Should education be focused on the disease or the person? On the mastery of universal scientific knowledge or the care of unique individuals? These polarities are not mutually exclusive, of course, but finding the right balance among them is an elusive and ever-changing task. The history of medical education is also characterized more recently by a conflict between educating a privileged male minority and opening medical education to women, immigrants, and racial and ethnic minorities.

This chapter sketches the history of these issues in medical education as they emerge in antiquity and evolve into the twenty-first century, focusing on Western Europe and the United States. Our principal interests are: (1) the shifting pedagogical balances of theory versus practice and the scientific versus the humanistic; (2) the evolving mix of gender, race, and ethnicity in medical student bodies over the last 150 years; and (3) the shifting and often unstable economic realities, incentives, and needs of teachers, students, and institutions.

THE BIRTH OF LEARNED MEDICINE

Traditionally, formally trained medical students came from privileged family backgrounds. In ancient India, for example, the *Charaka Samhita*, an Ayurvedic Sanskrit text from 300 BCE, advised teachers to seek students who associated with or came from a family of doctors. Teachers urged their students "to be chaste and temperate, to speak the truth, to obey ... in all things and to wear a beard."[2] In addition to a robust beard, discipline and integrity were essential. In ancient Egypt, medical students often lived under the strict supervision and direction of their teachers. One treatise demonstrates that some student recreational habits seem unaffected by history. "It has been reported to me," a teacher admonished a rare female pupil, Emena, "that thou neglectest thy studies and seekest only thy pleasure, wandering from tavern to tavern. But what profiteth the odour of beer?"[3]

Before the fifth century BCE, Greek medicine was characterized by two kinds of knowledge: secular traumatology (the care of wounds, injuries, and broken bones) and supernatural revelation (the wisdom of the gods). In the first case, a resident or wandering craftsman imparted knowledge orally and by practice, usually from father to son. The second kind of practitioner – the priest as physician – imparted religious wisdom to his initiates. This situation was altered when the Hippocratics (c. 400 BCE) separated medical from religious explanation and produced the first secular medical texts. Despite the influence of the Hippocratic Corpus, its pedagogical value was often called into question. Aristotle (384–332 BCE), whose father was a physician, commented on the perennial tension between textual and clinical learning: "Clearly you do not become a physician by books ... the writers of books try to describe ... the general ... methods of therapeutics. That would be useful for the skilled man but the untrained one gains no use from it."[4]

In 323 BCE, teachers at the world's largest and most famous library – the "Musaeum" at Alexandria – invented new educational formats that later became known as lectures and seminars. In medicine, competing sects produced rival educational forms. Herophilus of Chalcedon (335–280 BCE) undertook the first formal dissections of human bodies, which in turn became part of the education of physicians. In contrast, the empiricists claimed that the knowledge of internal human processes could only be learned from the experience of caring for patients. After Alexandria passed into Roman rule in 80 BCE, Roman hostility to Greek philosophy and science led to a shorter and less theoretical style of education. Roman physician Thessalus (c. 70–95), who popularized the study of medicine, claimed that he could transform a student into a physician in six months.[5]

During the Hellenistic Period (326 BCE–146 AD) an amalgam of Greek, Jewish, and Egyptian cultures yielded more open social norms and popular forms of medical knowledge. Some writers called for medical knowledge to be taught as part of general public education, leading to occasional public lectures and advice for laymen in need of sudden medical assistance. The term "iatrine" (meaning a woman physician) signified authority and jurisdiction that occasionally went beyond the traditional expectations of women as midwives. Male physician Heracleides of Taras, for example, wrote to a woman physician, Antiochis, addressing her as a colleague and providing clinical advice.[6] Slaves were also sometimes permitted to become physicians among the Romans. In general, however, the ideal physician was expected to be a healthy, courteous male from a lofty social position.

In the tradition of learned medicine, Galen's (131–201) ambiguous attitude toward books exemplified the perennial tension between textual and clinical education. On the one hand, he argued that books undermined the importance of seeing with one's own eyes. On the other hand, Galen wrote up to 600 treatises and employed scribes to write down his words. Indeed, the works of Hippocrates (c. 460–377 BCE) and Galen came to be regarded as infallible sources of medical knowledge – which both fostered and limited the growth of education and research – for more than 1,500 years.

After the fall of the Roman Empire in the fifth century, the urban life of antiquity was replaced by a medieval countryside that was dotted with castles and cathedrals. Learned medical practice and teaching virtually disappeared. Although some manuscripts were preserved and studied in European cathedrals and monasteries, the center of medical knowledge and learning shifted to the east. During the eighth century (sometimes known as the age of translations) scores of Greek texts were translated into Arabic, including Hippocrates' major texts and 129 of Galen's works.[7] The *Firdaws al-hikma*, a medical compendium by Ali ibn Rabban al-Tabari (838–870), contained Arab translations of not only Hippocrates, Galen, and other Greek writers but also texts from the Persian and Indian traditions. Arabic scholars thus preserved classical Western medical knowledge that would otherwise have been lost and made their own contributions as well.

In a largely rural European society, very few people read at all, let alone medical texts, which were written in Latin, scattered among monasteries and a few cities, and hand copied on parchment made from the skin of sheep and cattle. Aspiring medical students, however, were expected to possess knowledge of the classical liberal arts by the age of fifteen. From the ninth century, medical texts balanced classical philosophy with practical advice and observation. "From what signs do you diagnose melancholia?" asked one treatise. Answer:

> From a distaste for life and dislike of other people's company: from the sadness of the countenance, from the silence, suspicion and irrational weeping of the patient: from the inflammation of the precordia, from the coldness of the limbs accompanied by slight perspiration, from the thinness of the body and the general debility of the subject.[8]

This question-and-answer format implies the existence of a student-teacher relationship, although its nature and frequency cannot be documented. Medical texts often warned students against drunkenness, overeating, consorting with women of ill repute, or any activity that could damage one's mind.[9]

Formal medical education in the west appeared with the founding of universities at Paris (1110), Bologna (1158), Oxford (1167), Montpellier (1181), Cambridge (1209), Padua (1222), and Naples (1224). Padua and Bologna offered the most advanced medical education and attracted students from across Europe. Like the other learned professions of law and theology, medicine anchored itself in textual analysis. By the end of the twelfth century, medical education had become a process of learning set doctrines in unquestioned traditional texts. Learned physicians and church officials tended to disparage surgery, which was considered a "lower," less refined art. However, itinerant surgeons who practiced their craft daily were likely more skilled than those who taught from books and occasional practice.

THE RENAISSANCE CHALLENGE TO TRADITION

The rebirth of European intellectual and cultural life in the fourteenth and fifteenth centuries brought with it profound implications for both medical knowledge and ethical norms. As an interest in "all things Greek" suffused the field of medicine, scholars called for new translations of Hippocrates and Galen in order to avoid reading imperfect, second-hand texts from the Arabic or Latin. By 1531 most of Galen's work was available in both Greek and Latin. New translations of Galen, Hippocrates, and others not only reasserted the superiority of ancient medicine, they also contributed to a medical tradition rooted in book learning rather than in practice and observation. In the teaching of anatomy, for example, the teacher sat above students and read from Galen's *On Anatomical Procedures,* which included errors that no one challenged for centuries.[10]

Just as he questioned the method of Galenic anatomy, Andreas Vesalius (1514–1564) also contested the traditional pedagogical method of instruction through books. In his *De Humani Corporis Fabrica* (1543), which was immortalized by Jan van Calcar's (1499–1546) stunningly beautiful illustrations, Vesalius detailed the method in which the professor himself performed the dissection (known today as a prosection). Eventually, the Vesalian insistence on "seeing for oneself" became a fundamental tenet of the so-called "New Science." The same year that the *Fabrica* was published, Nicolaus Copernicus (1473–1543) used a telescope to demonstrate that the earth revolved around the sun. By the seventeenth century, the great English physician Thomas Sydenham (1624–1689) would insist that "the physician who earnestly studies, with his own eyes – and not through the medium of books – the natural phenomena of the different diseases, must necessarily excel in the art of discovering what, in any given case, are the true indications as to the remedial measures that should be employed."[11]

What a crowd! How many figures are there? Can you speculate about their age, profession, class status, and relationship to one another? Pay attention to their clothing, hairstyle, posture, gestures, and position within the frame. Which details are most helpful? Could some of the figures be representations of actual people?

You probably noticed immediately that the crowd is witness to the dissection of a female cadaver. On her right stands Andreas Vesalius, the creator of the book *De Humani Corporis Fabrica* (On the Fabric of the Human Body).

The *Fabrica*, as it is called, first published in 1543, is regarded as one of the most influential books on human anatomy. What instructions do you think Vesalius might have given to the artist, a student of the great Venetian painter Titian, to communicate the significance of his book?

Look at the overall composition and note that the crowd is divided into four sections by the skeleton's staff and the rail that separates the crowd into upper and lower levels. The cadaver seems to lie on Death's staff as if it were a sacrifice. What could be said about the relative positions of Vesalius and the skeleton? The entire scene is framed by fluted Roman columns. What sort of status do they add to the scene? How would the scene be different if the columns were simple wooden posts?

For comparison, look at two other pictures: *The School of Athens*, by Rafael (1483–1520), which accompanies Chapter 15 and was painted only twenty years before the publication of the *Fabrica*; and the *Portrait of Dr. Samuel Gross* (see Chapter 18), painted 300 years later. What elements do these three works of art share?

For further study, visit: http://vesalius.northwestern.edu.

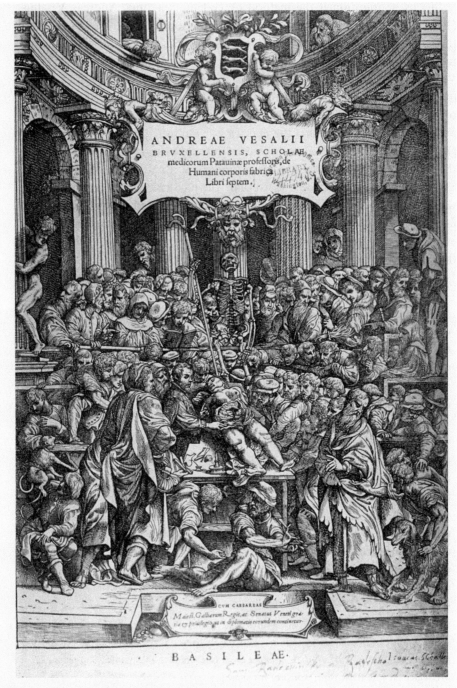

Figure 3. Vesalius performing dissection, title page of *De Humani Corporis Fabrica*, 1543, Courtesy of National Library of Medicine

Despite the growing emphasis on seeing for oneself, early modern medical educators often argued that seeing inside the human body had no necessary connection with clinical signs and symptoms of health and disease. In Anglo-American schools, anatomical dissection did not become a required part of the curriculum until the late eighteenth or even the nineteenth century.[12]

MEDICAL EDUCATION IN THE EIGHTEENTH CENTURY

For 500 years, both the content of medical education and the social class of teachers, students, doctors, and patients varied little. Medicine was largely understood as a learned profession that was studied in universities, conveyed in Latin, and divorced from the practical, hands-on work of surgeons, pharmacists, or other healers. In the eighteenth century, however, practical rather than theoretical training gained the upper hand, books were published in national languages, and hospital teaching took hold.[13] A physician's success now required a first-hand knowledge of health and disease *and* a mastery of new academic subjects – physiology, chemistry, botany, pathology, comparative anatomy, and therapeutics. By the end of the century, the gap between medical theory and practice had virtually disappeared.

Institutional forms of medical education varied across national lines. In Germany, clinical study was bound to the university, whereas revolutionary French reformers instructed students outside university walls. Eighteenth-century medicine in Europe was also taught in state-run practical schools, military schools, private medical colleges, and hospitals. In eastern Europe, specialized schools trained country practitioners, midwives, and bathkeepers.[14] In Great Britain, most university physicians were trained in Glasgow and Edinburgh, whose medical school was established in 1726 and soon became a leading institution throughout Europe.[15] Both Scottish medical schools offered a wide range of medical courses – including midwifery and surgery – along with practical clinical education.

In the early eighteenth century, many ambitious students from North America, which had no formal medical schools or European-style universities, studied at Edinburgh. As the absence of universities might suggest, American medicine left a good deal to be desired. Speaking with some hyperbole, one colonial doctor put it this way:

> In general, the physical Practice in our Colonies, is so perniciously bad, that excepting in Surgery, and some very acute Cases, it is better to let Nature under a proper regiment [*sic*] take her Course ... than to trust to the Honesty and Sagacity of the Practitioner.... Frequently there is more Danger from the Physician, than from the Distemper.[16]

The first medical schools in Canada and the United States were planned, developed, and staffed by graduates of Edinburgh. Americans John Morgan (1735–1789), William Shippen Jr. (1736–1808), and Benjamin Rush (1746–1813) – all graduates of Edinburgh – founded the medical department at the University of Pennsylvania in 1765. Following the model of Edinburgh, the Philadelphia school received its income from student fees, accepted a variety of students, and instituted qualifying examinations. Other schools sprouted up at Kings College of New York (later Columbia) (1767), Harvard (1782), and Dartmouth (1797).

However, even as university-based medical education developed in the United States, the number of their graduates was small, their effectiveness was limited, and their prestige and authority were challenged by a growing number of alternative healers. Elite physicians struggled to defend their privileged status against practitioners of lower socioeconomic status or less formal education (so-called quacks). During the Revolutionary War for, example, William Smith wrote that "Quacks abound like Locusts in Egypt, and too many have recommended themselves to a full Practice and Profitable Substance."[17] But in North America, the lack of training institutions, hospitals, or government involvement meant that apprenticeship – not university-based training – was by far the most common route to medical practice. Men of widely varied training identified themselves as doctors. Medical students of all types were considered a coarse, crude, rowdy bunch.[18] And while the line between professionally trained practitioners and popular healers was drawn legally after the Civil War, actual medical practices and theories continued to mingle until the great reform of medical education in the late nineteenth and early twentieth centuries.

MEDICAL EDUCATION IN THE NINETEENTH AND EARLY TWENTIETH CENTURIES

In the first half of the nineteenth century, medicine and health care in the United States encompassed a wide array of practices. Homeopaths, botanists, abortionists, midwives, and many others plied their trades in the exciting – and dangerous – world of patient treatment.[19] The formal medical education that *did* exist was woefully inadequate: so-called proprietary schools, which often had no formal admission process, were operated by self-appointed professors who supplemented their meager income obtained from the practice of medicine. The schools typically consisted of a lecture hall or another small space – perhaps a room above a store or a pharmacy. Perhaps seven or eight instructors taught primarily through lectures, without student participation in clinical work or scientific study in laboratories. After spending two sixteen-week terms learning from textbooks, students were often awarded a degree without having touched a patient.[20]

By mid-century, the American Medical Association and reformers such as Daniel Drake (1785–1852) were calling for improvements in both education and practice. No significant change took place until after the Civil War, which exposed an inept system of medicine whose therapeutics were still based in Galenic thinking. Union and Confederate soldiers succumbed to dysentery, malaria, measles, typhoid fever, smallpox, tuberculosis, pneumonia, bronchitis, scarlet fever, and scurvy – diseases that were aggravated or caused by squalid living conditions, unsanitary hospitals, and poor treatment. Doctors, clinging to humoral theory, exacerbated their patients' ailments through bloodletting or suppuration (removing pus from a wound, which was thought to be part of a natural healing process but actually led to terrible infection in the absence of antiseptic techniques). Amputations were often fatal. One historian estimates that 110,000 Union soldiers perished from battle wounds and 225,000 died from disease. For every Confederate soldier who died in battle, three died from disease. In the face of these maladies, doctors stood virtually helpless.[21]

Meanwhile, aspiring American doctors sought elite medical instruction in Europe, where the most advanced medical research and practice shifted from Edinburgh to France early in the nineteenth century and later to Germany. During the 1830s and 1840s, young, upper-class men from the East Coast – Oliver Wendell Holmes (1841–1935), H. I. Bowditch (1840–1911), and Lemuel Shattuck (1793–1859) among them – traveled to France in order to learn from the great Parisian teacher Pierre Louis (1789–1872), who pioneered statistical methods for evaluating the effectiveness of bloodletting.[22]

After 1850, the leading edge of medical science moved to Germany, where *Naturphilosophie* (a holistic philosophy of nature) was losing its intellectual dominance to the empirical sciences of biochemistry, physiology, experimental pathology, pharmacology, and bacteriology. Elite American students followed suit. "As regards scientific medicine," said John Shaw Billings (1838–1913) in 1881, "we are at present going to school in Germany."[23] In contrast to Parisian medicine, the Germans prized laboratory techniques and methods of experimentation over clinical and postmortem observation. Out of German laboratories came new discoveries in cell theory, modern physiology, cellular pathology, and microbiology. Between 1870 and 1914, at least 10,000 American students – along with students from all over the world – studied in Germany or in German-speaking medical schools in Austria or Switzerland.[24] Perhaps the greatest strength of German medical science was that its laboratories and medical schools were housed in modern research universities.

In the United States, the modern research university began to appear only after the Civil War, when an explosion of new knowledge clashed with the traditional pedagogy of American colleges and universities. Institutions of higher education were transformed from places for the transmission of relatively fixed bodies of knowledge into dynamic institutions committed to the growth of new knowledge. The traditional fields of theology, philosophy, classical languages, and mathematics faced competition from new disciplines in the natural and social sciences. As early as 1869, Charles Eliot (1834–1926), the president of

Harvard, argued that scientific studies should foster "the powers of observation, the inductive faculty, the sober imagination, the sincere and proportionate judgment. A student ... gets no such training by studying even a good text-book, though he really master it, nor yet by sitting at the feet of the most admirable lecturer."[25] The new, scientifically based research universities gradually assumed educational control over fields previously served by apprenticeship such as law, dentistry, pharmacy, and medicine.

Although medical schools had previously been housed in several American universities – Harvard, Penn, Yale, Dartmouth, and Michigan – they were not much the better for it. Kenneth Ludmerer (1947–) paints a dim picture of university medical schools before the reforms of the late nineteenth century. At Harvard, for example, admission in 1869 was open to all who could pay tuition. "Only 20% of students held a college degree, and one faculty member estimated that in 1870 over half the students could not write. As elsewhere, the curriculum consisted of two four-month terms of lectures." There were no written exams, no laboratory or clinical work, and only a loose association between the university and the medical school. One study described the school as "a money making institution, not much better than a diploma mill."[26]

Under Eliot, Harvard took its first steps toward reform. Beginning in the 1870s, leading university presidents used their financial and administrative power aggressively to promote the reform and development of their medical schools. The modern research university and with it the modern teaching hospital (which emerged in the same period), provided the scholarly and clinical infrastructure for the vast overhaul of American medical education between 1880 and 1920. In this period, inspired by a new model of medical education, university medical schools replaced proprietary schools. By the 1920s, American medical education and research had become the envy of the entire world.

What was this new model? And how did it come to dominate medical education? The initial changes were first introduced by a small but influential group of men who had studied in Germany and chose the arduous struggle for reform at Harvard, Michigan, Cornell, and the newly founded Johns Hopkins, which opened its hospital in 1889 and its medical school in 1893. At Johns Hopkins, William Osler (1849–1919) and his colleagues – Howard Kelly (1858–1943), William Halsted (1852–1922), Franklin Mall (1862–1917), William Howell (1860–1945), and the Dean William Welch (1850–1934) – stressed that students should be taken out of the lecture halls and placed at the bedside of living, breathing patients. As Osler put it, "To cover the vast field of medicine in four years is an impossible task. We can only instill principles, put the students[sic] in the right path, give him methods, teach him how to study, and early to discern between essentials and non-essentials."[27] Knowledge gained by experience at the bedside, in other words, was more reliable than knowledge gained through books or lectures. The new model of medical education envisioned a careful balance of teaching, research, and patient care – a balance that would prove impossible to maintain in the tumultuous economic climate of the later twentieth century.

While the new model of medical education was well developed by the early twentieth century, only a handful of elite schools could meet its standards or afford the costs of expanded faculties, laboratories, and clinical facilities. The catalyst for full-scale reform appeared in 1910, when Abraham Flexner (1866–1959) of the Carnegie Foundation published his report on American and Canadian medical education. (Not a single Canadian school was deemed inadequate.) Flexner surveyed, visited, and evaluated every medical school in the United States and concluded that most of them were substandard and underfunded. He recommended closing half of them. By then, many of his conclusions and recommendations were commonplace but had not yet been widely enacted. Flexner's report, together with the Carnegie Foundation's money and public outrage over the state of American medicine, transformed the reform of medical education into an effective social movement in the Progressive Era.

Flexner's severe judgment of proprietary schools led to state licensing laws that excluded for-profit schools from accreditation. He argued that medical schools should have an admissions process with minimum standards of a high school education and at least two years of college level or university science. Flexner also recommended that medical curricula be extended to four years (two years of basic sciences and two years of clinical study) and that medical schools be housed in modern universities and given control of clinical instruction in hospitals. Finally, he agreed with Osler that "doing," not thinking, should be the primary skill of the successful medical student.[28] Between 1910 and 1935, more than half of all American medical schools merged or closed. Of the sixty-six surviving MD-granting institutions in 1935, fifty-seven were part of a university. In some schools, senior faculty were fired and younger, scientifically trained faculty were hired to carry out the threefold mission of education, research, and patient care.

The Flexnerian model was appealing because it raised standards of training and improved quality of care. The motivations for reform, however, were not entirely altruistic, and the consequences were not all sanguine. Outside of surgery, orthodox medicine in 1910 actually had no new effective therapeutics to offer. Nevertheless, Flexner recommended excluding schools of osteopathy, chiropractic medicine, eclectic medicine, and homoeopathy (what is now called alternative complementary medicine) from accreditation. These reforms redounded to the economic self-interest of orthodox physicians, whose income and prestige rose considerably when other forms of medicine were excluded and licensing laws required the closing of proprietary schools.

Reform also had negative consequences. Rigid entrance requirements excluded many potentially good candidates. Others could not afford an expensive and lengthy university-based medical education, leaving student bodies composed of upper-class white males. In contrast, some small proprietary schools had previously accepted women, poorer students, and even African Americans (in the North). These graduates had subsequently provided care for people of color, residents of rural areas, and those who could not afford to pay.

In 1880, women represented approximately 5 percent of American doctors. Female physicians seemed to have gained a foothold in medical education and practice.[29] However, public opinion sternly resisted the idea of female medical practitioners, and medical school reform created barriers that were not dismantled until the 1970s. In 1892, aspiring women doctors had access to twenty women's colleges around the country.[30] Flexnerian reforms – especially the decision to link medical education with the university – caused a sharp decline in female enrollment. By the 1920s, only the Women's Medical College of Pennsylvania survived. Women's schools were sometimes closed in the belief that women would become better trained in university medical schools. Although Johns Hopkins was an exception, women were in fact largely excluded from admission to the new schools.

The Flexner Report accentuated similar, more severe barriers to the education of African American physicians. In 1900, a black student wishing to pursue a career in medicine could choose between ten schools across the country; by 1923, after the release of the Flexner Report, that same student could only choose between Meharry Medical College and Howard University The reduction can be attributed to Flexner's scathing review of black colleges and his general indifference to their lack of financial resources.[31] By 1950, the number of black practitioners in the United States continued to fall, reflecting the inability of the two existing schools to train enough students and to raise financial support. In 1972, African Americans made up 2.4 percent of American medical school classes, a percentage that gradually rose to 6.5 percent in 2011.[32]

MEDICAL EDUCATION SINCE WORLD WAR I: ADVANCES AND CHALLENGES

Thanks to the intellectual revolution of the late nineteenth century, a new class of teacher developed: the full-time professor. Professors with a PhD in one of the basic sciences focused on research and laboratory work with students. MD professors found their own balance of classroom teaching, clinical practice, and research. As medical knowledge expanded, it became clear that four years of medical education was not enough to produce a physician whose knowledge and clinical competence prepared them to practice at the expected standard of care. By the 1920s, the internship – one additional year of supervised hospital-based experience – became an expectation, if not a requirement for licensing for every physician. In addition, students entering a specialized field of expertise (by 1940, there were already fourteen specialties from anesthesiology to plastic surgery) were required to complete a residency composed of several additional years of supervised practical training.[33] Internships and residencies, like medical schools, remained largely the province of white men. African Americans, women, ethnic, and religious minorities – especially Jews – found the doors of postgraduate medical training closed to them. Through World War II, there was not a single surgery residency program that accepted women.

After the Flexner Report, American medical education witnessed an institutional revolution. Medical schools exploded in size, wealth, and complexity. Resources were abundant, classes were smaller, and the average student received far more attention than students in the overflowing medical classes of Europe. Budgets skyrocketed from an average of $100,000 (in 1910) to $1 million (in 1940) to $20 million (in 1965) to more than $200 million (in 1990).[34] Ever since American medical schools, universities, and teaching hospitals joined forces in the early twentieth century, medical educators have seen their mission as a three-legged stool: education, research, and patient care. The stool, however, has not always been well balanced. Changes of professional power, economic climate, political support, and public trust have affected sources of funding and the relative priority of education.

The history of medical education since Flexner falls into three basic periods: (1) In the first period, from the 1920s to the 1940s, medical schools saw themselves as primarily in the business of teaching; the needs of learners took precedence over research and patient care. Second, from World War II until the 1980s, research, fueled by the rapid growth of federal funds from the National Institutes of Health, replaced teaching as the most prestigious and valued aspect of medical schools. The final period, since the 1980s, witnessed the rise of managed care organizations and competition from corporate medicine and the need to generate income from faculty clinical practice, which reduced the funding and time available to educate students.

By the 1950s, medical schools had become an inseparable part of larger entities known as academic health centers (also known as health science centers or academic medical centers). Although no two are alike, academic health centers are best understood as geographic complexes that contain a number of contiguous, collaborating institutions – medical schools, hospitals, research facilities, and other professional schools. They transformed medical education by linking it to the education of other health professionals and by tying education to large, integrated systems of health care delivery. By the 1990s, there were more than 125 academic health centers, but declining federal funding, spiraling health care costs, and a competitive health care market put many of them in financial jeopardy.[35] "As the twentieth century was ending," Ludmerer writes, "a second revolutionary period in American medical education had begun. Major characteristics of this period included the erosion of the clinical learning environment, the diminishing of faculty scholarship, and the reemergence of a proprietary system of medical schools in which the faculties' financial well-being was placed before education and research."[36] Faculty who had previously been supported to teach and do research were told they had to devote their time to seeing increasing numbers of patients. The need to maximize productivity – to increase clinical income by seeing more patients in less time – displaced the personalized education of the student and the care of the patient.

Despite these trends, reform-minded educators and scholars since the 1970s have pressed the case for respecting the patient as a whole person through active listening, compassionate presence, and collaborative decision making. More recently, the need to educate and support the "whole student" has also become apparent. Evidence suggests that students, faculty, and physicians in general suffer from the financial pressures of academic health centers and the general dehumanization of modern medicine. These conditions contribute to significant rates of "burnout," a condition characterized by emotional exhaustion, depersonalization, and decreased sense of self-efficacy. In response, programs for faculty health and well-being have sprung up, and self-care has become an important but still underappreciated concern for faculty and students alike.[37]

CASE STUDY: A MEDICAL STUDENT'S PERSONAL NARRATIVE

In the following excerpt, Karen Kim discusses her frustration, in the first decade of the twenty-first century, with the demanding schedule of medical school – especially the lack of opportunities to explore students' own motivations and experiences.

"As pre-clinical students, we never have any forums in which we can learn about each other and the incredible wealth of experiences and accomplishments that we collectively bring to medical school. We have virtually no class time devoted to discussing the whole slew of motivations that brought us into medicine: belief (at least to some degree) in the biomedical model; a desire to combat poverty, disease, and racial disparities in care; a search for prestige or financial stability; personal experiences of prejudice and discrimination; commitment to our communities. With thirty hours a week of class time spent sitting in a lecture hall looking at PowerPoint slides, who has the time? As the workload and stress mount, discussion of anything outside the required basics becomes superfluous, unimportant, and an added headache. Virtually no one wants to attend a voluntary two-hour symposium on the ethics of transplanting embryonic tissue into the brains of Parkinson's patients – after all, who wants to spend extra time and energy caring about stuff we aren't tested on?"[38]

1. What seems to be the essential problem that Karen struggles with?
2. Can you identify with Karen's challenges? If you are a medical student, is your own experience similar to or different than Karen's?
3. Do you agree with Karen that medical education should promote student self-knowledge by attending to the "slew of motivations" that brings them to the profession?

In 2010, the Carnegie Foundation for the Advancement of Teaching – which sponsored the Flexner Report of 1910 – published another major study of medical education in the United States. The new report, based on research in eleven medical schools and three non-university teaching hospitals, named four key deficiencies in contemporary medical education. Its first finding reflects the limits of the Flexnerian model a century after its adoption: "Medical training," wrote the authors, "is inflexible, overly long, and not learner-centered."[39] A second finding described the poor coordination between excessive, formal "book" learning (during the first two years of basic sciences) and experiential learning (during the last two years of clinical work). The report's third finding noted the lack of holistic learning about patients' experiences and the absence of teaching about the "broader civic and advocacy roles of physicians." Finally, the report emphasized that the "pace and commercial nature of health care often impede the inculcation of fundamental values of the profession."[40]

The Carnegie Foundation's 2010 Report identified serious threats to humanistic forms of learning, knowing, valuing, and caring. These threats have become endemic in schools that must now function within a technocratic, reductionistic, and commercialized health care system. But they are not "new" or immutable. Before the Flexnerian marriage of medical education with teaching hospitals and the modern university, proprietary schools in the nineteenth century were run primarily as businesses. Likewise, today's concern about eroding professional values has its historical counterparts in eighteenth-century Britain and nineteenth-century America, when modern professional ethics arose to counterbalance rampant self-interest and competition for patients. And as we have seen, the tension between book learning and clinical learning is as old as Aristotle.

The new Carnegie Report is both a reflection of and an inspiration for a broad contemporary movement to reform medical education. The Report and the movement rightly call for the cultivation of professional identity formation – one of the key themes and purposes of this textbook. The Report also advocates a better connection between formal knowledge and clinical experience; facilitation of lifelong learning and critical thinking; more flexible, individualized, and outcome-based ways to advance toward completion of a medical degree; and more engagement with population health, patient safety, and quality improvement. Interprofessional education – that is, education involving health professional students from, for example, medicine, nursing, dentistry, pharmacy, and so on – is yet another key element in the reform of contemporary medical education. Learning to value and communicate with other professions and to work collaboratively in health care teams is increasingly viewed as essential to the highest quality of care.[41]

Since the late twentieth century, faculty and students – as well as patients – have become subject to damaging pressures in contemporary academic medicine and health care. Yet there are many encouraging responses, ranging from programs on faculty health and well-being to renewed emphasis on mentoring students and supporting development of their professional identity. Medical humanities attends to these issues by doing what it does best: facilitating active engagement with literature, history, ethics, the arts, and with spiritual/religious resources. Topics such as the ethics of health policy, the history of medicine, the experience of suffering, and the nature of healing help individuals address aspects of medicine and science where technical mastery is impossible, ethical problems are difficult, and existential meaning is hard to come by. Lectures, seminars, workshops, performances, and film screenings allow students and faculty to reflect, replenish, and renew themselves. We suggest that humanizing patient care in the future will require recovering and supporting the humanity of students and faculty.

SUMMATION

This chapter explored the history of medical education in the west. Beginning with a discussion of how medical knowledge was established and transmitted in antiquity, it examined how many important medical texts were translated into Arabic in the Middle Ages; how scholars rediscovered and rethought these texts in the Renaissance; how medical education evolved during the eighteenth and nineteenth centuries to include new academic subjects such as physiology and chemistry; and how, by the middle of the twentieth century, medical education came to be associated with academic health centers. Then, with a focus on a 2010 Carnegie Foundation Report, it considered some of the challenges facing medical education in the twenty-first century. Overall, it emphasized that medical education is influenced by a complex network of interests, and that learning about these interests can help us to evaluate how and why we are educating doctors.

EXERCISES FOR CRITICAL THINKING AND CHARACTER FORMATION

QUESTIONS FOR DISCUSSION

1. We have seen how the balance between "knowing" (book learning) and "doing" (hands-on experience) has changed over time. As a student, how do you strike a balance between these two ways of learning?
2. Do you think one form of learning is more important than the other?
3. How do you feel about the increasing role of specialization in contemporary medical education?
4. How do you think about your own needs as an undergraduate or medical student or as a physician involved in continuing medical education?

SUGGESTED WRITING EXERCISE

Imagine that you are training to be a doctor during the medieval period. What kind of healer would you like to be? Would you train to become a midwife? A barber? A learned physician? Write for seven to ten minutes on the potential difficulties that you might face during the period.

SUGGESTED VIEWING

The Interns (1972)
Scrubs (2001–2010)

Still Life: The Humanity of Anatomy (2001)

FURTHER READING

Arthur Hertzler, *The Horse and Buggy Doctor*
Sylvia Plath, "Two Views of a Cadaver Room," in *The Collected Poems*

Samuel Shem, *House of God*

ADVANCED READING

Kenneth Ludmerer, *A Time to Heal*
Kenneth Ludmerer, *Learning to Heal*

Solomon Posen, *The Doctor in Literature: Satisfaction or Resentment?*

JOURNALS

International Journal of Medical Education
Journal of Continuing Education in the Health Professions
Medical Education

ONLINE RESOURCES

ACGME: Accreditation Council for Graduate Medical Education
http://www.acgme/org
Alliance for Continuing Education in the Health Professions
http://www.acehp.org/imis15/acme/

Liaison Committee on Medical Education
http://www.lcme.org/
Society for Continuing Medical Education
http://www.sacme.org/
World Medical Association
http://www.wma.net/en/10home/index.html

4 Technology and Medicine

Man has, as it were, become a kind of prosthetic God. When he puts on all his auxiliary organs he is truly magnificent; but those organs have not grown on to him and they still give him much trouble at times.... Future ages will bring with them new and probably unimaginably great advances ... and will increase man's likeness to God still more. But ... we will not forget that present-day man does not feel happy in his Godlike character.[1]

– Sigmund Freud

ABSTRACT

This chapter explores the history of medical technology. Beginning with a discussion of the ancient and medieval distinction between medicine and surgery, it examines how, before the eighteenth century, doctors primarily obtained information from observation and from patients' narrative accounts of illness; how, by the nineteenth century, these accounts came to be supplemented by the invention of such new technologies as the stethoscope; and how the proliferation of medical technology in the twentieth century led to both great advances and serious ethical, political, and economic questions. Then, with a focus on contemporary molecular biology, genetics, and biotechnology, it considers some of the promises and challenges of medical technology in the twenty-first century.

INTRODUCTION

Advances in medical technology have led, as Freud predicted, to previously unimaginable diagnostic and therapeutic devices. Nevertheless, we are not always happy with our God-like inventions. Often we think of technology as an autonomous force that drives change of its own accord – sometimes leading to perfection, sometimes running roughshod over personal and cultural concerns. But technology is always used and defined in specific social contexts by individuals and institutions with their own values and interests. Choices are made. Technologies are adopted and resisted, causing unintended or unforeseen consequences.

This chapter traces the history of medical technology, following both its triumphs and its shadows. We define technology, following Stanley Reiser(1938–), as "material inventions developed to extend or replace human capabilities."[2] As early as the invention of the stethoscope in 1819, new technologies have – literally and figuratively – come between doctor and patient. By the early twentieth century, some patients and doctors were concerned that medicine had become impersonal. The 1960s made it clear that the life-saving technologies of medicine had outstripped the moral resources needed to use them wisely. Technology appeared to be the master rather than the servant of medicine and the health professions. New fields of scholarship and expertise emerged to wrestle with ethical issues in medical technology.

More recent advances carry similar promises and dangers. Genetic engineering seeks to prevent or cure inherited diseases as well as to enhance or select for certain "positive" traits. It also carries ethical dilemmas and religious concerns about control, access, and the consequences of altering the human genome or "playing God." Finally, we touch on the emerging digital revolution in medicine with its great potential for individualized health care and its unknown impact on costs, power, care, and confidentiality in the doctor-patient relationship.

MEDICAL TECHNOLOGIES FROM ANTIQUITY TO 1800

The earliest known form of surgery, performed more than 10,000 years ago in Russia and Neolithic Europe, was a brain operation known as trepanation. Practitioners apparently bored a hole into the skull of a "patient" with a sharp tool in order to expose the brain.[3] The purposes of this fascinating technique remain unclear: It may have been to relieve pressure on the brain that resulted from internal bleeding, to expel evil spirits from a sick person, or both. Whatever its precise aim, trepanning demonstrates that surgical techniques have been used to mitigate pain, suffering, and infection since the beginning of civilization.

Extant manuscripts from ancient India and Egypt reflect an impressive range of medical knowledge. The *Susruta Samhita* (800 BCE), an ancient surgical text, described the procedures of cutting for stone; removing cataracts; extracting arrowheads, splinters, or other articles of war; and examining human corpses.[4] Ancient Egyptian practitioners also had a plethora of instruments that were used for surgery and embalming: straight scalpels, lancets, curved knives, and sharpened stones.[5]

As we have seen, Greek and Roman medicine was organized around humoral theory, which viewed health in terms of balance and harmony. Although the Hippocratics preferred to restore equilibrium through a healthy environment and good lifestyle, doctors were nonetheless equipped with surgical instruments in case of emergencies. The practice of bloodletting, for instance, started with Hippocrates (c. 460–377 BCE) and became a mainstay of Galen (131–201), who wrote extensively of its benefits. In order to open a vein, practitioners used a lancet, or double-sided blade, to cut the patient. A more conservative method, "cupping," involved scratching the surface of the skin and applying a horn or cup to induce a vacuum, which gradually suctioned a portion of the patient's blood.[6]

While surgery and medicine are closely allied today, ancient and medieval surgery were considered more a trade than a profession, and surgeons were often more allied with barbers than with physicians. This ancient divide was reinforced by Pope Innocent II's (?–1143) religious injunction in 1139 that forbade the clergy's participation in surgery; it was also reflected in the reluctance of university-trained physicians to operate directly on the patient. The medieval barber had tools for bloodletting, amputation, treating war wounds, and stanching blood flow (the barber's pole, with red and white strips symbolizing blood and bandages, still survives today).

The authority of barbers and surgeons was a matter of considerable confusion and controversy. In medieval England and the German states, an alliance of barbers and surgeons led to a kind of hybrid occupation. In Paris, when the College of St. Cosme was established in 1210, physicians and surgeons united against barbers. When anatomy was introduced into the curriculum, a physician instructed from a Galenic text while a surgeon performed the dissection.[7]

In spite of the traditional divide, elite medieval surgeons whose texts have come down to us were at considerable pains to align surgery with learned medicine. Henri de Mondeville (c. 1260 –1316), for example, studied and lectured at Montpellier, Paris, and Bologna; he also served as a military surgeon to the French royal family. De Mondeville's views on bathing and healing of wounds drew ire from those who followed the Hippocratic therapy of creating and draining pus through wound salves made of plasters and powders. Guy de Chauliac's (1298–1368) *Chirugia magna* [*The Great Surgery*] (1363) was an encyclopedic work that contained thousands of references to other works in its attempt to demonstrate that surgery was a learned art. "The conditions necessary for the surgeon are four," wrote de Chauliac: "first, he should be learned, second, he should be expert, third, he must be ingenious, and fourth, he should be able to adapt himself. It is required ... that the surgeon should know not only the principles of surgery, but also those of medicine in theory and practice."[8]

Until the advent of anesthesia, a surgeon was required to "cut like an executioner," since the shock, pain, and blood loss of nightmarish amputations and operations led more often to death than to recovery. Nevertheless, despite a lack of anesthetic or antiseptics and a limited knowledge of human anatomy, medieval surgery had its share of successes.

While earlier scientists had experimented with magnifiers, Dutch scientist Cornelius Drebbel (1572–1633) presented the first compound microscope, which revealed phenomena that were previously invisible to the naked eye. By the end of the century, Italian physician Marcello Malpighi (1628–1694) used the microscope to produce elaborate descriptions of human microanatomy, including the structure of the lungs, spleen, and kidney.[9] Meanwhile, English scientist Robert Hooke's (1635–1702) *Micrographia* (1665) contained the first description of the cell and its biological structure.

Until the nineteenth century, the microscope largely remained an instrument used by scientists rather than physicians. It also had its share of medical critics – Thomas Sydenham (1632–1689) and John Locke (1602–1734) among them – who argued that the microscope distracted doctors from the primary task of tending to the patient.[10] Proper diagnosis, according to Sydenham, involved clinical observation and attention to the patient's descriptions of his or her symptoms, pains, and ailments. Indeed, before and up to the seventeenth century, the patient's narrative account of illness was the primary way doctors obtained data. Sometimes the patient gave his or her account in person; sometimes the patient sent a letter. Many letters resembled the one that John Symcotts (c. 1592–1662), an English doctor with a large practice in England, received from one of his patients:

Sir,

I have a great burning pain about the reins of my back, which strikes up to the top of my belly, and a wonderful ill scent arising from my stomach. I do desire your best advice. In my hankering for physic I have taken so much all ready and it has done me no good, and therefore I would desire you to send me no physic but some oil or some cooling thing, for I am very sore about my back that I cannot stand upright. The greatest pain of all is my left kidney.[11]

The focus of these letters is a story of the illness as experienced by the patient. If the patient's narrative was lost, as Sydenham and Locke feared, then the doctor's full capacity to heal might be lost with it.

Nevertheless, new diagnostic techniques and instruments led doctors to discount the value of the patient narrative. In 1761, Austrian physician Leopold Auenbrugger (1722–1809) discovered two methods of listening for chest disease that, in his opinion, would replace the patient's unreliable and imprecise account. The first method, called percussive diagnosis, involved placing one's ear to the patient chest and tapping lightly; the second method, "auscultation," involved listening to the patient's breathing by placing an ear on the patient's chest. In both cases the physician bypassed the patient's personal narrative in favor of his own aural senses, which could be used to make a diagnosis. In addition, as we have seen in Chapter 2, Morgnani's monumental *On The Seats and Causes of Disease* (1761) detailed the appearance of pathological lesions in the human body. For Morgnani, disease could only be understood if it was physically traced and observed on the postmortem human body. Taken together, Auenbrugger's and Morgnani's achievements anticipated the empirical method of modern science that would privilege the specialized opinion of the doctor over the subjective and unreliable accounts of the patient.[12]

THE BIRTH OF MODERN MEDICAL TECHNOLOGY

As we have seen, the practice of medicine long depended on the physician's observations and the patient's description of his or her symptoms. In the nineteenth century, physicians increasingly used manual diagnostic techniques, beginning with the invention of the stethoscope. The stethoscope, which French physician Rene Laennec (1781–1826) invented in 1816, allowed him to listen to heart sounds much more distinctly than when he put his ear to the patient's chest – a practice that was already impeded with female patients by the cultural norms of feminine modesty. Laennec coined the phrase "mediate auscultation," or indirect listening, to distinguish the use of the stethoscope from Auenbrugger's practice of "immediate auscultation," or putting one's ear directly on the patient's chest.

While the stethoscope represented a revolutionary aural method of diagnosis, the opthalmoscope, invented by Hermann von Helmholtz (1821–1894) in 1851, represented a similar advance in visual diagnosis. Thanks to this instrument, which could detect light rays entering and leaving the pupil, scientists and physicians could see a clear and detailed image of the retina.[13] By 1894, the American Medical Association mandated that Helmholtz's instrument, which detected astigmatisms and other visual disorders, be used for all patient examinations. The laryngoscope, designed by Dr. Ludwig Türck (1810–1868), allowed observation of the structure of the larynx. Whereas previous investigations of the vocal chords relied on sound – chronic hoarseness, coughing, or strained breathing – doctors could now peer into the patient's mouth and, with the aid of mirrors, observe the larynx. Just as Auennbrugger and Laennec had listened for disease, Helmholtz and Türck looked for it. By the 1860s, similar new devices appeared that allowed examination of the bladder, rectum, and stomach.

Other devices, all capable of analyzing the functions of organs and producing extensive graphs, represented a further shift away from subjective observations (pulse feeling, listening to the heart or the lungs) to objective data that could be recorded and organized. In 1835, the sphygmometer produced numerical results for blood pressure. The spirometer, arriving a few years later in 1846, recorded the amount of air inspired and expired by the lungs, while the kymograph, introduced in the 1840s, monitored blood pressure. By the turn of the century, the electrocardiograph, thermometer, and the galvanometer performed similar functions. The advent of data-storing machines undercut not only the personal accounts of the patients but also the clinical observations of the doctors themselves.

During the early nineteenth century, the pain experienced during surgery was often so excruciating that many patients chose possible death over certain agony.[14] But the development of anesthesia and antiseptics reduced the pain and infection of surgery. In the early 1800s, pharmacist Friedrich Sertürner (1783–1841) successfully separated morphine from opium. Morphine, while highly addictive, has become widely used in the treatment of acute and chronic severe pain. In 1846, American dentist William Morton (1819–1868) gave the first public demonstration of ether as a general anesthetic to a young man who suffered from a tumorous growth. Shortly after the operation ended, the patient declared that he had felt no pain.[15] Although the medical community was initially incredulous about the use of anesthesia – how, after all, could pain be separated from incisions? – Morton's successful demonstrations laid the groundwork for modern hospital surgery and the development of the new medical specialty of anesthesia.

To be sure, anesthesia was not a panacea. Its rapid diffusion did not mean the end of agonizing surgery for all patients. In addition, the great power of anesthesia created anxiety over its potential uses and abuses. What if anesthetics gave physicians too much power over their patients? The new discovery threatened to overturn the vital checks and balances governing professional authority. One possible danger was the loss of the patient's supervisory power over the operation; unanesthetized patients could protect themselves against medical carelessness, including the ability to make sure that the right tooth, growth, or limb was being removed.[16]

Just as anesthesia reduced pain, so did the discovery of antiseptics reduce infection. Joseph Lister's (1827–1912) *Antiseptic Principle of the Practice of Surgery* (1867) introduced antiseptics into surgery. Using carbolic acid as an agent of antisepsis, which destroyed the invading bacteria, Lister treated patients at an unprecedented rate of success: only one of his first eleven patients died and the others recovered.[17] He also urged doctors to use rubber gloves, thoroughly wash medical instruments, and shave the hair around surgical sites, all of which contributed to the dramatic decrease in wound infections and mortality.

The use of anesthesia and antiseptics also revolutionized birthing practices, which had long been plagued by painful deliveries and infection-related deaths. A particularly dangerous type of infection, puerperal (afterbirth) fever, accounted for about half of all deaths related to childbirth, and was second only to tuberculosis in killing women of childbearing age. What made matters worse were the unsanitary doctors themselves who brought the disease to birthing women. Gradually, doctors realized that they were endangering the lives of pregnant women and took pains to sanitize themselves while applying anesthesia. By the end of the nineteenth century, some form of anesthesia (ether or chloroform) was used in over half of medically attended births.[18]

Doctors were also eager to hospitalize birthing women, arguing that hospitals reduced the chances of infection. Reformers like Lister and the famous nurse, Florence Nightingale (1820–1910), stressed the importance of having a large space, much light, and fresh air. Doctors' arguments about the cleanliness of hospitals gradually carried more weight, and by the 1920s the site of childbirth was steadily shifting from the home to the hospital. Maternal mortality, however, did not decline until the 1930s.[19] While we might not consider hand washing and the use of sterilized gloves "technologies," these practices have saved far more lives than any other medical advance.[20]

The widespread use of photography in the nineteenth century, along with the trend toward visual representation of medical knowledge, were combined in the X-ray machine – a spectacular technology that German physicist Wilhelm Roentgen (1845–1923) invented in 1896. After becoming interested in cathode rays (later known as electrons), Roentgen discovered new forms of radiation that could pass through solid objects. These rays could then be captured on photographic plates, which he demonstrated with a bony image of his wife's hand. X-ray machines easily detected bullets, broken bones, and solid objects lodged within the body. In addition to its spectacular capacity to "see" inside the human body, X-ray images could also be viewed by a group. Whereas the opthalmascope and laryngoscope could be used only by one person at a time, the X-ray machine produced large photographic plates which allowed several people to observe, interpret, discuss, and teach what they saw.[21]

In American society, the X-ray machine took its place alongside the dazzling array of technological innovations in the late nineteenth and early twentieth centuries. The phonograph allowed people to listen to music without musicians; the telephone, the automobile, and the airplane enabled people to converse or travel rapidly across great distances; photographs made it possible to see family members who were not present. Culturally, the X-ray was seen as a form of beauty and prestige as well as an image of death and a threat to privacy. In Thomas Mann's (1875–1955) *The Magic Mountain* (1924), the character Hans Castorp cherishes the X-ray image of his lover: "He drew out his keepsake, his treasure ... a thin glass plate which must be held toward the light to see anything on it. It was Claudia's X-ray portrait ... How often had he looked at it, how often pressed it to his lips."[22]

X-ray machines also turned out to be a useful platform for allopathic physicians to assert their professional dominance over homeopaths, chiropractors, and other practitioners of health care. However, even among mainstream allopaths, the reception of the X-ray was far from uniform. Although many urban American hospitals purchased an X-ray machine within a few years, it took more than a decade to incorporate them into clinical care. Some medical authors argued that X-rays rarely provided useful information that could not be obtained through other methods. When President McKinley was shot in 1901, for example, his surgeons decided not to use X-rays to locate the bullet. Even in the diagnosis of fractures, the X-ray machine encountered skepticism. "No one will for a moment suppose," wrote one author, "that the vacuum-tube and induction-coil will, or ever can, displace the sense of touch guided by a well-balanced and experienced mind."[23] Other reasons for the slow adoption of X-rays in patient care were the absence of clinical X-ray units and storage space, the lack of physicians specifically trained to interpret results, and the lack of standardized forms for reporting them.

Technology, as we have seen, is not simply an impersonal force that drives historical change for better or for worse. For all its capacities, the X-ray machine did not simply burst on the medical scene like a diagnostic savior. The invention and uses of the X-ray, rather, were embedded in a complex social and cultural context – in power relationships within the healing professions, conflicting points of view among physicians, the social and administrative structure of the new scientific hospitals, and broader cultural meanings and responses.[24] The X-ray raised pressing questions: Who owned the new machines and images? Who was authorized to interpret them and bill for their creation and clinical use? And who had access to them?

TWENTIETH-CENTURY MEDICAL TECHNOLOGIES

At the turn of the twentieth century, American medicine shed its reputation as a decentralized institution dominated by country doctors and, instead, increasingly organized itself around hospitals. As we saw in Chapter 1, the number of urban hospitals grew rapidly from less than 200 in 1873 to almost 5,000 in 1923.[25] The availability of anesthesia, antiseptics, and record-keeping machines – not to mention medical experts – made hospital visits more attractive. By 1925, the urban hospital was actively and self-consciously based on science. Hospitals were becoming complex institutions whose spatial structure and organization were transformed. Ward laboratories near the patients' beds made it easier for house officers to test their patients; clinical laboratories were active day and night. The new hospitals built an elaborate and often bewildering structure of operating rooms, in-patient rooms, waiting rooms, and areas for consultation.

The patient's experience changed radically as well. Rather than seeing only one doctor, patients visited a greater variety of specialists. The ophthalmologist looked into patients' eyes; the dietitian decided what patients could eat for breakfast; medical students, busy learning their trade, questioned patients and listened to their hearts, probed their abdomens, and tested new scientific and therapeutic devices. Even the person who wheeled patients around to their various tests represented a new kind of worker.[26]

As hospitals increased in size and complexity, so too did the effort to establish sound patient records. Most hospital records (when they were even written down at all) were incomplete and confusing. Writing of her experience in European hospitals in the 1850s, Florence Nightingale had complained that "in all hospitals, even those which are best conducted, there is a great and unnecessary waste of life ... in attempting to arrive at the truth, I have applied everywhere for information, but in scarcely an instance have I been able to obtain hospital records fit for any purposes of comparison."[27] To make the problem worse, many doctors believed that a handwritten account of the doctor-patient encounter were laborious and unnecessary.

Massachusetts General Hospital in Boston was among the first to develop effective methods for systematically detailing and preserving patient records and began publishing "Case Records of the Massachusetts General Hospital" in 1915. In 1918, the American College of Surgeons (ACS) called for the reform and standardization of patient record keeping. In order to improve standards of care, those who applied for membership in the ACS were required to submit records of one hundred surgeries.[28] Raymond Pearl (1879–1940), a statistician from Johns Hopkins, aided the transition from the sketchy reports of nineteenth-century hospitals to the scientific, statistically oriented reports of the modern medical era. Thanks to quantitative measurements made possible by the new data-keeping machines, patient records could, in Pearl's opinion, grow into an exact science. But his plan was not foolproof. One significant problem involved the cost of hiring librarians and professional statisticians to compile and analyze increasingly complex data.

In the twentieth century, new machines aimed at prolonging patients' lives increasingly appeared within hospitals. The mechanical ventilator or, "iron lung," was invented in the 1920s in order to temporarily assist the respiration of patients who stopped breathing or whose breathing was severely compromised from drowning, electric shock, or an accidental drug overdose. These respirators, which required that patients be put into large iron tanks, were especially helpful to polio victims who were struggling to breathe. "Of all the experiences the physician must undergo," wrote J. L. Wilson of Children's Hospital in Boston, "none can be more distressing than to watch respiratory paralysis in a child with poliomyelitis – to watch him become more and more dyspneic [air hungry], using with increasing vigor every available muscle of neck, shoulder and chin – silent, wasting no breath for speech, wide-eyed, and frightened, conscious almost to the last breath."[29]

By the 1930s the iron lung assisted such children, most of whom could be weaned from the machine as their own lungs began functioning again. Meanwhile, anesthetists in operating rooms developed a new form of assisted respiration known as intermittent positive pressure ventilation (IPPV), a technique that involved cutting into the patient's windpipe, inserting a tube, and pushing air directly into the lungs. The procedure was dramatically expanded in 1952, when a polio outbreak swept through Copenhagen, infecting more than 900 people. The chief physician at Bledgdam Hospital ordered the use of manual compression bags to push air into the lungs of hundreds of patients. Thanks to the round-the-clock efforts of its doctors and medical students, the mortality rate dropped from 80 percent to 40 percent. Soon, machines known as respirators replaced manual compression and were operating throughout Europe and the United States.

The iron lung introduced unanticipated issues of access and cost that would increasingly plague medical technology throughout the twentieth century. An iron lung cost more than two thousand dollars in 1930, creating a shortage of machines in hospitals and burdensome costs for patients and insurance companies. During polio epidemics, which patients should receive treatment? Who should decide and on what criteria? These problems intensified with the development of the artificial kidney, which could pass blood through a membrane that separated body waste from blood cells, thereby preventing death from kidney failure. This procedure, known as dialysis, gradually moved from being a short-term treatment for patients in crisis to a long-term, far more costly procedure.

When the Seattle Artificial Kidney Center opened in 1961, expenses and patients far outnumbered machines and the capacity to treat – a situation mirrored across the country, where 5,000–10,000 patients needed dialysis. In the fall of 1972, Congress passed a bill authorizing Medicare payment for all patients with chronic kidney disease. While the bill solved the immediate ethical problem of who should receive a scarce medical resource, it also put the United States on the road to rising health care expenditures, which increased from one in twenty dollars in 1960 to one in six dollars in 2006.[30] These increases were not only unsustainable, they also threatened to reduce funding for other social needs such as education, infrastructure, and environmental protection. Paradoxically, the introduction of new medical technologies has actually led to fewer patients getting access to those technologies. Despite the belief that new medical technology saves more lives and makes us healthier, the introduction of such technologies has been coterminous with an increase in health disparities, which means that more expensive medical care has been delivered to fewer and fewer patients.[31]

In addition to problems of cost, health policy, and social justice, new technologies also ushered in highly controversial ethical problems of decision making at the bedside. When respirators came into widespread use in Europe and the United States, they became the core technology of what came to be called "intensive care" units, which included cardiac monitoring, intravenous lines, nasogastric tubes, catheters, and other devices. Physicians quickly learned when and how to use these technologies, but no one had any experience turning them off.

Compare this picture with the title page of the *Fabrica*. Have tubes and wires displaced the crowd that observed the cadaver? The artist has rendered the peculiarity of each device to a level of detail similar to the figures surrounding the dissection. But where is the human skill and expertise Vesalius represented? And where is the prospect of human mortality as poignantly represented by Death's skeleton?

Consider the difference in the point of view of this picture and the *Fabrica*. Vesalius's gaze is directed toward us; we have the privileged view of the dissection. The composition of the title page honors the viewer, the person to whom Vesalius dedicated his work, the Emperor Charles V, with these words:

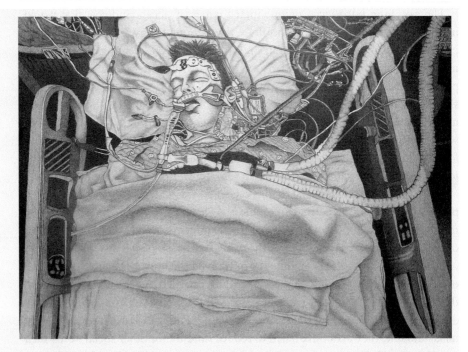

Figure 4. *Sleeping*, 2012, Michael Bise 1976–, Courtesy Moody Gallery, Houston, TX © Michael Bise 2012.

I beseech your imperial Majesty with all reverence on bended knee to permit this youthful work of mine … to remain in the hands of mankind under your leadership, splendor and protection . . . .

As we view Michael Bise's work, where are we, who are we, what is being asked of us? For artists today, medicine continues to be an aspect of humanity to explore. Michael Bise is represented by Betty Moody Gallery in Houston. In addition to galleries, resources for contemporary art include art museums – especially those with libraries with art magazines – as well as books and online resources.

In 1958, Dr. Bruno Haid, chief of anesthesia of surgical clinic at University of Innsbruck, consulted Pope Pius XII (1876–1958) for ethical guidance on the use of respirators. How should caretakers proceed when, after being saved from death, a patient lay unconscious in a respirator for weeks, months, or even years, suspended in limbo between life and death? What to do if a patient's family wished to remove him or her from life support? How is it possible to determine the precise moment of death? It was clear that there were no obvious answers to these dilemmas. The Pope concluded that, in cases of deep unconsciousness or when all hope for recovery was gone, neither physicians nor family members were obligated to keep the patient alive through artificial respiration.[32] The Pope's discussion ushered in a new era of religious and secular ethical thought and deliberation about the use of medical technology at the edges of life.

CURRENT AND FUTURE MEDICAL TECHNOLOGIES

At the dawn of the twenty-first century, medical research and the expansion of bioengineering continued apace in every direction. The advent of modern molecular biology, genetics, and biotechnology identified the genetic causes and potential treatments for many inherited diseases.[33] In therapeutic cloning, for instance, human embryos were cloned to extract stem cells that could be used to repair tissues and organs. In addition, the field of nanomedicine began devising innovative methods to fight cancer cells on the submolecular level. In one example, special gold-coated particles called nanoshells have been designed to absorb near-infrared light, causing the particles to heat up at specific frequencies that, in turn, kill cancer cells.[34]

The existence of these and other cutting-edge technologies, exciting as they are, may only hint at future possibilities. Some scientists argue that nanotechnology will be capable of building fleets of nanorobots that will remove obstructions in the circulatory system, battle cancer cells, or replace faulty body parts.[35] Other theorists of technology, most notably the controversial futurist Ray Kurzweil (1948–), envision a world utterly transformed by technology. Kurzweil argues that human-created technologies will culminate in a stage of human history called the "singularity" during which "the pace of technological change will be so rapid, its impact so deep, that human life will be irreversibly transformed.[36] If Kurzweil is correct, a host of unimaginable technologies will create a world in which distinctions between humans and machines, reality and virtual reality, or even life and death disappear completely. The union of man and machine would surely give new meaning to the "prosthetic man" that Freud (1856–1939) envisioned almost a century ago. For the time being, however, nanorobots and the singularity still exist in the realm of science fiction.

Partly because of biomedical breakthroughs in diagnosis and treatment, the technological problem of keeping patient records grew worse throughout the twentieth century for health care professionals and organizations from small, private clinics to large, public hospitals. Put simply, doctors and care providers suffered from too much information. In the 1960s, a veritable explosion of data came from exams, tests, histories, and medical specialists, all of which produced more information than could be meaningfully interpreted. There was a dire need to bridge the gap between the finite capacities of doctors and the influx of information that resulted in hefty, hundred-page case files.

The development of the computer in the second half of the twentieth century raised hopes that the glut of information could indeed be managed. By the 1980s, the electronic medical record, or EMR, was touted as a comprehensive health information system that stored, retrieved, and modified patient records. A 1991 report by the National Academy of Science's Institute of Medicine called for the transition from a private, paper-based method to a public, electronic system of record keeping. In his 2004 State of the Union address, President George Bush similarly called for a "health information technology infrastructure [that] reduces health-care costs resulting from inefficiency, medical errors, inappropriate care and incomplete information."[37] During the presidency of Barack Obama, the EMR had yet to deliver on all the claims made for it. Even with access to apparently endless electronic sources of information and hyperefficient applications (the iPad and smartphones) physicians continue searching for the best ways in which to preserve the medical information – and the confidentiality – of their patients.

Among the most far-reaching changes in medicine and health care are those being driven by the digital revolution. In *The Creative Destruction of Medicine*, cardiologist and visionary Eric Topol hails the "superconvergence" of digital technologies that he believes have only begun to transform medicine and health care.[38] Since the 1970s, several major digital advances have revolutionized daily life: the cell phone, the personal computer, the Internet, digital devices, and social networks. Topol sets these technologies alongside their medical counterparts – wireless sensors, genomics, imaging, and information systems. He foresees a radically new individualized medicine that will empower patients and create better and less expensive health care. In the second decade of the twenty-first century, smartphones, for instance, are already combining diverse functions from telephone, e-mail, text messaging, web surfing, picture taking, and storing to library, translator, and flashlight. And they are just beginning to be "loaded for medicine," using wireless sensors to display vital signs, conduct laboratory analyses, create ultrasound images, and convey this information to both patients and their physicians.

Another example of digital, wireless medicine is the pocket-sized mobile echocardiogram which Topol uses to examine all of his patients instead of a stethoscope. At minimal cost, this device immediately produces images and data that can foster discussion between doctors and patients. Here, it seems, is a technological change that can create communication rather than distance between patient and doctor. Many questions remain, however. With so much information about themselves at their fingertips, will patients become more equal partners in medical decision making? Or will they be overwhelmed by a glut of data, leaving them as dependent as ever on medical expertise?

Topol's view is based on the notion that it is now possible to digitize human beings in various ways. It is not only that medicine can determine the molecular sequence in each person's genome. It can also remotely and continuously monitor blood pressure, body temperature, brain waves, oxygen concentration, and create three-dimensional images of organs, bones, and tissues. The problem with Topol's notion of digitizing human beings, however, is that it leaves out the moral and spiritual dimensions of being a person. One cannot digitize the experience of suffering or the telling of a life story or the need for meaning. It remains to be seen whether, once doctors routinely digitize a patient's anatomy and physiology, they will be able to care for them as individuals.

In this brave new world that blurs the lines between humans and technology, medicine will face many questions. What, for example, happens to the relationship between doctor and the patient? How do hospitals adopt new technologies without losing sight of the humanity of those who need care? How do governmental institutions even begin to regulate burgeoning and controversial new technologies? How do doctors and patients use the knowledge gained from the digital revolution mindfully and justly? These questions have no clear answers. Nonetheless, they need to be raised continually. In a report on emerging biotechnologies, the president's Council on Bioethics put the matter succinctly by reminding us that, in order enjoy the benefits of biotechnology, "we will need to hold fast to an account of the human being, seen not in material or mechanistic or medical terms but in psychic and moral and spiritual ones."[39]

SUMMATION

This chapter explored the history of medical technology. Beginning with a discussion of the ancient and medieval distinction between medicine and surgery, it examined how, before the eighteenth century, doctors primarily obtained information from patients' narrative accounts of illness; how, by the nineteenth century, these accounts came to be supplemented by the invention of new technologies such as the stethoscope; and how the proliferation of medical technology in the twentieth century led to both great advances and serious ethical, political, and economic dilemmas. Then, with a focus on contemporary molecular biology, genetics, and biotechnology, it considered some of the promises and challenges of medical technology in the twenty-first century. Overall, this chapter emphasized that medical technology is often a double-edged sword, and that we must pay attention to the moral and spiritual dangers of an unreflective use of it.

EXERCISES FOR CRITICAL THINKING AND CHARACTER FORMATION

QUESTIONS FOR DISCUSSION

1. How would you define a "technology"?
2. How is the stethoscope a metaphor for the role of technology in medical practice?
3. Do you use your iPhone for your health? If so, how? If not, can you think of some ways in which smartphones could be used to regulate health?
4. What kinds of tests and technologies do you see in your doctor's office? How have they affected your relationship with your doctor or doctors?

SUGGESTED WRITING EXERCISE

Respond to Freud's quote at the beginning of the chapter. Do you think technology has the potential to "solve" the problem of aging and other ailments, creating a society envisioned by Aldous Huxley or Ray Kurzweil? Or do you believe, with Freud, that we will never achieve an entirely seamless union with technology?

SUGGESTED VIEWING

Alien Resurrection (1997)
Gattaca (1997)

To Age or Not to Age (2010)
Transcendent Man (2010)

FURTHER READING

Aldous Huxley, *Brave New World*
Florence Nightingale, *Notes on Hospitals*

H. G. Wells, *The Island of Doctor Moreau*

ADVANCED READING

Rafael Campo, "Technology and Medicine" in *The Other Man Was Me: A Voyage to the New World*
Aubrey de Grey, *Ending Aging: The Rejuvenation Breakthroughs That Could Reverse Human Aging in Our Lifetime*
Raymond Kurzweil, *The Singularity is Near: When Humans Transcend Biology*

Judith Leavitt, *Brought to Bed: Childbearing in America 1750 to 1950*
Stanley Reiser, *Medicine and the Reign of Technology*
Sheila M. Rothman and David J. Rothman, *The Pursuit of Perfection: The*
Promises and Perils of Medical Enhancement
Eric Topol, *The Creative Destruction of Medicine: How the Digital Revolution Will Create Better Health Care*

ONLINE RESOURCES

The Advanced Medical Technology Association
http://www.advamed.org/MemberPortal/
American Medical Technologists
http://www.americanmedtech.org/default.aspx
Health and Life Sciences Partnership
http://www.hlsp.org/

Ray Kurzweil
http://www.kurzweilai.net/
The SENS Foundation (Strategies for Engineered Negligible Senescence Foundation)
http://www.sens.org/

5

The Health of Populations

[T]he Fury of the Contagion was such at some particular Times, and People sicken'd so fast, and died so soon, that it was impossible and indeed to no purpose to go about to enquire who was sick and who was well.[1]

– Daniel Defoe

Weep not for me; think rather of the pestilence and the deaths of so many others.[2]

– Marcus Aurelius

ABSTRACT

This chapter explores the history of public health. Beginning with a discussion of the health of populations in prehistory and antiquity, it examines how religious institutions of the medieval period took on the obligation to care for the poor, the needy, and the sick; how public health officials responded to plague outbreaks in the early modern period; how infectious disease devastated New World populations; how a democratic, person-centered view, which established health as a right of citizenship, arose in the eighteenth and nineteenth centuries; and how various states have dealt with the health of populations since then. Then, with a focus on some contemporary issues such as climate change, it considers some of the challenges facing public health efforts in the twenty-first century.

INTRODUCTION

It is tempting to view the history of public health as a story of triumph and progress. In this "heroic" narrative, exemplified by George Rosen's classic study *History of Public Health*, the modern nation state and health reform liberate society from the bondage of disease.[3] Scientific knowledge triumphs over ignorance and superstition, while enlightenment triumphs over barbarism. On the other hand, scholars in the last quarter of the twentieth century have offered an "antiheroic" view of public health history. In a challenging body of work, Michel Foucault (1926–1984) claimed that the entire state apparatus of medicine and public health has been positively repressive.[4] As medicine and public health were used to police health and illness, sickness was turned into a form of deviance.

There is much truth in both the "heroic" *and* "antiheroic" narratives. Due in part to the conquest of many devastating infectious diseases, people in modern Western societies live considerably longer and healthier lives than those who lived before 1750. It is also true that state control can be found everywhere: in forms of health surveillance, quarantine, vaccinations, standards of drinking water and clean air, building codes, and many other measures. However, neither the heroic nor the antiheroic narrative alone does justice to the complexities, triumphs, and coercions of modern public health reform. Following Dorothy Porter, this chapter defines the history of public health as the "history of collective action in relation to the health of populations,"[5] focusing on responses to the epidemic diseases that have periodically swept through local and regional populations and devastated millions of people. As we will see, one constant holds true across history and geography: Poverty is the primary reason why epidemic and endemic diseases are able to flourish within human populations.

DISEASE BEFORE AGRICULTURE AND THE BEGINNINGS OF URBAN LIFE

Surprisingly, epidemic disease does not seem to have afflicted the earliest human societies. After the invention of clothing and the domestication of fire, hunters and gatherers emerged from Africa and wandered the earth. These early humans seem to have escaped epidemic diseases because (1) they lived in a cold climate that was inhospitable to the parasites and disease organisms that flourished in a tropical environment; and (2) because they lived in small, isolated groups that prevented parasites from moving rapidly from person to person.[6]

This early freedom from infectious disease would not last. The Neolithic Revolution, which in some regions began as early as 10,000 BC and as late as 5,000 BC, marked the transition from subsistence hunting and wandering to a sedentary lifestyle of agriculture and the beginnings of urban life. For microbial diseases, these more concentrated human populations offered unprecedented opportunities for infection. The presence of domesticated herd animals also facilitated the transmission of disease from animals to humans. As urban civilization spread throughout Eurasia, a host of infections established themselves in these communities. Waterborne, insect-borne, and skin-to-skin infections flourished within city environments, setting the stage for the perpetual struggle between human populations and epidemic disease.[7]

PUBLIC HEALTH IN ANTIQUITY

Despite the transition from a nomadic to a sedentary lifestyle, the world of classical antiquity remained largely rural. Most people lived in small villages of a few thousand people that, in general, were too scattered to allow for frequent and widespread outbreaks of epidemic disease. It is not surprising, then, that Athens and Rome – cities filled with hundreds of thousands of people – were frequented by infectious diseases. Historians have puzzled over the origins of the Plague of Athens, which struck three times from 440–430 BCE. Typhus, smallpox, and measles are the main suspects. The Antonine Plague (165–180 CE), which may have resulted from an outbreak of smallpox or measles, ravaged Rome, decimated the Roman army, and spread across the entire Empire. The Antonine Plague is sometimes known as the Plague of Galen (131–201), named after the great Roman physician who ironically fled its ravages and lived to describe it.

Ancient authors and public officials attended to public as well as individual health. The Hippocratic text *On Airs, Waters, Places* (400 BCE) stressed the effects of winds, waters, and seasonal conditions on an individual's constitution – factors that today would be known as environmental determinants of disease.[8] As Greek civilization expanded westward toward Italy, Sicily, and Spain, this Hippocratic text advised colonizers to build their settlements on elevated areas that benefited from fresh breezes and ample sunlight. Itinerant physicians also used the text as a reference to deal with local disease.

The large, well-organized government of the Roman Empire brought major public health advances. By the second century CE, roads were built throughout the Empire and fresh water was carried into Rome by aqueducts. Aesclepian shrines reputedly contained an impressive temple area filled with baths, theaters, gymnasiums, and sleeping quarters for their guests. The Romans also established *valetudianarias*, or infirmaries, for sick slaves, as well as military hospitals for wounded soldiers.[9] These places aimed at sending slaves and soldiers back to work quickly. There was, however, no similar motivation to care for those who were poor and sick. By the fifth century, as the decline of the Roman Empire led to a subsequent disintegration of public health, the care of the sick shifted to the communal efforts of the medieval church.

RELIGION, CARE OF THE SICK, AND THE BLACK DEATH

The rise of Christianity during the reign of Constantine (272–337 CE) brought with it a new religious obligation to care for the poor, the needy, and the sick. The resulting institutions – the first hospitals – were organized and supervised by local bishops in the eastern Mediterranean, which had been spared the devastation of the barbarian invasions that had destroyed the Roman Empire. Some hospitals were multifunctional, while others contained teaching facilities, homes for the aged, leper houses, and women's hospitals. By the sixth century, Jerusalem boasted a hospital (*nosokomeia*) with 200 beds while Constantinople possessed hostels (*xenones*) that housed the poor and the sick.[10]

The first Islamic shelter or hospital was established in the capital city of Damascus, Syria, around 707. It was founded in conjunction with Syrian Christians who had already built their own charitable institutions, and was modeled after the *xenones* and *nosokomeia* that were built centuries earlier throughout the urban centers of the Byzantine Empire. Islamic rulers gradually established more hospitals, or *bimaristans*, throughout Cairo (874), western Baghdad (918), eastern Baghdad (981), Damascus (1156), Cairo (1284), and Granada (126). In contrast to Christian shelters, which were smaller and more prevalent, Islamic *bimaristans* were impressive structures that stood as symbols of political and economic power. Extravagant rather than functional, these imperial showcases had little effect on public health.[11]

In the high Middle Ages (1000–1300) the welfare of the needy was taken up by Christian philanthropists. In 1145, Guy of Montpelier (1160–1209) founded the Holy Ghost Hospital, while Pope Innocent built a hospital of the Holy Ghost in Rome in 1204. Knightly groups, especially the Hospitallers and the Knights of St. John, set up hospitals from Malta to Germany. The Hospitallers' Hospital of St. John in Jerusalem (1023) was located literally at the center of the Christian world. The hospital was primarily devoted to needy Christian pilgrims, but Jews and Muslims could also be accepted – a significant gesture given the contentious era of religious strife and the Crusades. Medieval hospitals thus stood not only as a shelter for the poor and the sick, but also as symbols of civic pride, religious faith, and progress.[12]

One of the great trials for early public health officials was, of course, the Black Death of the mid-fourteenth century (see Chapter 2). Although the miasmatic or "bad air" doctrine was still popular among those medieval medical practitioners who had been reared on Galenism, others rejected this explanation as insufficient and believed that the disease was somehow contagious. Descriptions in Boccaccio's *Decameron* (1350), for example, imply that the plague might be spread from person to person: "the sick communicated it to the healthy who came near them, just as a fire catches anything dry or oily near it."[13] Various city officials frantically established methods of quarantine – the process of segregating the sick from the well – by refusing to allow ships with plague victims to land in their ports. The bodies of the victims were shunned, thrown over town walls, and hastily buried in mass graves while their clothes were burnt.[14] The public, led by church authorities, performed rites of penance and supplication. Pope Clement VI ordered public flagellations as an act of contrition; when these public spectacles spiraled out of control, Clement gave the order to hang and burn numerous flagellants.[15] Still, the plague raged on.

While the worst ravages of the plague took place between 1340 and 1350, new public health measures were prompted by later outbreaks. By 1486 in Venice, three officials were annually elected to a Commission of Public Health. Two important forms of public health control were established: citywide quarantine and isolation of the diseased victims. Within the affected town, the families of plague victims were confined to other houses. Food and supplies were passed into the houses from the outside, while objects used by the sick and the deceased were seized and burnt.[16]

EPIDEMICS IN THE NEW WORLD AND COLONIAL AMERICA

Europeans gradually gained immunity from certain infectious diseases. With each epidemic eruption of smallpox, for example, some people survived and passed on antibodies to the next generation. When Europeans arrived in the New World, carrying germs that thrived in dense, semi-urban populations, the indigenous people of the Americas were helpless. Scholars believe that small-pox arrived in the Americas in 1520 on a Spanish ship sailing from Hispaniola, carried by an infected African slave.[17] As soon as the party landed in Mexico, the infection began its deadly voyage through the continent. Even before the arrival of Pizarro, smallpox had already devastated the Incan Empire, killing the Emperor Huayna Capac and unleashing a bitter civil war that distracted and weakened his successor, Atahualpa.

The Spaniards' dominance over the Incas can be attributed not only to the physical ravages of the disease, but also to psychological factors. The Incas were surely unhinged by a disease that killed only their own people and left Spaniards unharmed. For the Incas, such partiality could only be explained supernaturally: God was on the side of the Spaniards, and each new outbreak of infectious disease imported from Europe (and soon from Africa as well) renewed the lesson.[18] European diseases, especially smallpox, decimated the native population of the Americas, which in 1500 may have been between 50 and 100 million. By the middle of the seventeenth century, that number had fallen below 10 million – and perhaps below 5 million – reducing its population by up to 90 percent.[19]

The arrival of new infectious disease was no less devastating to native populations in the northern hemisphere. In some cases, the transmission of disease was a deliberate act of war. During a 1763 conflict between the Pontiac Indians and the British in Pittsburgh, one British commander, Jeffrey Amherst, proposed that troops send smallpox-infested blankets to the Indians. The other officer, Bouquet, assented: "I will try to inoculate [today's word would be "infect"] the bastards with some blankets that may fall into their hands, and take care not to get the disease myself."[20] Amherst responded favorably, writing, "You will do well to inoculate the Indians by means of blankets, as well as every other method that can serve to extirpate this execrable race."[21]

In early America, there was little awareness of epidemics. Public health, when organized at all, was a strictly local concern.[22] However, the yellow fever outbreak of 1793 to 1806, which ravaged a number of eastern cities, forced Americans to confront epidemic disease. The virus was transmitted during the massive transatlantic slave trade between England, Africa, and the Americas. While its causes would not be discovered until the twentieth century, what was known, and known all too well, was the general progress of the disease: headaches; painful sensitivity to light; fevers up to 105 degrees; terrible aches; internal hemorrhaging and vomiting of black blood; red blood running from the eyes, nose, and gums; and skin turning gold and the eyes yellow, culminating in death.

The yellow fever outbreak prompted strict quarantine regulations and the appointment of public health committees. At first, sanitary reform and state medicine were based on a belief in the environmental determinants of disease – the "miasma" of antiquity. Benjamin Rush (1745–1813), for instance, believed that a rotting cargo of coffee had caused the 1793 outbreak of yellow fever.[23] Others acted on contagionist assumptions. At times, when city officials were especially alarmed, they hedged their bets by employing both contagionist and anticontagionist measures at once: enforcing strict quarantines and, at the same time, cleaning up hazardous sections of the city that were deemed unsanitary.

MODERN HEALTH OF POPULATIONS

In the eighteenth and nineteenth centuries, the mercantile, state-oriented approach to health gave way to a democratic, person-centered view that established health as a right of citizenship. Nation-states in the Western world collected scientific information, developed educational campaigns, passed regulations, and built public health bureaucracies. French revolutionaries added health to the Rights of Man and asserted that health citizenship should be a characteristic of the modern democratic state. While citizens of the United States never took such a collective stance, Thomas Jefferson provocatively declared that sick populations were the product of sick political systems.[24] By this logic, despotism produced disease while democracy created health. But since government bureaucracies increasingly determined public measures to prevent disease, some revolutionaries opposed them. Quarantines, for instance, could be interpreted not as public protection but as state suppression of individual liberty. For some Enlightenment thinkers, medical policing and quarantines symbolized all that was wrong with the traditional, autocratic regime: its tyranny, corruption, and superstition.[25]

Public health measures also required a new social scientific analysis of health. Endemic infections of malaria, smallpox, gout, and cholera flourished in urban settings and were increasingly understood not as divine mysteries but as knowable diseases to be eradicated. Victorian Britain best illustrates the evolution of public health as a response to rapid urbanization and industrialization. In 1801, 800,000 people lived in London; by 1841 – less than half a century later – the city's population had more than doubled to 1.8 million,[26] among them a growing class of factory workers who lived in poverty and squalor. These conditions spawned devastating epidemics of typhus and cholera.

Public health controversy in nineteenth-century England centered on whether diseases – especially cholera – were caused by contagion or miasma. Were they transmitted from one individual to another? Or were they caused by poisonous particles in foul-smelling air in dirty and unsafe environments where poor people lived? Neither position explained epidemic outbreaks entirely: If a miasma was responsible, why did cholera strike some people in one area of town and not others? If cholera was contagious, why did it suddenly appear in a previously unaffected section of town? And why did it not affect those who treated the sufferers? In 1853, writing of cholera's uncertain origin, Thomas Wakley, editor of *The Lancet*, admitted that "all is darkness and confusion, vague theory, and a vain speculation. Is it a fungus, an insect, a miasm, an electrical disturbance, a deficiency of ozone, a morbid off-scouring from the intestinal canal? We know nothing; we are at sea in a whirlpool of conjecture."[27]

British physician John Snow (1813–1858) helped resolve this mystery by demonstrating that cholera was spread by sewage in water supplies. Questioning miasmatism, he argued that cholera could not be spread by a poison in the air since it affected the intestines, not the lungs. In 1854, after noticing a lethal cluster of cholera cases in a single neighborhood in London, Snow learned that many cholera victims drew their water from a single pump on Broad Street. The pump, it turned out, drew its water from a polluted section of the Thames River. Once local authorities removed the pump, cholera disappeared from the area. Snow's demonstration radically challenged the miasmatic theory of disease and ushered in a new era of sanitation and public health that focused on the cleanliness of the water supply, living conditions, and the urban environment.

Still, many scientists – especially the miasmatists – were reluctant to accept his claim that cholera derived from a specific, if unknown, waterborne disease. In 1854, the same year that Snow investigated the water supply in London, Italian physician Filippo Pacini (1812–1883) isolated the bacterial cause of cholera (*Vibrio cholerae*). His finding was not widely known until the 1880s when Robert Koch (1843–1910), unaware of Picini's work, rediscovered the vibrio bacillus along with the bacteria responsible for tuberculosis and anthrax.

As debates raged over the cholera outbreak, the study of epidemics relied increasingly upon statistics and objective data. Facts, not opinions, were the answer for the great sanitarians, for whom cholera served as a measuring stick in the ongoing struggle to eradicate disease. In his famous *Report on the Sanitary Condition of the Labouring Population* (1842), which outsold many novels of the time, British utilitarian reformer Edwin Chadwick (1800–1890) argued for a major correlation between disease and an unclean environment. "The annual loss of life from filth and bad ventilation," he declared, "is greater than the loss from death or wounds in any wars in which the country has been engaged in modern times."[28] Chadwick's *Report* was a passionate piece of propaganda aimed at goading the government into reform. In 1848, the British Parliament passed a Public Health Act that empowered local boards of health to build sewers, pave and clean streets, enforce drainage of cesspools, inspect housing and burial grounds, and control the water supply.[29] By the second half of the century, cities in Britain and elsewhere had implemented Chadwick's system, which greatly improved sanitation and health.

HEALTH AND THE MODERN STATE

The population explosion in the nineteenth century, coupled with industrialization and the rise of science, radically changed public health in the twentieth century. Western nations turned to epidemiology and the study of population health to help gauge the strength of the state. Many pressing questions emerged. What constitutes a "healthy" society? How should the government care for its most poor and downtrodden citizens? What type of welfare state should be implemented? At the end of the nineteenth and the beginning of the twentieth centuries, nation-states turned to Charles Darwin's (1809–1882) evolutionary theory to strengthen the health of their populations. One result was the morally troublesome social philosophy and science of "eugenics," which advocated the control of reproduction in order to produce more people with "desirable" traits.

While its sources were diverse, the eugenics movement coalesced around the ideas of Darwin's cousin, Sir Francis Galton (1822–1911). Galton believed that the mental, moral, and temperamental characteristics of human beings were wholly determined by heredity. He coined the term "eugenics" to refer to "the study of agencies under social control which may improve or impair the racial qualities of future generations."[30] Eugenics emerged, in part, from the desire to reconcile the contradiction between narratives of progress – a belief in the eventual "perfectibility" of society – and the stark realities of urban poverty and disease. In short, it offered a way to "purify" racially undesirable citizens in order to create a healthier society. Consider, for instance, the rhetoric of the leading British socialist Sidney Webb (1859–1947):

> In Great Britain at this moment, when half, or perhaps two-thirds, of all the married people are regulating their families, children are being freely born to the Irish Roman Catholics and the Polish, Russian and German Jews .... This can hardly result in anything but national deterioration; or, as an alternative, in this country gradually falling to the Irish and the Jews. Finally there are signs that even these races are becoming influenced. The ultimate future of these islands may be to the Chinese![31]

Webb articulated the widespread fear that the population explosion at the turn of the century, if gone unchecked, would lead to a nation composed not of Anglo-Saxons but of ravenous, diseased, degenerate hoards from other racial, ethnic, and national groups. Eugenics, in other words, was a means by which dominant groups improved their health and maintained their social position.

From the early to the mid-twentieth century, various eugenics practices were widely accepted and practiced in the United States. Many states enacted legislation prohibiting marriage between individuals who had epilepsy or who were deemed "imbeciles" or "feeble-minded." Anti-miscegenation laws were on the books in all southern and some western states until the Supreme Court declared them unconstitutional in 1967. Margaret Sanger (1879–1966) advocated birth control measures or sterilization for poor women. Whereas Sanger left these decisions to individual women, some states enacted compulsory or forced sterilization for criminals, various institutionalized populations, and others thought to be "unfit" or "undesirable."[32] Since women actually produced children, they were disproportionately sterilized (especially poor and black women) in eugenic efforts to regulate birth rates, to "protect" white racial health and weed out the "defectives" of society. Other methods used in the eugenicist vision of health included restrictions on immigration from southern and eastern Europe and even euthanasia.[33]

American eugenic policies were adopted with a vengeance when the Nazis, whose entire social and political agenda hinged on obsessions of racial supremacy, came to power in Germany in 1933. The Nazi agenda called for the active extermination of the unwanted racial members of society: Jews, gypsies, or indeed, anyone non-Aryan. But it was also applied to categories within the Aryan population: the privileging of men over women, the young over the old, the strong over the weak, straight over gay, the "sane" over the "insane." Nazi psychiatrists, for instance, lumped the mentally ill into the same category as "racial undesirables." Between 1940 and 1942, 70,000 mentally ill patients were gassed, chosen from lists of those whose "lives were not worth living" according to nine leading professors of psychiatry and thirty-nine physicians.[34]

Anxieties over the purity and putative health of populations in other European countries led white, male political leaders to take a new interest in maternal and child welfare. As policymakers began to see family support as a key function of welfare, maternalism and child welfare became the central platform of social policies. Once again, this concern was especially pronounced in Nazi Germany, where the attempt to breed an Aryan race was supported through financial and tax incentives for early marriage and the production of large families among "Aryan types."[35]

At the beginning of the twentieth century, modern states played little part in the delivery and organization of medical care. But with the rise of the "classic welfare state," as historians of public health call it, governments were expected to ensure the health of their citizens.[36] The *execution* of this lofty ideal has varied considerably from nation to nation. Throughout Europe, for instance, most nations established social insurance systems after World War I, which eased the extreme poverty of its most destitute citizens. The second phase of this process, enacted after World War II, created new forms of social security that went beyond basic subsistence wages to include income security, health insurance, and provision for the elderly.

Public health legislation in the United States has taken a very different form. Reformers in the Progressive Era (ca. 1900–1920) tried with some success to establish state legislation enacting workers' compensation, retirement benefits, and health care insurance. In 1935, a national system of social insurance was established by the Social Security Act, which set up programs providing old-age assistance, old-age retirement benefits, unemployment compensation, aid to dependent children, maternal and child welfare, and aid to the blind. Health insurance was not among its provisions. In the second half of the twentieth century, the United States was the only major Western country without a national system that provided health care for all its citizens. In the early 1970s, after Medicare and Medicaid provided health insurance for the aged and the poor, roughly 10–12 percent of citizens remained without insurance coverage. As of 2009, this figure had risen to 16.7 percent, or to 50.7 million.[37] The Affordable Care Act (2010) aimed at providing health care insurance coverage for almost all those without it, but the role of government in the provision of health and welfare remains a matter of strenuous debate in the United States.

In addition to the problem of uncertain political support for health policies, public health advocates and officials also faced new disease challenges in the second half of the twentieth century and into the new millennium. By the 1970s, many infectious diseases in developed countries had been defeated through advances in public health, nutrition, living conditions, vaccines, antibiotics, and other medical interventions. This trend, known as the "epidemiological transition," marked a shift in causes of deaths from infectious to chronic disease.[38] As attention shifted to chronic disease, public health officials faced a new challenge: there was no consensus or strategy about preventing or curing cancer, heart disease, stroke, chronic obstructive pulmonary disease, or diabetes. There was also little agreement about how other important etiological factors – nutrition, occupation, and the environment – influenced one's susceptibility to disease. Many public health leaders suggested that the new problems represented by chronic disease called for the long-overdue union of preventive and curative medicine.[39] If chronic disease could not be cured, they argued, then it could be controlled through screening, education, and medical supervision.

In 1954, American physicians created a new specialty – preventive medicine – to address this gap in the care and control of chronic, occupational, and environmental diseases. Preventive medicine, which focused on the health of individuals, communities, and defined populations, occupied a middle ground between public health and hospital-oriented clinical specialties.[40] In addition to clinical training in disease prevention, preventive medicine specialists were also trained in traditional subject areas of public health: biostatistics, epidemiology, environmental and occupational medicine, planning and evaluation of health services, management of health care organizations, research into causes of disease, and injury in population groups.[41] In the latter twentieth century, academic medicine, public health, and government in Western countries joined hands to promote healthy lifestyles. Through advertising, marketing, and public relations, the idea of "healthy living" was cultivated to reduce or prevent disability and chronic diseases associated with an aging population – in particular cardiovascular disease, stroke, chronic obstructive pulmonary disease, cancer, accidents, Alzheimer's disease, and diabetes. Nonetheless, despite recommendations about diet, exercise, and smoking that Galen would have made 2,000 years ago, rates of diabetes and obesity in the United States and around the world continued to rise.

THE CONTEMPORARY CHALLENGES OF GLOBAL HEALTH

The epidemiologic transition has occurred largely among developed nations where it is uncommon to die from infectious disease and common to live past seventy. In Third World nations, in contrast, infectious diseases remain the chief causes of death. Cholera and tuberculosis, for instance, kill large numbers in South Asia, China, and Africa. As we have seen, infectious disease remains largely a function of poverty and living conditions. As of 2002, 1.2 billion people, a fifth of the world's populations, were living in "extreme poverty" and nearly 2.4 billion people lacked access to sanitation.[42] For example, following a devastating earthquake in Haiti in 2010, an outbreak of cholera revealed a developing nation that possessed neither a public health infrastructure nor the medical facilities and personnel to battle a disease that, in developed nations, had long been vanquished.

Despite the epidemiologic transition in Western and developed countries, infectious diseases have by no means been eradicated. Contrary to the high hopes spawned by the invention of antibiotics, a host of new and resurgent infectious diseases threaten all areas of the globe.[43] On the one hand, many "older" pathogens that were thought extinct – notably tuberculosis and malaria – have successfully mutated and become immune to the drugs that previously killed them off. On the other hand, more than thirty highly lethal viral and bacterial diseases have emerged since 1950, in developed and as well as undeveloped nations.[44]

When text accompanies an image, you have reason to expect it to be instructive or a message of some sort. The title of Eric Avery's print tells us that the terms surrounding the frame, "Cholera," "drug resistant bacteria," and "West Nile fever," among others, are among the emerging infectious diseases confronting humankind.

One also has reason to expect the image to depict some aspect of those diseases. Avery depicts caregiving to both patients suffering from infectious diseases and to one who has died in a clinic-like setting. How would you describe the quality of care?

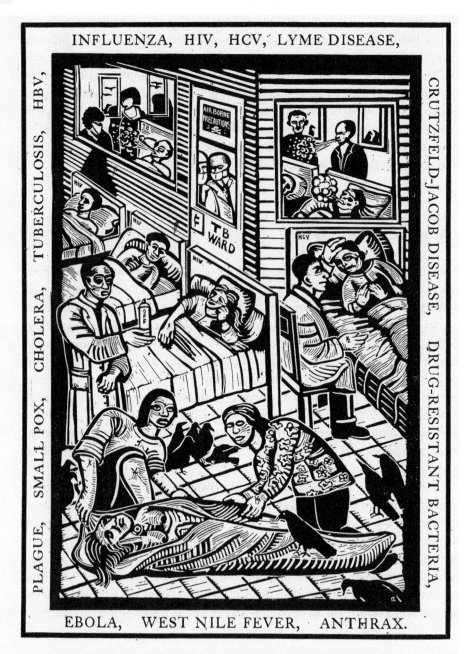

Figure 5. *Emerging Infectious Diseases,* 2000, Eric Avery, MD, 1948– © Eric Avery, MD 2000.

This is representational art – that is, it depicts recognizable objects. At the same time, though, the style is almost crude: the poses and gestures of the figures are stiff and even cartoonish. In keeping with the style, Avery rendered the three-dimensional space of the clinic in a rough approximation of classical perspective. Notice how he drew the beds progressively smaller, as if the patients extended beyond the edge of the picture, toward the vanishing point of infinity.

What other messages can we glean from the image? What might the black birds symbolize? Can you imagine an abstract image of infectious diseases? Something like the symbol for radiation hazards? Are any of the caregivers in lab coats women? What roles do women have? Why would Avery draw the corpse in the foreground? Is the gaze of the women preparing the corpse directed at the viewer, at us?

For forty years Eric Avery has not only made prints that explore issues such as human rights abuses, and social responses to disease, death, sexuality, and the body; he has also worked as a physician and psychiatrist. To learn more about Eric Avery's work, visit http://www.docart.com/index.html.

One of these "new" diseases, HIV/AIDS, first appeared in Los Angeles within the gay community, where victims appeared to have a particularly virulent form of cancer that was exacerbated further by pneumonia. By 1982, the media, still lacking a name for the disease, called it "the gay plague." As Susan Sontag (1933–2004) pointed out, the label of "plague," with its connotations of sinfulness, came readily to those who stigmatized gays.[45] Just as lepers had been considered sinners and those with cholera had been considered punished, so too gay men were considered to be punished for their actions. The underlying disease turned out to be not cancer but an unknown virus (HIV or human immunodeficiency virus) which often develops into AIDS (acquired immunity deficiency syndrome). This especially devastating, sexually transmitted infectious disease has afflicted both straights and gays and killed millions of people throughout the world, reaching epidemic proportions in Africa. Since the 1990s, new antiviral medications have transformed AIDS from an inevitably fatal disease into a more chronic, manageable disease for those with the ability to pay for medication in developed countries.

As public health scholars, clinicians, and officials have repeatedly made clear, the human contest against disease will depend – as it has always depended – on our ability to understand the complex interrelationship between disease, the environment, and human behavior. While global climate change has become the most pressing environmental concern of the twenty-first century, this concern is rarely expressed in terms of the real and potential costs in human lives and suffering. The World Health Organization estimated recently that, in 2000 alone, floods due to climate change were responsible for 166,000 deaths and 5.5 million years lived with disability.[46] The numbers are staggering and the prognosis is grim. Effective change will require political will and an improved understanding of the often indirect, long-term, and complex consequences of climate change for human health.

As public health looks ahead into the twenty-first century, researchers and policymakers debate whether questions of justice and health policy should extend beyond national boundaries. Do developed countries, grappling with chronic disease, have an obligation to assist developing nations that suffer under the pall of infectious disease and the health effects of climate change? The answers will depend largely on whether *public* health becomes widely understood as *global* health and whether global health is seen as an obligation to a global community.

SUMMATION

This chapter explored the history of public health. Beginning with a discussion of the health of populations in prehistory and antiquity, it explored how religious institutions of the medieval period took on the obligation to care for the poor, the needy, and the sick; how public health officials responded to plague outbreaks in the early modern period; how infectious disease devastated New World populations; how a democratic, person-centered view, which established health as a right of citizenship, arose in the eighteenth and nineteenth centuries; and how various states have dealt with the health of populations since then. Then, with a focus on some contemporary issues, such as climate change, it considered some of the challenges facing public health efforts in the twenty-first century. Overall, this chapter emphasized the importance of understanding the complex interrelationship between disease, the environment, and human behavior.

EXERCISES FOR CRITICAL THINKING AND CHARACTER FORMATION

QUESTIONS FOR DISCUSSION

1. Does public health policy affect your life? How?
2. If you were writing a history of public health, would your narrative be heroic or antiheroic?
3. How did Hippocrates' *On Airs, Waters, Places* contribute to early understandings of public health?

4. In your opinion, do developed nations like the United States have a responsibility to provide for the well-being of developing world nations?

SUGGESTED WRITING EXERCISE

Imagine that you are one of the public officials in a medieval city when the Black Plague arrives. The debate centers on the problem of quarantine versus the persistence of an unclean environment, or "miasma," in certain areas of the city. Write for five–ten minutes on which public health policy you would implement. State the benefits and disadvantages of each policy, and explain your decision about which policy to adopt.

SUGGESTED VIEWING

28 Days Later (2002)
Apocalypto (2006)
Blue Gold: World Water Wars (2008)
Contagion (2010)

The Dallas Buyers Club (2013)
God's Children (2002)
Super Size Me (2004)

FURTHER READING

Albert Camus, *The Plague*
Daniel Defoe, *Journal of the Plague Year*
Tracy Kidder, *Mountains Beyond Mountains: The Quest of Dr. Paul Farmer, a Man Who Would Cure the World*

Thomas Mann, *The Magic Mountain*
José Saramago, *Blindness*

ADVANCED READING

Michel Foucault, *Madness and Civilization: A History of Insanity in the Age of Reason*
Howard Markel, *When Germs Travel: Six Major Epidemics That Have Invaded America since 1990 and the Fears They Have Unleashed*
William McNeill, *Plagues and Peoples*

Dorothy Porter, *Health, Civilization and the State: A History of Public Health from Ancient to Modern Times*
Guenter Risse, *Mending Bodies, Saving Souls: A History of Hospitals*
George Rosen, *A History of Public Health*

JOURNALS

American Journal of Public Health
European Journal of Public Health

International Journal of Environmental Research and Public Health

ONLINE RESOURCES

The Clinton Foundation
http://www.clintonfoundation.org/
The Hastings Center for Bioethics and Public Policy
http://www.thehastingscenter.org/
The Medicine and Public Health Initiative
http://medph.org/
National Environmental Health Association
http://www.neha.org/index.shtml
Pan American Health Organization
http://new.paho.org/index.php

Partners in Health
http://www.pih.org/
Public Health and Social Justice
http://www.publichealthandsocialjustice.org/
Public Health Foundation
http://www.phf.org/Pages/default.aspx
The World Federation of Public Health Associations
http://www.wfpha.org
World Health Organization
http://www.who.int/en/

6 Death and Dying

*The physician should be the minister of hope and comfort to the sick, that by such cordials
to the drooping spirit, he may soothe the bed of death, revive expiring life, and counteract
the depressing influence of those maladies which often disturb the tranquility of the most
resigned in their last moments.*[1]

– The 1847 American Medical Association Code of Ethics

ABSTRACT

This chapter explores the social and cultural history of death and dying in the west.
Beginning with a discussion of how life and death were understood in antiquity, it examines
the medieval ideal of the "tame death"; the plague's contribution to early modern images
of death as the "king of terrors"; the eighteenth-century Enlightenment's growing interest
in the precise, scientific nature of death; the nineteenth-century Victorian romanticization
of and denial of death; and the increasing "medicalization" of death in the twentieth century. Then, with a focus on contemporary end-of-life issues in America, it considers some
of the questions facing us when we think about how we die and what it means to die in the
twenty-first century.

INTRODUCTION

Death, as Frank Kermode (1919–2010) once observed, is a "fact of life and
a fact of the imagination, working out from the middle, the human crisis."[2]
Experiences of dying and perceptions of death, that is, are matters of cultural and personal meaning that are shaped by their historical, social, and
cultural contexts: religious frameworks, social institutions, rituals, the state
of medical knowledge, and technology. This chapter examines the cultural
and social history of death and dying in the west, focusing on the increasing role of medicine in the United States in the modern period. Three basic
themes thread their way through this history: (1) the search for definitions
of death and for signs that determine biological death; (2) cultural constructions of "good" and "bad" deaths; and (3) the medicalization of death – that

is, the role of medicine and physicians in trying to ease the dying process or to defeat death.

No account of the history of death can afford to ignore Philippe Ariès' (1914–1984) groundbreaking contributions to the field.[3] Ariès' primary contention is that, from the early Middle Ages to the twentieth century, Western civilization went from being familiar with death to denying its existence and banishing it from sight. This chapter makes use of Ariès' interpretive framework, but addresses its two major limitations: (1) a tendency to overlook the medicalization of death, which has accelerated since the eighteenth century; and (2) more recent movements – which have largely emerged since the publication of his work in the 1970s – of palliative care and the right to die that have brought death back into the open and challenged aspects of high-tech rescue medicine in hospital care of the dying.[4]

ANCIENT UNDERSTANDINGS OF DEATH

What is death? Where is it located? How can it be understood? Throughout medical history, doctors, philosophers, and bioethicists have debated these fundamental questions. While contemporary definitions of death have grown increasingly complex, the answer prior to the eighteenth century was surprisingly consistent: the cessation of the heart indicated the clinical sign of death.[5] As Aristotle (384–322 BCE) wrote, the orifices of the heart "are the springs of man's existence; from them spread throughout his body those rivers with which his mortal habitation is irrigated, those rivers which bring life to man as well, for if they ever dry up then man dies."[6] Life was thus understood as "possession," or the condition of having vitality. Death, on the other hand, was understood as privation – that is, as a non-entity that designated the absence of vitality, having no positive content of its own.[7]

Just as doctors and philosophers debated the nature of life and death, so too did they scour the body for indications, or *signa*, of actual death. These signs included stopping of the pulse or breathing, pallor, coldness, lack of sensation, cadaverous spots, eye signs, relaxation, rigor mortis, and (the most reliable of all) putrefaction, or the foul-smelling decay of the body.[8] Even as they searched for indications of death, Hippocratic physicians did not see themselves as miracle workers who saved the dying from the clutches of death. Nor were the Hippocratics concerned with either immediate or distant causes of death, which was understood as an existential mystery rather than a medical problem. Many philosophers, especially the Stoics, kept an agnostic attitude toward death. "What is to come," advises Seneca, "is uncertain." Stressing the boundary between gods and humans, he goes on to say:

> Life is the gift of the immortal god.... [Death] has an evil reputation. Yet none of the people who malign it has put it to the test. Until one does it's rather rash to condemn a thing one knows nothing about. And yet one thing you do know and that is this, how many

people it's a blessing to, how many people it frees from torture, want, maladies, suffering, weariness. And no one has power over us when death is within our own power.[9]

As we have seen in Chapter 2, medical thought in the ancient western world was shaped by a fundamentally religious worldview, which was particularly expressed in care of the dying. As the sick, impoverished, aging, or mortally wounded entered the Aesclepian temple or the early hospital (the *xenodocheion*) they expected to take comfort in these places and to make peace with their community and their gods.

MEDIEVAL AND EARLY MODERN DYING: FROM "TAME DEATH" TO THE "KING OF TERRORS"

How could medieval practitioners and healers tell if a sick person was going to die? One method, apparently recommended in France around the year 800, was to "take the tick of a black dog in the left hand and go into the sick room, and if, when the sick man sees you, he turns himself towards you, *non euadit* [he's 'a goner']." Alternatively, one might wipe the sick person with a lump of lard and throw it to a dog. If the dog eats the lard, the patient will live.[10]

These anecdotes, along with many others, present the world of medieval healing as superstitious, anti-medical, and comically inept. This picture, however, is not entirely accurate. Literate medieval medical practitioners borrowed from and reproduced the early instructions of Hippocrates (c. 460–377 BCE), Pliny (61–112), and Dioscorides (40–90). These medieval texts described the *signa mortifera* – literally the death-bearing signs – of small eyes, sunken cheeks, dryness of the face, sharpening of the nose, distortion of the earlobes, insomnia, diarrhea, and vomiting. At the same time, these traditional medical ways of discerning death intersected with religious or magical beliefs and practices. *Lunaria*, for example, involved predicting the outcome of disease according to the day of the lunar cycle on which the patient fell sick. Another practice, known as "onomancy," converted the sufferer's name into a numerical value in order to determine the day on which he or she would die.[11] The available forms of prognosis – clinical observation, astrology, and divination – thus spanned medicine, religion, and magic, categories not considered mutually exclusive.

In the early Middle Ages, according to Aries, "tame death" emerged as an ideal of the good death. In this ideal, one went to death as one goes to sleep: peacefully, silently, without a fight.[12] Aries argued that this attitude of familiarity and acquiescence persisted through much of the medieval period. Rich literary and liturgical traditions – especially the Arthurian legends – offer poignant images of knights, warriors, clergy, and peasants who settled their worldly affairs and submitted to death and the afterlife. After he is mortally wounded in combat by Sir Lancelot, Gawain tells his uncle, King Arthur, to preserve his memory: "Dear uncle, I am dying. Send word to Lancelot that I salute him and that I beg him to come and visit my grave after I am dead."[13] A feeling of renunciation pervades the scene: the dying person, Gawain, accepts both defeat and death before commending his soul to God. The unified vision implied here – between fathers and sons, friends and foes, the individual and the community, the earthly life and the afterlife – suggests a oneness between the living and the dead. In the medieval ideal, physicians are nowhere to be found.

"I am the Resurrection and the life," Jesus said. "He that believeth in me, though he were dead, yet shall live."[14] In spite of the ideal of a "tame death" and the Christian promise of a new body and a new life beyond death, fear haunted late medieval Europe. It appears to have reached a peak during the terrible diseases of the fourteenth and fifteenth centuries. As we saw in Chapter 3, the Black Plague epidemic of 1348–1350 took the lives of up to one-third of the population; it also wreaked havoc with traditional rituals and images of dying and burial. As death tolls rose and the dead were stacked up before the doorways of houses, traditional funeral processions and ceremonies had to be forbidden in many cities. Burial, when it was even possible, was hasty and unceremonious; in many cases, family members simply fled the scene.

The collective psychic trauma of the Black Plague contributed to a terrifying vision of death as the "king of terrors." During the late Middle Ages, the imagery of the *Danse Macabre* (dance of death) and *Ars Moriendi* (the art of dying) accentuated the physical horrors of death and deterioration. Tombs were covered with sculptures of the dead in advanced stages of decomposition. Life-size images of the dead were commonplace in churches and public places.[15] In spite of the image of death as the "king of terrors," medieval Christianity preached contempt for worldly suffering and jubilation over salvation of the soul. At the same time that the literature of the *Ars Moriendi* depicted the physical agonies of death, it offered consolation and practical guidance for the dying, whose prescribed prayers, actions, and attitudes would be rewarded in the next world.

Although the medieval period is known as the era of plague and leprosy, epidemic outbreaks persisted into the Renaissance and Reformation, culminating in the plagues of 1576–1577 in Italy that cast a long, dark shadow over western Europe. Dread and anxiety about death also made their way to the New World among colonists who settled in New England in the seventeenth century, when as many as one-quarter of all children did not live to see their tenth birthday. The New England colonists' Calvinist theology did not assuage this anxiety and may actually have heightened it. For them, faith in God's goodness and in his covenant offered hope, but no assurance of salvation or resurrection. They walked a tightrope between perfection and punishment, seeing death as both purification – the bestowal of a new body – and as the gateway to hell, the ultimate punishment of the unregenerate.[16] As late as the eighteenth century, theologian and pastor Jonathan Edwards (1703–1758) preached this message:

> Death temporal is a shadow of eternal death. The agonies, the pains, the groans and gasps of death, the pale, horrid, ghastly appearance of the corpse, its being laid in a dark and

silent grave, there putrifying and rotting and become exceeding loathsome and being eaten with worms (Isaiah 66:24) is an image of hell, and the body's continuing in the grave and never rising in this world is to shadow forth the eternity of the misery of hell.[17]

THE ENLIGHTENMENT, ROMANTICISM, AND MODERN MEDICAL CARE OF THE DYING

Despite Edwards' lingering Baroque imagery, the eighteenth century marked a period of increasing longevity, a reduction of devastating epidemic disease, and the advent of less frightening imagery and beliefs about death. Many Protestant theologians, ministers, and churchgoers came to the view that salvation and resurrection were guaranteed to those who believed in the divinity of Jesus Christ, reducing the anxiety embedded in the Calvinist views of uncertainty about one's eternal fate. Cherubs, angels, and other heavenly images replaced death's heads and depictions of hell in religious art and on cemetery headstones.

As European and colonial American demography and culture came to enjoy some relief from death as the king of terrors, medicine gradually came to play a more important role in care for the dying. For the most part, dying remained the province of the clergy until well into the nineteenth century. Physicians were instructed to "abstain from visiting the dying," in the words of Friederich Hoffman (1660–1742), author of the manual *Medicus Politicus* (*The Politic Physician*), published in 1738.[18] Nevertheless, the intellectual roots of a new medical approach to care of the dying had already been articulated over a century earlier, when Francis Bacon (1561–1626), also credited as "father" of the scientific revolution, redefined the duties of the physician. Bacon called on physicians to "acquire the skill and to bestow the attention whereby the dying may pass more easily and quietly out of life. This part I call ... *outward Euthanasia*, or the easy dying of the body to distinguish it from that Euthanasia which regards the preparation of the soul."[19]

Bacon's charge had profound implications for the relationship between religious and medical care of the dying. In the late eighteenth century, Scottish physician John Gregory (1724–1773) condemned physicians who abandoned the dying: "Let me here exhort you against the custom of some physicians who leave their patients when their life is despaired of, and when it is no longer decent to put them to further expense. It is as much the business of a physician to alleviate pain and to smooth the avenues of death, when unavoidable, as to cure diseases."[20] Over the next 250 years, however, medical advances led to a strong and enduring tension between this ideal of easing the physical agonies of dying and a new biomedical and technological ideal of saving lives. In the process, the term "euthanasia" was transformed from its original meaning of a "good death" to that of actively taking of a life – a crime against humanity in the context of

Nazism – and a moral-legal battleground for end-of-life care in the era of high-tech medicine.

During the Enlightenment, scientists and physicians took an ever-increasing interest in the precise nature of death. Fear of premature burial and concern about apparent death (e.g., from drowning or seizures) versus actual death prompted the question: How could one accurately determine when a patient had died? The modern scientific debate (which continues today) over the signs of death began in 1740 with the publication of Parisian anatomist Jacques Winslow's (1669–1760) *The Uncertainty of the Signs of Death and the Dangers of Precipitate Interments and Dissections.* Winslow claimed that he himself had twice been abandoned as dead, only to revive and discover that he had been placed in a coffin. He concluded that the traditional heart-lung criteria, pinpricks, and even incisions were inconclusive, leading to the view that putrefaction (the foul-smelling decomposition of the body) was the only sure sign of death. Many contemporary medical, legal, and social procedures – death certificates completed by a physician, the delay of burial, and resuscitation techniques – are indebted to the Enlightenment fear of premature burial and obsession with determining the accurate *signa* of death.[21]

In the nineteenth century, medical care of the dying was integrated into professional ethics. British physician Thomas Percival (1740–1804), echoing the words of Francis Bacon (1561–1626), insisted that it was the physician's responsibility to "obviate despair, alleviate pain, and sooth mental anguish."[22] By 1847, when the American Medical Association wrote its Code of Ethics, the care of the dying was considered an essential obligation: "The physician should be the minister of hope and comfort to the sick, that by such cordials to the drooping spirit, he may soothe the bed of death, revive expiring life, and counteract the depressing influence of those maladies which often disturb the tranquility of the most resigned in their last moments."[23] These words, some of which were taken directly from Percival's classic text *Medical Ethics* (1803), hinted that the doctor might displace the clergyman rather than work together with him.

Despite these pronouncements of the medical profession, care of the dying throughout the nineteenth century was carried out primarily by families who were as concerned about the eternal fate of the soul as they were about the physical condition of the body. Many could not afford the services of physicians, who were few and far between, often late or unreachable, and who in any case could actually do very little. Although morphine was isolated in 1816, not until the development of the hypodermic syringe in the 1850s did physicians have the means to deliver a powerful analgesic that in some cases reduced pain and eased labored breathing as a patient expired.[24]

Through the middle of the nineteenth century, the most influential vision of a "good death" was penned by Anglican bishop Jeremy Taylor (1613–1667), whose *The Rule and Exercise of Holy Dying* (1651) instructed his Protestant readers to remain lucid, resign themselves to God's will, and demonstrate stoicism in the face of physical pain and emotional suffering.[25] Even as families prayed and looked for signs of spiritual readiness, care of the body was a strenuous task. "Men and especially women," writes Emily Abel (1942–), "administered medications ... applied poultices, watched for dangerous symptoms, changed dressings and cleaned up vomit, excrement, pus and blood; after death occurred, friends and family sat by bodies, washed them and laid them out."[26]

Gradually, middle-class culture rejected Calvinist theology and its frightening imagery of death; in its place, Anglo-Americans held a romanticized attitude toward death. As one English author put it in 1899, "Death is regarded no longer as a king of terror, but rather as a kindly nurse who puts us to bed when our day's work is done. The fear of death is being replaced by the joy of life. The flames of hell are sinking low, and even heaven has but poor attraction for the modern man. Full life here and now is the demand; what may come hereafter is left to take care of itself."[27] Death also provided an opportunity both for conspicuous consumption and for sentimental excess, especially in funeral planning. The bleak, sparse spaces of Puritan graveyards gave way to ornate "garden cemeteries" filled with manicured shrubbery and sentimental statues.[28]

The Victorian romanticization of death was a double-edged sword. While it may have softened one's encounter with death or loss, it also offered a partial – and hence an inauthentic – account of the realities of dying. This evasiveness is captured in Leo Tolstoy's (1828–1910) masterful story *The Death of Ivan Ilych*. Ivan Ilych is a Russian government official who, by any external standard, leads a successful life. He is married with a family, enjoys professional success, and is well-liked by his peers. Over the course of a few months, however, Ivan falls ill and grows keenly aware that he is not only sick – he is dying. As he reflects on the ultimate meaning of his life, Ivan despises the refusal, among his family, friends, and doctors, to talk openly about the fact of his impending death:

> What tormented Ivan Ilych most was the deception, the lie, which for some reason they all accepted, that he was not dying but was simply ill, and he only need keep quiet and undergo a treatment and then something very good would result.... The awful, terrible act of his dying was, he could see, reduced by those about him to the level of a casual, unpleasant, and almost indecorous incident (as if someone entered a drawing room defusing an unpleasant odour), and this was done by that very decorum which he had served all his life long.[29]

What torments Ivan, in other words, is the unwillingness of his doctor, his wife, and his friends to call death by name – and, even more radically, to turn death into a sort of fiction by calling it a temporary "sickness." Ivan is also haunted by the realization that he has lived a shallow life, one measured by the outward appearance of success and empty of deep, loving relationships. *The Death of Ivan Ilych* raises a number of questions that remain relevant in contemporary society. What is the role of the physician in end-of-life care? What are the goals of care? What is the place of truth telling? How should one talk to or care for a dying friend? How should one organize one's own life during its final hours?

CASE STUDY: THE DEATH OF IVAN ILYCH

In this concluding scene from Tolstoy's *The Death of Ivan Ilych*, Ivan lies on his death-bed after three days of intense agony and despair. He suddenly realizes, with a flash of insight, that his life is not what it should have been. But if my life has not been lived correctly, Ivan asks himself, then what *is* the right way to live?

This occurred at the end of the third day, two hours before his death. Just then his schoolboy son had crept softly in and gone up to the bedside. The dying man was still screaming desperately and waving his arms. His hand fell on the boy's head, and the boy caught it, pressed it to his lips, and began to cry.

At that very moment Ivan Ilych fell through and caught sight of the light, and it was revealed to him that though his life had not been what it should have been, this could still be rectified. He asked himself, "what *is* the right thing?" and grew still, listening. Then he felt that someone was kissing his hand. He opened his eyes, looked at his son, and felt sorry for him. His wife came up to him and he glanced at her. She was gazing at him open-mouthed, with undried tears on her nose and cheek and a despairing look on her face. He felt sorry for her too.

"Yes, I am making them wretched," he thought. "They are sorry, but it will be better for them when I die." He wished to say this but had not the strength to utter it. "Besides, why speak? I must act," he thought. With a look at his wife he indicated his son and said: "Take him away ... sorry for him ... sorry for you too." He tried to add, "forgive me," but said "forgo" and waved his hand, knowing that He whose understanding mattered would understand.[30]

1. Ivan realizes that "his life was not what it should have been." What, specifically, do you think that Ivan wishes he could have done differently? What do Ivan's interactions with his wife and son suggest about his regrets?
2. Ivan also believes that, even in his final moments, his life can be "rectified." What does the final scene tell us about Ivan's (and Tolstoy's) beliefs about the proper response to life and death?
3. Do you think that a "correct" way to live exists for all persons? Or does the answer depend on the person and his or her situation?
4. Does Ivan's attitude toward death resemble any of the death attitudes from this chapter? As a twenty-first century reader, can you identify with Ivan's struggle? Is any of it recognizable in our own culture?

MODERN MEDICAL CARE AND CULTURAL IDEALS OF DYING

In the first half of the twentieth century, the Victorian romanticization of death evolved into the denial of death. Like Ivan Ilych's doctors, American physicians refused to discuss diagnoses of cancer and terminal illness, even with dying persons. Death, in short, was swept under the rug. As Geoffrey Gorer (1905–1985) observed in his classic discussion on the subject in Britain, death replaced sex as an unspeakable, "pornographic" topic.[31] From the late nineteenth to the mid-twentieth century, the denial of death shaped care of the dying, which moved largely from the home to the hospital and increasingly took the form of a battle for survival. After the 1970s, however, reformers, patients, and their families rebelled against dying in highly technological intensive care units.

In general, new scientific hospitals of the early twentieth century strenuously avoided any association with mortality. Hospital landscapes and buildings were designed to minimize the visibility of death. As they do today, most hospitals identified themselves as saving lives rather than caring for the dying, a point driven home in marketing campaigns. "Incurable cases,"[32] such as tuberculosis and cancer patients, might be denied admittance to private hospitals, which often transferred dying patients to almshouses to keep their mortality statistics low – a strategy that, in turn, inflated the mortality rates of public hospitals. Death of the poor was an especially offensive presence for patients in the new private hospitals and challenged the hospitals' financial health. Along with overcrowding, hospital employees often expressed prejudice against the poor, a point illustrated by a Philadelphia intern's comments about a patient close to death: "The unfortunate being certainly has suffered horribly, and would arouse everyone's sympathy did he not also call up feelings of utter disgust for his character."[33] These comments, which appeared in 1908, could just as easily have been made about "drug abusers," "bouncebacks," and "noncompliant patients" in public hospitals over a century later.

In 1910, the vast majority of Americans still died at home. Over the next fifty years, as rates of death in hospitals rose dramatically, patients became increasingly isolated from family and friends and suffered the loss of power over their dying as well. Medical attitudes toward care of the dying were typified by avoidance and detachment. In 1929, physician Alfred Worcester criticized his colleagues for their impersonal approach. "Those who are interested only in the diseases of their patients," he wrote, "find little that is noteworthy beyond the mere fact of fatality and the possible opportunity of verifying their diagnoses."[34] Even nurses, who performed the actual daily care of the terminally ill, were not instructed in compassionate care of the dying. By the early twenty-first century, roughly 25 percent of Americans died at home while 75 percent died in some form of institution (hospital, nursing home long-term care facility).[35]

As new technologies preserved the lives of patients who would otherwise have died, dying in hospitals became both more common and more problematic. As we saw in Chapter 4, during a 1952 polio epidemic, Copenhagen physicians developed a new ventilation technique (IPPV) that pushed air into the lungs through an endotracheal tube inserted through the mouth or nose.[36] Soon, machines known as mechanical ventilators or respirators spread throughout Europe and the United States and became the core of new "intensive care" units. Modern ICUs were designed to maintain normal bodily functions for patients with the most severe illnesses and injuries. In addition to mechanical ventilators, ICUs came to contain cardiac monitors, external pacemakers, defibrillators, dialysis equipment, various intravenous lines and nasogastric tubes, suction pumps, catheters, and a wide array of drugs for curative treatment and pain relief.

For all their success in saving lives, mortality rates in ICUs ranged from 10–20 percent, creating the frightening prospect of patients dying alone in a faceless medical institution, connected to machines and separated from loved ones. In some public hospitals in the 1960s, it was not uncommon for staff to virtually abandon the dying and to discourage communication between dying patients and their families.[37] In one of history's painful ironies, medicine's great success in keeping people alive also had the effect of prolonging dying and suffering. Critics argued that the high-tech "rescue" mentality of modern medicine was distorting the process of dying and denying its inevitability. The hospice movement, founded in 1967 by English nurse, social worker, and physician Cicely Saunders (1918–2005), aimed to increase awareness of death as a natural process, to relieve unnecessary suffering, and to "restore dignity to the dying."[38] Saunders' vision was to create institutions that would provide compassionate care for those with incurable diseases. "When we chose that ancient word 'hospice,'" she wrote,

> we joined a long tradition of offering hospitality and care which dates, in Europe, from the 4th century of the Christian era. At that time a welcome was given to pilgrims and travellers as well as to the sick and destitute. There was a strong tradition of honour for 'Our Lords the Sick' as saluted by the Knights Hospitallers of the Order of St John of Jerusalem in their statutes of the 12th century. Those who needed care were to be welcomed and served with honour and respect.[39]

Following Saunders' lead, the National Hospice Organization was founded in 1978; by 1997, more than 2,800 hospices existed throughout the United States.

The development of hospice was part of a broader cultural movement to break through the denial of death and humanize care of the dying. Among those activist critics and practitioners, none was more instrumental than Elizabeth Kübler-Ross (1926–2004), the physician and psychiatrist whose influential *On Death and Dying* (1969) found that hospitals overtreated dying patients, separated them from their families, and abandoned them when they were most needy. "Death has become a dreaded and unspeakable issue to be avoided by every means possible," she wrote of American society, and continued: "other societies have learned to cope better with the reality of death than we seem to have done."[40] In secular terms reminiscent of the medieval "tame death" and *Ars moriendi* traditions, she adds: "if we can learn to view death from a different perspective, to reintroduce it into our lives so that it comes not as a dreaded stranger but as an expected companion to our life, then we can learn to live our lives with meaning – with full appreciation of our finiteness, of the limits of our time here."[41] In her well-known five-stage theory, Kübler-Ross sees the onset of death as a great opportunity for growth, as a time of personal transformation and even triumph. If we talked more about death, she argued, then it would become less frightening.

Both the modern hospice movement and Kübler-Ross's five steps were driven by the desire of individuals to regain control over the dying process. But what happened when a person lost the ability to make decisions? Or when medical technology prevented death only by keeping the individual barely alive, in an unconscious "vegetative" state? A host of new technologies, from mechanical respirators to the development of organ transplantation, brought new and confusing ethical problems with them as well. One problem was how to determine when a person had died. In 1963, a young British man suffered severe brain damage and was put on an artificial respirator. With consent from his wife, his kidney was removed for transplant; shortly afterward, the respirator was removed and his heart and lungs ceased functioning. An inquest found that, since the time of death had occurred after the kidney was removed, the transplant violated the "dead donor rule," which requires patients to be declared dead before the removal of life-sustaining organs for transplantation.[42]

A more famous case involved South African surgeon Dr. Christiaan Barnard (1922–2001), who performed the first heart transplant in 1967. Like other transplants, the procedure required that the donor organ be removed as quickly as possible to maximize the likelihood of a successful transplant. To gain time for removing and transplanting the heart of a brain-injured and comatose patient, Barnard took her off life support. Rather than wait for her heart to stop beating, he injected potassium into her heart and paralyzed it, rendering her technically dead by the whole-body standard. Did Barnard kill her? Did he simply withdraw treatment from a woman who was dying? Was she virtually dead? Or already dead?

These transplant cases raised troubling ethical questions: What did the terms "alive" and "dead" really mean in circumstances of artificial respiration? Could a patient who seemed to be "alive" actually be "dead"? When could a ventilator be turned off? When could an organ be "harvested"? These questions prompted physicians and others to challenge the traditional cardiopulmonary criteria of death and move toward a new definition known as "brain death." In 1968, a Harvard committee recommended that a patient in an irreversible coma could be considered dead if he or she: (1) is unaware of and unresponsive to all external stimuli; (2) exhibits no muscular movement or breathing (when the respirator was turned off for three minutes); (3) shows no pupil reflexes when a light is shone into the eye; (4) exhibits a flat line when tested for brain activity on an electroencephalograph (a test recommended but not required).[43] This was later known as the whole-brain definition of death.

The Harvard committee's recommendations were widely endorsed yet hotly debated. Others put forward the notion of "higher-brain" death, which considers a person dead when the cerebellum – the neural basis of consciousness – is destroyed, even if the lower brain (brain stem) is still functioning.[44] Recognizing the need for consistency, a presidential commission in collaboration with the National Conference of Commissioners on Uniform State Laws, the American Medical Association, and the American Bar Association used the whole-brain standard to draft a state law to determine death in all circumstances. This 1981 law, known as The Uniform Determination of Death Act (UDDA), states that "An individual who has sustained either (1) irreversible cessation of circulatory and respiratory functions, or (2) irreversible cessation of all functions of the entire brain, including the brain stem, is dead. A determination of death must be made in accordance with accepted medical standards."[45] Although the Uniform Determination of Death Act is accepted as law in all states, there are still religious groups that consider a person alive until every cell in the body is dead.

As public interest moved from defining death for purposes of organ transplantation to clinical care of the dying, the stakes grew much higher. In the 1970s, medicine came under increased scrutiny for scandals in experimentation with human subjects.[46] Journalists revealed that physicians in prominent hospitals were making unilateral decisions about withholding or withdrawing treatment from premature or damaged infants. The public rebelled. In 1974, an array of popular newspaper articles and academic symposiums explored the topic, and a U.S. Senate committee listened to three days of testimony on the subject of "death with dignity."

But the event that transformed the cultural landscape and sparked what became known as the right-to-die movement, took place in 1975, when Joseph and Julia Quinlan asked that their comatose daughter, twenty-one-year-old Karen Ann, be taken off a respirator. After Karen Ann's doctor and the hospital administration refused to disconnect the machine, her parents petitioned the Supreme Court of New Jersey, which ruled in their favor. When the respirator was finally removed, Karen lived in an unresponsive condition for nine years before she finally died. All the while, the case occupied the national consciousness and sparked fierce debate. As a comatose young woman who was tethered to a breathing machine, Quinlan was a new sort of person – not fully alive but not yet dead. Discussions raged on about who is in charge of a person in a coma, who authorizes death, and what to do about someone who, like Karen Ann, occupies the bizarre state of "death in life."[47]

In these debates, there were those who advocated "euthanasia," which by then had come to mean active mercy killing. The term, however, smacked of Nazism and of the early twentieth-century American eugenics movement and in any case did not attract broad support. Thus, in 1974 the Euthanasia Society of America changed its name to the Society for the Right to Die, signifying the crucial distinction between active hastening of death and foregoing or withdrawing treatment. In the Netherlands, euthanasia and assisted suicide have been openly tolerated since the 1980s. In 2002, a Dutch law took effect specifying the conditions under which these ways to hasten a patient's death were legally acceptable. In contrast, neither the medical profession nor the American public widely supported the active taking of another's life, although this practice took (and still takes) place quietly in cases of extreme pain or hopelessness. In contrast, as of 2013, three states permitted physician-assisted dying, reflecting the conviction that self-determination includes the right to take one's own life. In Oregon, for instance, where doctor-assisted suicide has been legal since 1994, one doctor explained the significance of this right for her patient Cody, who suffered from terminal cancer: "Cody taught me that 'do no harm' is going to be different for every patient. Harm, for her, would have meant taking away the control and saying, 'No-No-No, you've got to do this the way your body decides,' as opposed to the way you, as the person, decides."[48] The rallying cries of "death with dignity" and the "right to die" marked an urgent personal and political search for a "good death."

Perhaps the most controversial and highly visible actor in the controversies over end-of-life care was the pathologist Dr. Jack Kevorkian (1928–2011), who claimed to have helped as many as 130 terminally ill patients to die – both by giving them the means to end their lives (assisted suicide) and by injecting a lethal dose of medication at their request (voluntary euthanasia). In 1999, Kevorkian was convicted of second-degree murder for his role in a euthanasia case and served eight years in prison. The legal response to Kevorkian's activities indicated that a minority of Americans, under strictly defined circumstances, were open to physician-assisted suicide but opposed to euthanasia. As of 2013, the American Medical Association was opposed to both.

What, then, was the status of death and dying in the second decade of the twenty-first century? In the United States at least, the medical and technological imperative to cure disease continues to trump the moral imperative to provide low-tech care and support to those who are dying, often after long and agonizing periods of chronic illness. Despite the Patient Self-Determination Act of 1990, relatively few people take advantage of the legal means to direct their end-of-life care after they lose capacity. Studies continue to show that pain control is often inadequate and that physicians often do not understand the needs and desires of dying people. In contrast, hospice care is rapidly expanding, paid for by both Medicare and private insurance companies as well as by individuals.

Culturally speaking, dying is in general more visible, less formally religious, and more individualized than in the past. A profusion of hopeful narratives address death both personally and publicly: in illness narratives (known by scholars as "pathographies," see Chapter 7); through news or reality shows charting the struggle of the sick or dying; among an assortment of grief specialists or "bereavement counselors"; and in popular books and films about death, grief, and loss. Whether the subject is treated with compassion, as in *Tuesdays with Morrie* (1997), or with black humor, as in the British comedy *Death at a Funeral* (2007), death is no longer hidden or "pornographic." At the same time, while many death practices are still informed by religion or a religiously inspired ethos, not all Americans subscribe to the traditional, Christian version of a "good death." Indeed, in recent years persons planning funerals have abandoned traditional classical music, like "Amazing Grace" or Mozart's *Requiem*, in favor of more modern songs like "Highway to Hell," "Stairway to Heaven," or Frank Sinatra's "My Way." American death practices have even seen the rise of virtual forms of grieving: some websites offer a "virtual cemetery" in which a deceased's loved ones can log on and contribute photographs, stories, poems, and memories – a sort of Facebook for the dead.[49] Today, it seems, there is no single way to die well.

Does he know he's dancing with Death? Death looks pretty energetic, don't you think? Would you have pictured Death as being so lively? Would you have pictured Death as a female skeleton? Would you have pictured death as personified in any way?

Death is represented as a skeleton on the title page of Vesalius's *Fabrica,* published in 1543, so we know this convention goes back almost 500 years. Also, as noted in this chapter, the *danse macabre* began to appear after the plagues of the fourteenth and fifteenth centuries. *Baile* is clearly of our time. Compare the settings: the *Fabrica* skeleton stands in an institution of some type, indicated by the elaborate columns, while *Baile* offers no architectural context. To lend it a setting, one might think of a dance hall or honky-tonk.

Since it depicts a dance, it's appropriate that *Baile* is full of dynamic, active lines. Can you find any lines in the *Fabrica* as lively as the curving edge of Death's skirt? Notice how the figures break out of the ground of the image, the man's right elbow and foot in particular. Even the tonality, the distribution of light and dark areas is lively, especially when compared with the uniform tonality of the *Fabrica.* In fact, the lights and darks in the two pictures are reversed. *Baile* almost appears to be an x-ray of the action.

Returning to the introduction of this chapter, how does *Baile* represent death as "a fact of the imagination," as "a matter of cultural and personal meaning?"

Search the web for the personification of death, images of the "dance of death," and the works of *Luis Jiménez* (1940–2006).

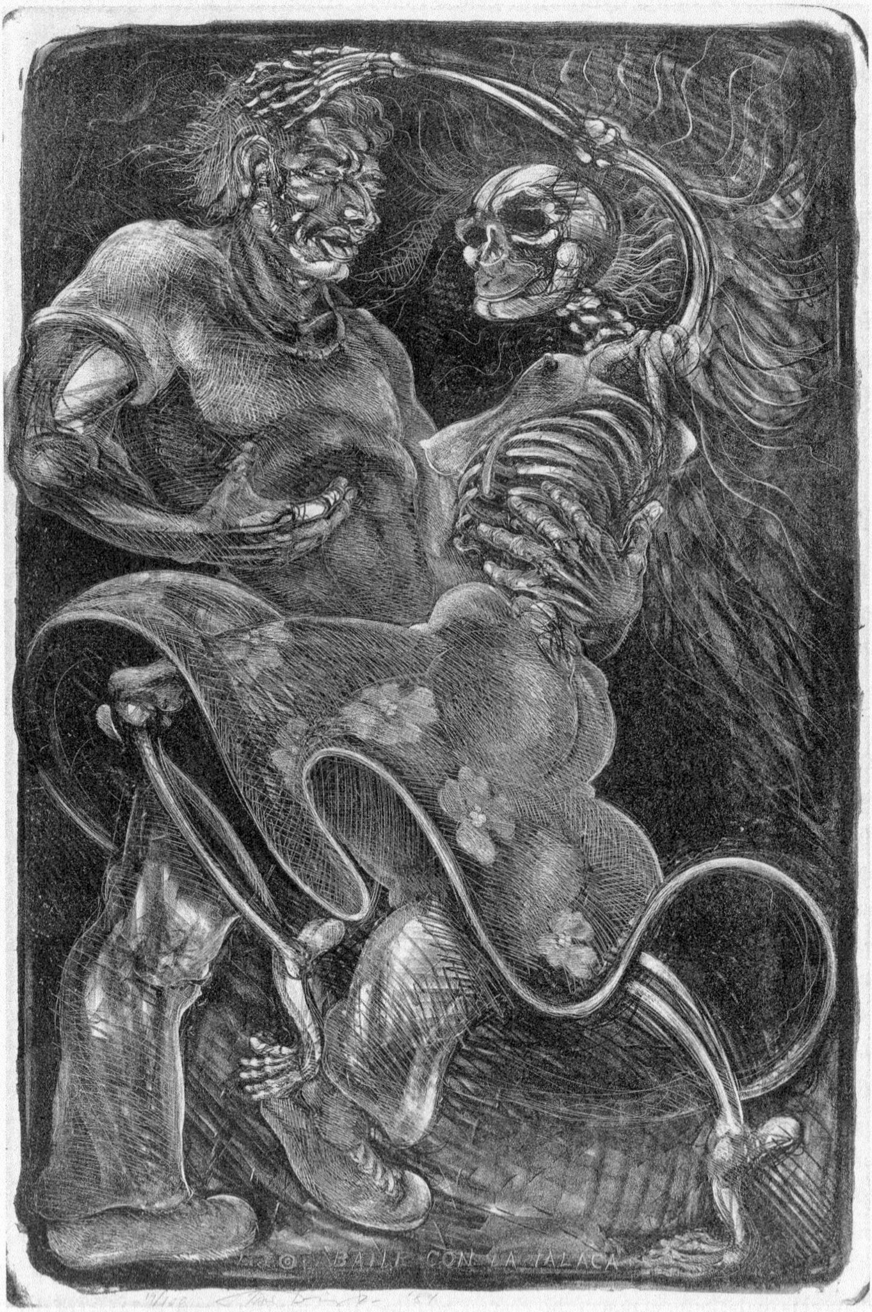

Figure 6. *Baile con la Talaca* (Dance with Death), 1984, Luis Jimenez 1940–2006, The Museum of Fine Arts, Houston, Gift of the Estate of Frank Ribelin © 2013 Estate of Luis A. Jimenez Jr./Artists Rights Society (ARS), New York.

SUMMATION

This chapter explored the social and cultural history of death and dying in the west. Beginning with a discussion of how life and death were understood in antiquity, it explored the medieval ideal of the "tame death"; the plague's contribution to early modern images of death as the "king of terrors"; the eighteenth-century Enlightenment's growing interest in the precise, scientific nature of death; nineteenth-century Victorian romanticization of and denial of death; and the increasing medicalization of death in the twentieth century. Then, with a focus on contemporary end-of-life issues in America, it considered how we might address some of the questions facing us when we think about what it means to die in the twenty-first century. Overall, this chapter emphasized that the meaning of death and dying has changed throughout history, and that a greater awareness of this history can help us understand and enhance our thinking about death and dying today.

EXERCISES FOR CRITICAL THINKING AND CHARACTER FORMATION

QUESTIONS FOR DISCUSSION

1. Has a close friend or anyone in your family died? If so, how and where were they cared for at the end? How did it affect you?
2. What do you consider an ideal or "good" death?
3. Is your ideal similar to any of the attitudes toward death in this chapter?
4. The twentieth century has seen a renewed interest in definitions of death. How are these definitions relevant to the controversial area of organ transplantation?

SUGGESTED WRITING EXERCISE

Imagine the ideal circumstances of your own death and write for five to ten minutes. Where would you die? Who would be present? Who would deliver the eulogy? What would they say?

SUGGESTED VIEWING

Grave Words: Tools for Discussing End of Life Choices (1996)
How to Die in Oregon (2011, Documentary)
Million Dollar Baby (2004)
Ikuru (1952)
Please Let Me Die (1974, Documentary)

The Savages (2007)
The Secret Garden (1993)
Six Feet Under (2001, Television series)
The Undertaking (2007)
You Don't Know Jack (2010)

FURTHER READING

Mitch Albom, *Tuesdays with Morrie*
Simon Critchley, *The Book of Dead Philosophers*
Charles Dickens, *A Christmas Carol*
C. S. Lewis, *A Grief Observed*

Thomas Lynch, *The Undertaking: Life Studies from a Dismal Trade*
Philip Roth, *Everyman*
Leo Tolstoy, *The Death of Ivan Ilych*

ADVANCED READING

Philippe Ariès, *The Hour of Our Death*
Peter Filene, *In the Arms of Others: A Cultural History of the Right-To-Die in America*
Elizabeth Kübler-Ross, *On Death and Dying*
Jessica Mitford, *The American Way of Death Revisited*

Sherwin Nuland, *How we Die: Reflections on Life's Final Chapter*
Mary Roach, *Stiff: The Curious Lives of Human Cadavers*

ORGANIZATIONS

The Association for Death Education and Counseling, The Thanatology Association
www.adec.org
The Compassionate Friends: Supporting a Family after a Child Dies
www.compassionatefriends.org

Compassion & Choices
www.compassionandchoices.org/
National Association for Home Care and Hospice
www.nahc.org

JOURNALS

Omega: Journal of Death and Dying

PART II
Literature, the Arts, and Medicine

PART OVERVIEW
Literature, the Arts, and Medicine

The term "the arts" derives its meaning from the context in which it is used. "Fine arts" refers to activities and products of the imagination such as music, painting, and sculpture, which appeal to a sense of beauty. Branches of learning such as history, languages, literature, philosophy, and religion are traditionally known in academic parlance as liberal arts. "Arts and sciences" distinguishes the humanities, also known as human sciences, from natural sciences and social sciences. Similarly, in an older idiom, "letters and sciences" draws the same distinction but gives literary learning pride of place in the humanities. And there are "arts of," as in martial arts and healing arts. This section explores some contemporary connections between humanistic study and the healing arts, giving special attention to relationships between visual and verbal meaning.

Art both mirrors and challenges our settled perceptions. John Berger (1926–) writes, "Seeing comes before words ... [and] the way we see things is affected by what we know or what we believe. We only see what we look at. To look is an act of choice. As a result of this act, what we see is brought within our reach."[1]

Conversely, visual images also shape the way we think.[2] Being bombarded with images, as we are, is not conducive to reflection. Pausing to look questioningly at a painting or photograph, or to critically view a film or television show prompts us to think more deeply about what we are seeing. In a discussion of her experience teaching medical students utilizing a range of visual materials, Mary Winkler describes how asking students to look carefully at "artworks that treat such subjects as death, pain, aging, fear, bureaucratic indifference, and poverty," and then asking them to consider the question "What do you see?" elicits empathy and "reinforce[s] the idea of our common humanity and the vulnerability that we all share."[3] You will find images not only in this section but throughout this text book that encourage you to reflect, probe for deeper meanings, articulate personal reactions.

As with images, the written word, too, can shape us by inclining us to introspection and circumspection and by inviting us into the lives of others.[4] Reading narratives of illness and stories of doctoring extends the reach of our minds and sensibilities, and deepens fellow feeling. This is important because, as Clifford Geertz (1926–2006) observes, "the reach of our minds, the range of signs we can manage somehow to interpret, is what defines the intellectual, emotional and moral space in which we live."[5] Vicariously experiencing, through the prism of poetry and the medium of memoir, what others have been through illuminates that space and makes it more capacious.[6] We know more and understand more fully for having experienced, at one remove, what it is like to hurt or heal.

What is more, we gain self-knowledge at the level of feeling. "The power and charm of the arts is that in them we discover the life of feeling that might sleep in us unregarded without their help .... It is as though we don't understand our own feelings until we are confronted with a contrived state of affairs that isn't a direct rendering of our feelings but somehow expresses their tone and form."[7] Literature and the arts, as they relate to medicine, are a learning laboratory wherein aspirants to the helping professions enter the lives of the ill where the hurt and anxiety are imaginatively real, to vicariously probe and ponder under the tutelage of poetry and story, memoir and moving picture.

In this section, we will ask why sickness prompts us to storytelling; how popular media influences our views about what it means to grow old or live with a disability, or to practice high-tech hospital medicine; how poetry makes language care; why it's important for doctors to strive to merge medical and humanistic sensibilities; and how student-teacher relations affect the moral formation of future health care professionals. In considering these questions, we will be looking closely and reading inquiringly for practical wisdom, heeding Nietzsche's counsel that to read well means "to take time ... to read slowly, deeply, carefully, considerately, with doors left ajar, with delicate fingers and eyes. ..."[8]

7   Narratives of Illness

All sorrows can be borne if you put them into a story or tell a story about them.[1]
— Isak Dinesen

ABSTRACT

This chapter explores how we narrate our experiences of illness. Beginning with a discussion of how narrative shapes our experience of brute fact into intelligibility and meaningfulness, it examines four narratives of illness: Oliver Sacks's *A Leg to Stand On*, William Styron's *Darkness Visible*, Lucy Grealy's *Autobiography of a Face*, and Aaron Alterra's *The Caregiver*. Then, with a focus on the relationship between narrative interpretation and our encounters with illness, it considers how reading narratives of illness attentively, expectantly, and reflectively can heighten our powers of perception, deepen our self-knowledge, and thicken our understanding of what it's like to suffer through an illness or cope with an injury.

INTRODUCTION

This chapter discusses a type of illness narrative known as "pathography," a subgenre of autobiography and biography. And it offers "readings" of four such narratives, each with a different focus – loss of bodily integrity, mental collapse, disfiguring cancer, and incurable degenerative disease – and all authored by professional writers.

Why do we tell stories? How can we not? We are born storytellers or, better, we live our stories before we tell them. Each of us is born into a family, a community, a culture from which we derive our initial sense of self and of what life is like. Without realizing it, we assimilate and live by stories that rescue us from a sequence of disconnected happenings. Over time, as we experience other ways of seeing the world and thinking about things, we may question and begin rewriting some of these taken-for-granted storylines according to our own lights. But as long as all goes well with us, we tend to live our story without giving it much thought. It is only when we ask *why* things happened the way they did that a narrative impulse is triggered. Serious illness and injury are especially powerful events that interrupt the largely unself-conscious flow of our lives and prompt the impulse to emplot them, that is, shape them into a livable story, a narrative of an experience of illness that scholars call a pathography.[2]

Pathographies, whose numbers expanded rapidly in the final decades of the twentieth century, first appeared in the middle of the century and coincided with the rise of heroic rescue medicine. John Gunther's (1901–1970) memoir, *Death Be Not Proud*, for example, chronicles the fifteen-month-long saga of surgery and medical treatments aimed at curing his sixteen-year-old son's ultimately fatal brain tumor.[3] In *Death of a Man*, Lael Tucker Wertenbaker (1909–1997) tells the story of her husband Wert's struggles with incurable metastatic colon cancer and her vow to help him die by his own hand when suffering became unbearable and the end was near.[4]

Well into the 1970s, narratives of illness continued to focus principally on living with life-threatening conditions and care of the dying. Among them are Stewart Alsop's (1914–1974) *Stay of Execution*,[5] Betty Rollins's (1936–) *Last Wish*,[6] and Stephen S. Rosenfeld's (1932–2010) *The Time of Their Dying*.[7] Beginning in the 1980s, the genre expanded. Memoirs of dying continued to predominate but were now augmented by accounts of living with maladies of mind and body, soul and self.

The study of pathography, as with medical humanities generally, is part of a larger narrative turn that has characterized the humanities and interpretive social sciences in recent decades.[8] Anne Hunsaker Hawkins writes, "Pathographies interpret experience, and they do so in a way that discloses certain important mythic attitudes about illness and treatment. Mythic thinking of all kinds becomes apparent in that delicate autobiographical transition from 'actual' experience to written narrative, since this transition is one that constructs necessary fictions out of the building blocks of metaphor, image, archetype, and myth."[9]

Hawkins's book is a treatise on the ways in which authors of illness narratives, in the process of recording what they have been through, rewrite their story in the light of received wisdom captured in metaphors of journey and battle, and myths of death and rebirth, thereby taking their story from brute fact to intelligibility and meaningfulness. The premise of Hawkins's project is that studying pathographies promises to restore the patient's voice to patient-physician encounters. Moreover, studying illness narratives positively contributes to shaping students' emotional, intellectual, and moral capacities – "not a bad start," as Robert Coles (1929–) has remarked, "for someone trying to find a good way to live this life: a person's moral conduct responding to the moral imagination of writers and the moral imperative of fellow human beings in need."[10]

In a related analysis, Arthur Frank proposes a tripartite typology of cultural narratives – the restitution story, the chaos story, and the quest story – which illuminate and shape the composition of pathographies as authors construct an account of their unique experiences. Frank believes that awareness of these typologies may help health care professionals to attend more carefully to patients' stories of illness.[11] Elsewhere he further argues that "Knowing illness as a series of dramas enhances the capacity of the ill to find meaning in their plight."[12] There is the drama of genesis that concerns itself with the origin and cause of an illness. There are dramas of fear and loss, of meaning, and of self, this last portraying the sick person's struggle to recognize his or her "new" self once the worst is over.

A Leg to Stand On

Oliver Sacks's (1933–) *A Leg to Stand On* is one such account and is notable for its marvelous mixture of neurological observation, psychological insight, mystical experience, and speculative vision.[13] Throughout, music is the metaphor of action, and acknowledgement of the uncanny is the intuitive counterpart of body facts. The book begins with the author's accident and injury, proceeds through a meticulous account of the experience of illness and convalescence, and ends with provocative reflections on the need for "a neurology of the soul."[14]

We are incarnate and we experience ourselves as embodied. Bodily injury threatens to undermine our sense of who we are. So it was for Sacks when, having survived a harrowing hiking accident, a new horror began to dawn in the form of a radical breach in his settled perception of this own body. The relation between his left leg, which dangled "like a piece of spaghetti," and the rest of his body was obscure and puzzling. It was not simply that the quadriceps had visibly atrophied beneath the cast following surgery, but that the muscle was completely atonic. Try as he might, the patient could not contract the muscle. The frustration attendant upon physical incapacity was compounded by a sense of impotence and futility.

Still more troubling was the thought that beyond this physical incapacity was a vacancy of mind where once there had been tacit knowledge of how to flex the muscle. "I had the feeling that something had happened ... to my power of 'thinking' – although only with regard to this one single muscle ... I had 'forgotten' something ...."[15] And no strenuous effort of will availed in retrieving that lapsed memory.

Then Sacks's experience took an uncanny turn. The patient was awakened from nightmarish sleep by an alarmed nurse to find that unbeknownst to him the "dead" left leg had fallen half off the bed. He could not believe his eyes. He could see that the "cylinder of chalk" had moved, but he had no *sense* that that was so. "*I knew not my leg.*"[16] It was as if, absent its familiar feeling and function, the leg had become an unrecognizable member of the body commonwealth.

Sacks decided to explore this experience of alienation in all its detail, or rather to peer into the hole in his personal reality where once there had been a leg to stand on. Medically, his condition continued to improve. Anatomically, healing was occurring predictably. But personally, existentially – the leg remained lifeless and alien. Sacks came to the conclusion that he was dealing not with a problem that required a solution but rather with a mystery which he had to face. Mendelssohn's Violin Concerto provided an early clue to fathoming the mystery. Music promised renewal and indeed seemed "the very *score* of life."[17]

Attempts at rehabilitation advanced falteringly, and the mystery remained. Eventually, "with the return of my own personal melody which was somehow elicited by, and attuned to, the Mendelssohnian melody,"[18] Sacks remembered how to walk – not by calculation or deliberation but by recollection. The mystery, though not dispelled, was displaced by grace, "the prerequisite and essence of all *doing*."[19] Now convalescence was possible – putting behind the moral infancy of patienthood, returning to fluency of motion, and celebrating the sacrament of thanksgiving.

One great merit of Sacks's pathography is that it richly reintroduces the patient and his experience of ailing into a drama of injury and recovery that prompts a reconsideration of the diagnostic art. Confronted with an experience of severance, of absence, analysis is of limited use. Needed in addition to the dissecting, disconnecting activities of analysis are painstaking attentiveness to the detail and pattern of experience, appreciation for nuance in that experience, and constructive imagination, even in the face of the uncanny.

Darkness Visible

Of several illness narratives that appeared in the 1990s, three are particularly noteworthy: William Styron's (1925–2006) *Darkness Visible: A Memoir of Madness*,[20] Lucy Grealy's (1963–2002) *Autobiography of a Face*,[21] and Aaron Alterra's (1913–2013) *The Caregiver: A Life with Alzheimer's*.[22]

Borrowing a phrase from John Milton's (1608–1674) *Paradise Lost* as the title of his "memoir of madness," William Styron takes the reader into the depths of a serious depressive illness that nearly killed him. Prize-winning author of critically acclaimed novels, Styron enters a months-long descent into "despair beyond despair."[23] The onset of severe depression that stretched well beyond the doldrums of everyday life was marked by self-loathing and "gloom crowding in on me, a sense of dread and alienation and, above all, stifling anxiety."[24]

Shortly prior to departing for Paris in the autumn of 1985 to accept a literary award, and feeling that something was seriously wrong with him, Styron made an appointment with a psychiatrist. For several months he had attributed his increased irritability and anxiety to his having abruptly sworn off whiskey following forty years of heavy drinking. Lately, however, he had begun to fear that his "mind was dissolving."[25] With the encouragement of the psychiatrist, Styron made the trip, but once in Paris he became confused and his behavior turned erratic.

Back at home, he slipped ever further down the spiral of "anxiety, agitation, [and] unfocused dread,"[26] suffering "a veritable howling tempest in the brain."[27] His body became sluggish, his responses slowed, his voice turned wheezy and nearly disappeared. Libido vanished, and food was taken merely for sustenance.

Sleep was bought with the tranquilizer Halcion, to which he became addicted. "Death was now a daily presence ... blowing over me in cold gusts."[28]

CASE STUDY: WILLIAM STYRON ON DEPRESSION

In the following passage, Styron describes his encounter with depression – especially the difficulty of rendering it comprehensible to anyone who has not experienced depression for themselves.

"Depression is a disorder of mood, so mysteriously painful and elusive in the way it becomes known to the self – to the mediating intellect – as to verge close to being beyond description. It thus remains nearly incomprehensible to those who have not experienced it in its extreme mode, although the gloom, "the blues" which people go through occasionally and associate with the general hassle of everyday existence are of such prevalence that they do give many individuals a hint of the illness in its catastrophic form. But at the time of which I write I had descended far past those familiar, manageable doldrums. In Paris, I am able to see now, I was at a critical stage in the development of the disease, situated at an ominous way station between its unfocused stirrings earlier that summer and the near-violent denouement of December, which sent me into the hospital ....

For those who have dwelt in depression's dark wood, and known its inexplicable agony, their return from the abyss is not unlike the ascent of the poet, trudging upward out of hell's black depths and at last emerging into what he saw as "the shining world." There, whoever has been restored to health has almost always been restored to the capacity for serenity and joy, and this may be indemnity enough for having endured the despair beyond despair.[29]

E quindi uscimmo a riveder le stele.

And so we came forth, and once again beheld the stars."

1. How would you describe depression? Do you think it can be expressed in words? In images? Do you think it is even possible to describe depression – or any illness?
2. Why do you think Styron chooses to write about his illness? How might the act of writing have the potential to heal?
3. Styron concludes his pathography with a line from *Dante's Inferno*. What do you think that line means? What mythic or metaphorical image does it make use of?

Neither psychotherapy nor medication were effective in treating Styron's symptoms, which now included an acute fear of abandonment and fantasies of suicide, taken to the point of locating the means to accomplish it. Styron methodically prepared to dispose of the valued notebook in which over the years he had committed ideas and observations for his writing. With the future slipping rapidly away, Styron engaged in a foreshadowing of his self-destruction by meticulously preparing the notebook for burial, assembling "the new roll of Viva paper towels to wrap the book, the Scotch-brand tape I encircled it with, the empty Post Raisin Bran box I put the parcel into before taking it outside and stuffing it deep down within the garbage can, which would be emptied the next morning. Fire would have destroyed it faster, but in garbage there was an annihilation of self appropriate, as always, to melancholia's fecund self-humiliation. I felt my heart pounding, and knew that I had made an irreversible decision."[30]

Unable to sleep and watching a scene in an old movie filmed in a music conservatory, Styron hears a contralto voice singing a soaring passage from Brahms's *Alto Rhapsody* and, overwhelmed by a flood of emotion at the thought of all that he was about to abandon, wakes his wife, Rose, and plans are made for his hospitalization. Over the course of the ensuing seven weeks, Styron's condition steadily improved. He attributes this slow retreat from the precipice on which he had stood at the time of his admission to a crucial adjustment in his medication, the compassion of the staff, and, importantly, to the hospital itself which for him was "a way station, a purgatory,"[31] "a sanctuary where peace can return to the mind," "a refuge,"[32] "my salvation."[33]

On the mend and able to return to his writing, which had been defunct, Styron reflects on the near-fatal calamity he had suffered. His review of the psychiatric literature impressed him with the idiopathic nature of clinical depression and "the malady's all but impenetrable mystery."[34] As to what triggered his crisis, he wonders whether alcohol withdrawal may have played a role, or turning sixty, "that hulking milestone of mortality."[35] Dissatisfaction with his work? His father's battle with depression? Any and all of these seemed plausible.

In the end, Styron is most drawn to the likelihood that the death of his mother when he was thirteen, and his subsequent inability to mourn her loss, had shaped his life and work in ways that seemed to him now to make eminent sense. "Loss," he writes, "in all of its manifestations is the touchstone of depression – in the progress of the disease and, most likely, in its origin."[36] Moreover, he ventures, the repressed rage over the loss of his mother may have both precipitated his life-long self-destructive behavior (his heavy drinking and, later, thoughts of suicide) *and* fueled his desire to overcome it: "my own avoidance of death may have been a belated homage to my mother. I do know that in those last hours before I rescued myself, when I had listened to the passage from the *Alto Rhapsody* – which I'd heard her sing – she had been very much on my mind."[37]

Recalling Hawkins's analysis of mythic dimensions of illness and Frank's typology of cultural narratives, we hear in *A Leg to Stand On* echoes of epic battle followed by restoration of bodily integrity, accompanied by the metaphor of music. And following Styron's story may be usefully enhanced by invoking metaphors of chaos and the threat of death, and eventual restitution to a settled state of mind.

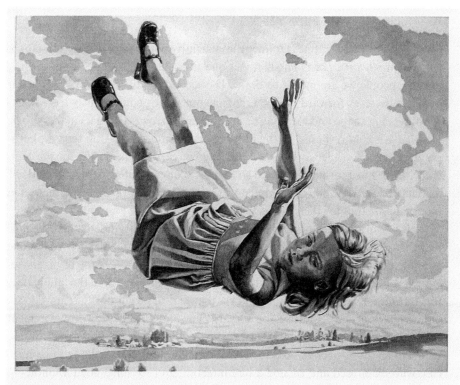

Figure 7. *Fallen, Fallen, Light Renew*, 2005, Mary McCleary, 1951–, Courtesy Moody Gallery, Houston, TX © Mary McCleary 2005.

The relationship between a work of art and its title is not always so direct as it is for Eric Avery's *Emerging Infectious Diseases*. Title and work can be in dialogue or in tension. Mary McCleary's *Fallen, Fallen, Light Renew* creates a connection between light and a falling figure. Let's begin with the picture and the topic of this chapter, Narratives of Illness.

As we learn in this chapter, we turn to narrative to make sense of events that disrupt the unselfconscious story that we tell about who we are. The young girl in McCleary's painting certainly appears to be experiencing a frightening event, even if it's only a dream. Can you remember a time when you "fell" into a new situation? Look carefully at her face. Can we interpret the look on her face as the dawning of self-consciousness and – considering her possible age – the shock of adolescence?

The title seems to support this interpretation. It's taken from the poem *Introduction to the Songs of Experience*, by the English poet and artist William Blake, who also wrote *Songs of Innocence*. Blake intended for the two series of poems to be read together in order to show "the two Contrary States of the Human Soul."

McCleary demonstrates that painting can explore contrary states as provocatively as poetry or prose. Try to identify with the young girl's dawning awareness of her situation. Go back to *The Doctor*, the picture that accompanied Chapter 1. How might *Fallen, Fallen, Light Renew* represent the young patient's experience of illness?

To see more works of Mary McCleary, visit: http://www.marymccleary.com/.

For the works of William Blake, visit: http://www.poetryfoundation.org/bio/william-blake#poet.

Autobiography of a Face

Two evocative early lines frame the narrative of Lucy Grealy's memoir, *Autobiography of a Face:* The first is a question: "how do we go about turning into the people we are meant to be?"[38] The second, an observation: "While our bodies move ever forward on the time line, our minds continuously trace backward, seeking shape and meaning as deftly as any arrow seeking its mark."[39] The *question* arises in response to the author's recollection of having seen a photograph of herself while working at a party in her early teens, posing for the camera with her head turned and tilted so that her hair camouflaged the right side of her face. The *observation* is prompted by Grealy's memory of the event that set in motion her search for the significance of her troubled life journey.

It all began with a painful blow to the jaw in a fourth-grade game of dodge ball that left her momentarily stunned but not incapacitated. Later that same evening, however, a bothersome toothache made itself felt. A litany of diagnoses ensued. Lockjaw, her brothers said. Probably a fracture, ventured the family doctor. But the x-rays revealed a dental cyst that had to be surgically removed. Six months later, a lump appeared on Grealy's jaw and a bony growth was evident on a follow-up x-ray. The dental surgeon assured Mrs. Grealy that it was nothing to worry about. Unconvinced, she took her daughter back to the family physician who diagnosed and treated a bad infection and recommended a follow-up consultation with a leading head and neck surgeon.

During this consultation, a detailed medical history was taken and a physical examination done, including blood tests and a chest x-ray. Grealy was admitted to the hospital where she underwent a bone marrow test and diagnostic scans. Throughout this extensive workup, she remembered feeling perfectly fine. In fact, it was all something of an adventure: "There were definite problems to face here, but to me they seemed entirely manageable: lie still when you're told, be brave."[40]

She was nine years old when she was told she had a malignancy – Ewing's sarcoma – and that she was going to have a big operation. Sometime later, after several more surgeries, someone in her family casually mentioned Lucy's cancer, which came as a shock to Lucy: "In all that time, not one person ever said the word *cancer* to me, at least not in a way that registered as pertaining to me."[41] Later still, while working in a library in her teenage years, she looked up Ewing's sarcoma and discovered that it carried a 5 percent chance of survival.

Recovery from surgery to remove a tumor and a third of her jaw was slow and arduous, and the radiation and chemotherapy treatments, for two and two-and-a-half years, respectively, were extremely taxing. Chemotherapy, especially, induced waves of vomiting. Her hair fell out. The oncologist was inconsiderate and lacking in empathy.

In spite of it all, Grealy still believed her jaw was fixable. However, it was beginning to dawn on her that she might look much worse than she had supposed:

"More than the ugliness I felt, I was suddenly appalled at the notion that I'd been walking around unaware of something that was apparent to everyone else. A profound sense of shame consumed me."[42]

Throughout her teens Grealy endured taunts, bore the burden of isolation, and experienced "the deep, bottomless grief I called ugliness." She invented various stratagems for coping with her sense of foreignness, none of which had any lasting effect. In her mid-twenties, after nearly thirty operations, she still could not reconcile the person she felt herself to be with the imposter in the mirror: "It wasn't only that I continued to feel ugly; I simply could not conceive of the image as belonging to me."[43]

A year passed during which the habit of refusing to look in mirrors or at other reflecting surfaces provided some relief. It was then that she came to the realization that what she was up against was a matter of perception. For years she had been holding on to an *image* of her "'real' face, the one I was meant to have all along ... my 'original' face, the one free from all deviation, all error."[44] Consequently, she had never become acquainted with the face she actually had, nor developed a relationship with the person she actually was. With that simple but hard-won insight, she set out "to see if I could, now, recognize myself,"[45] and begin what the author calls her long "journey back to my face."[46] In light of Hawkins's analysis of mythic attitudes and Frank's cultural typology, the journey metaphor is clearly dominant in Grealy's story. It is not a journey that leads to restoration but one that continues a quest for self-recognition.

Theorizing stories, as Hawkins and Frank do, may add to our appreciation of narratives of illness, but only if they are used sparingly and judiciously. Theories are abstract and aim for generalizability, whereas the strength of stories lies in their singularity and particularity. Typologies deal in idealized types and thus risk reification, mistaking an idea of, in this case, an experience of illness, for the writer's rendering of that experience. Abstractions and ideal types have their place in interpreting illness narratives, but only when used heuristically to support reading unmediated by prefabricated categories. It is careful, expectant reading that reveals vital connections between the written word and everyday experience. When one adopts an attitude of knowingness, of reading with a preconceived idea of what one is looking or listening *for*, one sacrifices the possibility of discovering something new in the narrative, and forfeits the opportunity to have one's mind changed and one's spirit enlarged, by what one reads. Knowingness is the enemy of imagination.[47]

The Caregiver

Approximately 40 percent of all deaths in the United Sates occur following an often-prolonged period of increasing frailty and dementing illness. Approximately one-third of Americans live beyond the age of eighty-five and, of these, roughly half suffer major cognitive impairment. Caring for these dependent elders is mainly the responsibility of family members – as Aaron Alterra (a pseudonym) discovered while trying to keep pace with subtle changes in his wife's behavior. It was more than momentary memory lapses or forgetfulness or loss of words that he noticed. Stella (not her real name) seemed increasingly unable to see connections between things, and often was hesitant about what to do next. At times she looked blank and absented herself. Alterra talked with their daughter and son and their spouses, and the family physician. He consulted the *Merck Manual of Geriatrics* and quickly concluded that "the word 'dementia' was ludicrous for the essentially normal woman Stella was."[48]

Aaron continued to take Stella to see Dr. Loughrand, her primary care physician, who ordered tests to rule out other possible causes of Stella's symptoms and confirmed the likelihood that she was suffering from Alzheimer's. He urged Aaron to consider starting her on the only drug that was showing any promise of slowing the progress of the disease. As the evidence mounted, Aaron had to face the fact that his wife had an incurable, disabling, degenerative disease of which she was unaware. On the advice of his daughter, he contacted a psychologist who gave him what in retrospect was invaluable advice. "It might be helpful if you thought of yourself as the physician and Loughrand as somebody you respect enough to consult on major decisions .... Alzheimer's is not usually a doctor-intensive disease. It's more aide-and-caregiver intensive."[49]

Armed with the startling insight that he himself, and not medical professionals, was the primary caregiver, Alterra doggedly explored every conceivable option for Stella's care. A neurology consult? A psychiatry consult? Aaron opted for both. The director of the local affiliate of the Alzheimer's Association suggested clinical trials in which his wife might enroll. Stella was started on the drug Dr. Loughrand had mentioned and, when her body proved unable to tolerate it, Aaron took the initiative in getting her enrolled in a clinical trial. But while Stella regained her physical balance (an eligibility requirement for entering a research study), weeks passed and other capacities steadily declined.

Once Stella became a subject in the study to determine the experimental drug's efficacy, Aaron tried to persuade the clinical manager to tell him whether his wife was assigned to the group receiving the drug or to the placebo group. Learning that the research staff in a double-blind study is unaware of who is getting what, Aaron took a sample of the substance Stella was given to the hospital lab for testing, only to find that the lab outsourced its work to another lab in a distant city. Aaron called that lab and was told that they did not do testing for private individuals. Intent on leaving nothing to chance, he took his case to the local police lab where no active ingredient was found in the substance. Aaron withdrew Stella from the study and enrolled her instead in an observation program with assurances that she would be getting the best available medicine.

All this time Aaron cared for Stella at home with the help of a housekeeper who was intuitively attuned to his wife's moods and needs. But as Stella's disorientation mounted, her speech became less and less intelligible, and her ability to walk without assistance deteriorated, Aaron became distraught. Stella and Aaron were in their early eighties at the time. Aaron recalls, "I have rarely felt as entirely helpless in my life as I did then. Stella was slipping out of my hands."[50]

Aaron signed Stella and himself up for separate support group meetings at the Alzheimer's Association office. There he met kindred spirits whose shared experiences reminded participants that they were not in this alone. Practical tips were exchanged and confessions made. Seeking absolution for his guilt over having behaved badly toward Stella, Aaron recounted for the group an incident in which he had become uncontrollably angry at his wife for having pulled the bedroom blinds off their rollers and, in her bewilderment at what had happened, left them billowing across furniture and floor. As he berated her, Stella had uncharacteristically begun to cry. Aaron came to his senses, embraced her, and apologized. And then, "Consumed by guilt, I went to her and again apologized. She had no idea what I was talking about .... It was all gone from her memory."[51] The other members of the caregiver support group understood and sympathized, seared as they too had been by shame over similar experiences of their own.

Months, then years, of slow decline crept relentlessly along. When walking became an insurmountable challenge, Stella became wheelchair bound. Eating became ever more difficult even after Aaron happened onto an infant feeding siphon that allowed him to squirt an ounce or two of nourishment into Stella's mouth without a struggle. In time, urinary incontinence became a problem. Aaron would arise every day at four in the morning: "I turn on a low light, tell her why I am disturbing her, and raise her enough to draw out the top absorbent mat, leaving the dry undermat in place. I slip out her more personal gauze pad and replace it with another, kiss her on the cheek, tell her I'm done and to go back to sleep. Five minutes. She probably had not really awakened."[52]

So it went, day after day, until in year five when Aaron returned from a few days away, Stella didn't register his absence. What is absent is not real – a saddening fact that Aaron has trouble acknowledging. And yet, he writes upon reflection, when he was with her, which was most of the time, and "when she says, 'Love you, dear,' as she says one way or another every day without it staling – words, a glance, a hand held – it is not pro forma. It is not calculated – she has no calculation in her – the moment is transcendent."[53]

The title of Aaron Alterra's memoir, *The Caregiver*, signals that the primary focus will be on the author's experience. In one sense, that is the case. The climactic moment in the narrative is reached when Alterra realizes that it is *he* who is his wife's main caregiver. From then on, he becomes Stella's awareness, her protector from harm and custodian of her rights, her guide in the wilderness that her once-familiar world had become, and a steadfast presence in her otherwise bewildering circumstances. But because caring happens *between* people, the narrative necessarily becomes no longer his but *theirs*.

CONCLUSION

Narratives do not come from nowhere but are re-presentations of earlier stories, themselves often versions of earlier stories still. In the construction of narratives of illness, the writer strives to make existential sense of an experience by placing it in the context of a larger narrative of suffering and loss or healing, and then, in that light, giving a plausible account of what is happening now. Narrative enhances understanding by retelling received stories – some grand, others commonplace – bearing practical wisdom. In this way, each of the interpretive re-presentations introduced in this chapter highlighted moments of experiential significance and existential insight in the lives of the pathographers.

We read for a variety of reasons – for information, inspiration, insight. Reading narratives of illness attentively, expectantly, and reflectively can heighten our powers of perception, deepen our self-knowledge, and thicken our understanding of what it's like to suffer through an illness or cope with an injury, not abstractly or in the aggregate, but experientially and in particular – all prerequisites for humanistic clinical care.[54]

SUMMATION

This chapter explored how we narrate our experiences of illness. Beginning with a discussion of how narrative shapes our experience of brute fact into intelligibility and meaningfulness, it examined four narratives of illness: Oliver Sacks's *A Leg to Stand On*, William Styron's *Darkness Visible*, Lucy Grealy's *Autobiography of a Face*, and Aaron Alterra's *The Caregiver*. Then, with a focus on the relationship between narrative interpretation and our encounters with illness, it considered how reading narratives of illness attentively, expectantly, and reflectively can heighten our powers of perception, deepen our self-knowledge, and thicken our understanding of what it's like to suffer through an illness or cope with an injury. Overall, it emphasized that the *meaning* of illness is created through stories, and that reading these stories can help us to become more sensitive and humane caregivers.

EXERCISES FOR CRITICAL THINKING AND CHARACTER FORMATION

QUESTIONS FOR DISCUSSION

1. What is it about illness that prompts the impulse for reflection?
2. In *Darkness Visible*, what does Styron believe causes his depression? What, in his opinion, caused its remission?
3. What are some potential benefits of writing about illness?
4. How, and in what ways, does narrative have the potential to heal?

SUGGESTED WRITING EXERCISE

Susan Sontag writes, "Illness is the night-side of life, a more onerous citizenship. Everyone who is born holds dual citizenship, in the kingdom of the well and in the kingdom of the sick. Although we all prefer to use only the good passport, sooner or later each of us is obliged, at least for a spell, to identify ourselves as citizens of that other place." Responding to this quotation, write, for about twenty minutes, on your own experience with illness or that of someone close to you. You may write in any form that suits your purposes – an essay, a letter, a first-person account, etc. Whatever your approach, try be specific about your thoughts, emotions, and responses to your illness.

SUGGESTED VIEWING

Amour (2012)
Awakenings (1990)
Dialogues with Madwomen (1993)
The Diving Bell and the Butterfly (1997)

The Doctor (1991)
Out of the Shadow (2006)
Waltz with Bashir (2008)

FURTHER READING

Cortney Davis, *I Knew a Woman: Four Women Patients and Their Female Caregiver*
Kay Jamison, *An Unquiet Mind: A Memoir of Moods and Madness*
Audre Lorde, *The Cancer Journals*

Nancy Mairs, *Carnal Acts*
Jay Neugeboren, *Imagining Robert: My Brother, Madness, and Survival, A Memoir*
Stephen S. Rosenfeld, *The Time of Their Dying*

ADVANCED READING

Howard Brody, *Stories of Sickness*
Rita Charon, *Narrative Medicine: Honoring the Stories of Illness*
Arthur Frank, *The Wounded Storyteller*
Anne Hawkins, *Reconstructing Illness: Studies in Pathography*

Ruth Nadelhaft and Victoria Bonnebaker, eds., *Imagine What It's Like: A Literature and Medicine Anthology*
Danielle Ofri, ed., *The Best of the Bellevue Literary Review*

JOURNALS

Journal of Literary and Cultural Disability Studies
Literature and Medicine
Narrative

ORGANIZATIONS AND GROUPS

The International Society for the Study of Narrative
http://narrative.georgetown.edu/

Program in Narrative Medicine at Columbia University Medical Center http://www.narrativemedicine.org/

8

Aging in Film

Age has long been Hollywood's nightmare.[1]

– Sally Chivers

ABSTRACT

This chapter explores portraits of aging and old age in film. Beginning with a discussion of early Hollywood's cult of youth, it examines the slow emergence of aging characters in the 1950s and 60s; the themes of intergeneration and regeneration that frequently drove the plots of films depicting old age in the 70s and 80s; and the variable and complex images of aging presented in more recent age-related films. Then, with a focus on issues such as late-life sexuality and the trope of the "aging cowboy," it considers some of the ways that contemporary film has challenged negative stereotypes and images of old age.

INTRODUCTION

In the last quarter of the twentieth century, western societies entered an unprecedented era of mass longevity and aging. Most people could expect to live into their seventies in reasonably good health, while those eighty-five and older became the fastest-growing age group in the population. Yet as we have seen in Chapter 5, "The Health of Populations," the dark side of this triumph was an epidemiological transition in which chronic disease replaced infectious disease as the primary cause of mortality. Mass longevity came with a price tag: many older people now experience periods of disability, frailty, dementia, pain, and may suffer a prolonged death in intensive care units. In addition, western (and especially American) culture remains plagued by ageism – a pattern of prejudice and discrimination toward older people and old age, analogous to sexism and racism. Ageism and hostility toward the aging process are clearly reflected in the contemporary medical and popular ideal of "anti-aging" – the notion that one can grow old without aging. Despite our cultural illiteracy about how to grow old, the modernization of aging has generated a host of existential and moral questions that are largely suppressed in popular culture: Is there an intrinsic purpose to growing old? Is there anything really important to be done after children are raised, jobs left, careers complete? What are the avenues of spiritual growth in later life? What are the roles and responsibilities of older people? Who should care for old people who are frail and sick? Is wisdom an illusion or an accomplishment of those who pursue it? Is there such a thing as a "good old age?"[2]

Film, this chapter suggests, offers a valuable point of departure for exploring these and other age-related questions in popular culture. Until recently, the study of aging in film – like the study of aging in general – was largely neglected.[3] But as film scholars look back over the last century, they are identifying a variety of themes and characters. In the first half of the twentieth century, Hollywood rarely featured older characters; when it did, they were marginal, stereotyped, and often pathologized. Beginning in the 1950s, a few classic films featured older protagonists who challenged the limited portraits of the twenties and thirties. In the 1980s, men and women in their sixties or older appeared in cinema in closer proportion to their presence in the population. By the turn of the twenty-first century, a profusion of age-focused plots and characters came onto the scene, often featuring older actors who were familiar to audiences because of their youthful fame.

We begin with the premise that cinematic representations of aging both reflect and challenge prevailing cultural attitudes – in particular, ageism and fears of growing old.[4] The films discussed here contain positive as well as negative stereotypes of older people, tending to focus on: (1) old age as pathology, (2) intergeneration and regeneration, (3) caregiving, (4) sexuality, and (5) masculinity. Finally, we identify individuated older characters who transcend traditional cultural images and categories of aging. We hope that critically engaging these cinematic images and themes will encourage readers to challenge prevailing attitudes, to learn from and empathize with older characters, and to discover alternative perspectives on old age.

PATHOLOGIZING AGE: EARLY HOLLYWOOD'S CULT OF YOUTH

In the opinion of film scholar Sally Chivers, "Age has long been Hollywood's nightmare."[5] The "nightmare" of aging in early cinema took root in the 1910s and 1920s, when the birth of Hollywood coincided with a gradual, yet fundamental shift in American attitudes toward aging.[6] With increasing industrialization and a consumer culture that advertised diet products, exercise machines, and cosmetics, a pathologized conception of aging gained prominence from the late nineteenth century into the turn of the twentieth. Between 1909 and 1935, social reformers, academics, and physicians often stereotyped old people as sick, poor, and unable to support themselves.[7] Old age and its many negative associations – ugliness, poor health, decay, dependence – became a stage of life to be avoided or segregated.

By 1920, Hollywood had become the center of the cinematic universe and epitomized the quest for youthfulness that characterized much of modern American culture. As Heather Addison puts it, "Hollywood and the Industrial Age became close partners in the creation of a youth-oriented consumer culture. Hollywood, with its spectacular moving images of elegant bodies, romantic interludes, and extravagant living standards ... promot[ed] the new standards of behavior, appearance, and lifestyle to which the public was to aspire."[8] Young Hollywood stars – especially those whose lives had been tragically cut short, like Jean Harlow, James Dean, or Marilyn Monroe – were immortalized as unchanging models of youth, beauty, and permanence.[9] Looking mainly for young men and "girls" to perform, the Hollywood system equated vitality with youth. In these early decades of the twentieth century, filmmakers rarely even allowed an older person onto screen. When they did, the treatment of aging was belittling and marginalizing; older actors were used as comic bait or stock characters.[10]

THE EMERGENCE OF AGING CHARACTERS IN THE 1950s AND 1960s

By the mid-twentieth century, gains in life expectancy and an emerging academic study of old age known as gerontology, provided fertile ground for films to explore the lives of older protagonists. During the 1950s, a number of older actors and age-related issues found their way onto the silver screen. It is perhaps not surprising that male filmmakers began to imagine new, more interesting roles for older men. Japanese filmmaker Akira Kurosawa's *Ikiru* (1952), for example, tells the story of a retired city clerk who, after discovering that he has terminal cancer, devotes his remaining days to an act of benevolence. After reflecting on the many lost opportunities to be close to his family, he devotes his time to cleaning and completing a city park. In the final scene, Watanabe sits on a swing gazing through snowflakes on the completed playground, at peace with himself and the world.

Another classic film of old age and generational relations is Swedish filmmaker Ingmar Bergman's *Wild Strawberries* (1957). The plot follows Isak Borg, a lonely retired physician who is driving with his daughter-in-law Marianne to receive an honorary degree in Lund, Sweden. As both Robert Butler (1927–2010) and Erik Erikson (1902–1994) have pointed out, Borg's trip is the occasion of a life review that contains dreams and memories of failure, guilt, arguments with his elderly mother, and fear of his mortality.[11] Borg's emotional crisis reaches its peak when he and Marianne stop at the family's summer home, where he spent the first twenty years of his life. He has a vision of his first love, Sara, picking wild strawberries, flirting with his older brother, and reflecting on her choice of

Borg as her lover. Throughout these moments of recollection and reminiscence, Borg is reminded of his limitations, his lack of intimacy with others, and his feelings of inadequacy. Finally, he confesses to Marianne, "I'm dead although I'm alive." When he reaches Lund, however, Borg is surrounded by young people, reunited with his son, and lauded during the award ceremony. The film ends with another waking dream as Borg revisits his youth, watches his parents, and finds satisfaction that otherwise had been denied him throughout his life.

This chapter discusses the aging and identity of Dr. Borg in Ingmar Bergman's *Wild Strawberries* (1957). How much of Dr. Borg's emotional and psychological crisis is captured in the single frame that depicts Dr. Borg and his daughter-in-law Marianne driving to Lund? Where are they looking? What expressions are on their faces? What might these features of the image reveal about their relationship?

The composition of this frame also captures a powerful theme of the film – the relationship of old age to youth – by closely confining an old man and a young woman in the interior of a car. Simply putting a frame around two figures or objects gives them a rough equality, but compositional elements create important distinctions.

In this case, the young woman, Marianne, dominates the frame, filling the left half. She sits upright, her head reaches to the top of the frame, her shoulder overlaps the left edge, and the bottom of the frame runs just below her shoulders. She wears a white long-sleeve blouse under a sleeveless dress with a V-neck. The black dress and the white blouse are sharply

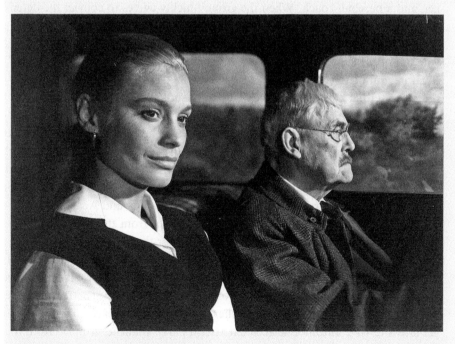

Figure 8. *Wild Strawberries* (single film frame), 1957, Director: Ingmar Bergman. Wild Strawberries © 1957 AB Svensk Filmindustri, Still Photographer: Louis Huch.

focused and contrast dramatically. She gazes down and to her right, outside the frame and away from her companion, as if lost in thought.

The angle of the camera puts Borg, the old man, farther back in the frame, making him appear smaller and slightly out of focus. His position is further diminished by posture and tonality. He slumps in the seat and his rumpled clothes are muted grays. Only the white collar of his shirt mirrors Marianne's costume. In contrast to Marianne's withdrawn gaze, Borg gazes directly and intently out the windshield.

Bergman's compositional choices raise a number of questions. Youth dominates old age and is more sharply focused, for youth life is composed of blacks and whites rather than grays. But can youth's gaze find an object outside itself? Old age moves a person into the background of life, with few sharp contrasts and lack of focus. However, old age can reflect on life as lived. Looking at the film frame again, could it be that Marianne is a projection of Borg's gaze, a projection of his youth as much as an actual person?

Thanks to Kurosawa's and Bergman's influence, American cinema also began to feature older male characters. *12 Angry Men* (1957) features an older character (played by Joseph Sweeney) who plays a pivotal role in the judicial trial of an accused murderer. Convened for the sentencing a youngster from a crime-filled neighborhood accused of murdering his father, the jury is comprised of conventional, middle-class Americans: a bank clerk, a small-time businessman, a garage owner, an architect, a construction worker, a copywriter, a stock exchange broker, and a baseball coach. When the group quickly agrees to convict the defendant, only one member of the jury – the old man – refuses to make a judgment so rashly. Himself a social outsider, the old man explains that he changes his vote out of principle, because "it is not easy to stand the ridicule of the others." Breaking out of the conformism that governs the group, he leads them to question their verdict and eventually acquit the defendant.

While *Ikiru*, *Wild Strawberries*, and *12 Angry Men* feature nuanced and sympathetic portraits of male protagonists, older women did not fare so well. In the 1960s, the beautiful, young actresses of the 1930s had been forgotten, relegated to marginal roles, or – in Bette Davis's and Joan Crawford's cases – featured as disabled, repulsive figures. Davis was regarded as one of Hollywood's finest actresses in the thirties, appearing on both Broadway and Academy-award-winning films. Crawford was also a famous flapper from the twenties. By the 1960s, however, both actresses were considered over-the-hill at fifty years old.

Whatever Happened to Baby Jane (1962) flashes back to the early success of the vaudevillian child star Baby Jane and her older sister Blanche, also a famous actress. In the film's present, Blanche (Joan Crawford) and Jane (Bette Davis) are retired from their careers and live together. One night after a party, the two sisters get into a terrible automobile accident after a party. Blanche, crippled from the accident, is usually holed up in her bedroom watching old movies on television. Jane is a shadow of her former self, still drinking and wearing caked-on makeup while she insistently talks to her toy doll. Blanche's wheelchair and Jane's out-landish behavior subtly link aging with both physical and mental disability, sug-gesting that older women – and by implication older people – are obsolete and ineffectual. While Crawford and Davis revitalized their careers at an age thought too old for starring female actresses, their fame came at a price. By playing has-been stars who gazed longingly back at a time when they were young and beau-tiful, their roles mirrored the declining trend of their own careers.

Whatever Happened to Baby Jane suggests that, disabled or not, older women are physically and mentally less capable than younger characters or their youn-ger selves.[12] Even into the twenty-first century, older women on the silver screen appear less active and attractive than old men, and old men are generally paired in romances with much younger women. Except for widely recognized stars like Maggie Smith, Judy Dench, or Shirley MacLaine, this bias against aging women in Hollywood culture remains pronounced. Increasingly unable to land regular work, even a star like Melanie Griffith has lamented her marginal role in Hollywood: "I wish that I could make more movies. The fact that I have some lines on my face, that's it. It's not because I lost my talent or I became deformed. It's only because I'm older."[13]

THEMES OF INTERGENERATION AND REGENERATION

After the 1970s, Hollywood films with strong older characters grew more fre-quent. Many of their plots revolved around the themes of *intergeneration* and *regeneration*.[14] *Intergeneration* refers to meaningful interactions between the old and the young – family bonds, grandparenting, friendship, and mentoring. The old are usually depicted as wise, nurturing mentors, and both the young and the old change dramatically based on the intensity and honesty of their inter-actions. The theme of *regeneration*, which is closely linked to *intergeneration*, features older characters who find closure, who resolve significant conflicts, and restore or create some kind of emotional or spiritual wholeness in their lives.[15] *Regeneration* often concerns one's relation to place, which grounds the old per-son in the tradition, values, and the reassurance of a stable community and home. As older characters feel the physical constraints of their changing bodies, they often undertake a "life review" that involves travel: a trip to or away from home, the return to one's roots or to see one's friends.

Harry and Tonto (1972), for example, follows Harry Coombs, a widower who lives in an Upper West Side apartment in New York City. When the building is condemned and Harry is forced out of his apartment, he initially stays with his son's family in Long Island. Soon, however, Harry begins a compelling cross-country trip (with his cat "Tonto" along for the ride) that leads to a series of intergenerational adventures. Always gregarious and curious, Harry brings his charm to every conversation. As he travels across the country visiting his children, he is reminded of their significant personal problems, which he has never been able to solve. But Harry is a good father to them nevertheless, remaining supportive and available. Harry's journey ends on the West Coast when Tonto dies, symbolizing the end of one stage of life and the beginning of another. Harry begins a new life with friends and his son.

In *The Trip to Bountiful* (1985), old Mrs. Carrie Watts also embarks on an elder journey that provides closure and a deepened perspective on her family history. Trapped in a small apartment in 1940s Houston, Mrs. Watts sneaks away from her son and her hostile daughter-in-law to return to Bountiful, the small Texas town in which she grew up. Cashing in her Social Security check for a bus ticket, Mrs. Watts undertakes a desperate journey to return to her roots.[16] Along the way, she meets two guides: a young woman who reminds Carrie of her own youthful passions and a kind, middle-aged sheriff who drives her to Bountiful when she is stranded in a nearby town. Although the town of Bountiful no longer exists, Mrs. Watts, in a struggle similar to those of Borg and Harry, finds resolution in her journey. She visits her old, long-abandoned house, muses on the fleeting nature of all life, and achieves new peace with her son and daughter-in-law, who arrive to bring her back to Houston.

CASE STUDY: THE TRIP TO BOUNTIFUL

In this scene, old Mrs. Watts sits on the front porch in Bountiful with her son, Ludie. As mother and son look outward to the fields and the forest, Carrie reflects on her life and the life that she left behind.

"Mrs. Watts [crying]: What has happened to us? How did we come to this?

Ludie: I don't know, Mama.

Mrs. Watts: Should have stayed and bought the land, it would be better than this!

Ludie: Yes'm.

Mrs. Watts: Pretty soon I'll just be gone. Twenty years, ten ... this house ... me ... you.

Ludie: I know, Mama.

Mrs. Watts: But rivers will still be here. The fields. The trees. And the smell of the gulf. I always got my strength from that. Not from houses. Not from people. So quiet ... so eternally quiet. I've forgotten the peace. The quiet. Do you remember how my papa always had that field over there planted in cotton?

Ludie: Yes, Mama.

Mrs. Watts: You see, it's all woods now. But I expect someday people will come and cut down the trees, plant the cotton, and maybe even wear out the land again. And then their children will sell it and move to the cities. And then trees will come up again.

Ludie. I expect so, Mama."

Mrs. Watts: And we're part of all that. We've left it, but we can never lose what it's given us.

Ludie: I expect ... I expect so, Mama.

1. Why does Mrs. Watts want so desperately to return to Bountiful?
2. Why are the woods and the cotton fields important to her? How does she understand them in relation to her family history?
3. What do Ludie's responses reveal about his relationship to his mother?
4. How does Mrs. Watts reconcile herself to returning to Houston, where she will live in the same situation she fled from?

Films from the 1980s do not attempt to tackle the psychological and social struggles of old age, but rather shield viewers from its harsh and ugly side. The film *On Golden Pond* (1981), for example, features seventy-eight-year-old Henry Fonda as Norman, a retired professor who has grown frustrated with the process of aging. "Do you think it's funny being old? My whole damn body is falling apart!" he complains to his wife Ethel (played by Katharine Hepburn). At the beginning of the film, Norman loses his way in the woods, facing temporary amnesia and a sense of horror that he has lost his way. At their cabin in Maine, the couple is visited by their divorced daughter, her boyfriend, and his son. What follows is a serene, almost reverent film in which reconciliation between generations softens the terrors of memory loss and weakness. It should be noted that Harry and Norman are idealized portraits of old age. For the most part their experiences end well, and their interactions with previous generations, from their children to their grandchildren, are positive and fulfilling.[17] They are also more or less healthy and enjoy financial independence. Old age, consequently, appears as a time of freedom, creativity, and a sense of fulfillment, which counters the negative stereotypes of aging in early Hollywood.

VULNERABILITY, DISEASE, AND CAREGIVING

The twenty-first century brought with it a panoply of films that featured aging as a central concern. Actors who enjoyed fame in their youth – Jack Nicholson, Meryl Streep, Robert Redford, Clint Eastwood, Sylvester Stallone, Jack Lemmon, Judy Dench, Julie Christie, and many others – are featured in roles that explore the process of growing old. While many of these films do little to challenge common attitudes toward growing old – aging is still seen as a state to be avoided, or at least delayed – they do offer variable and complex images of aging, including nuanced treatments of caregiving, terminal disease, sexuality, and intergenerational relationships.

Dad (1989), a story about intergenerational relations and caregiving, revolves around three generations of men: the grandfather Jake (played by Jack Lemmon), his son John (played by Ted Danson), and his grandson Billy (played by Ethan Hawke). When Jake goes to the hospital for diagnosis and eventual surgery, his physician, Dr. Santana, is faced with the dilemma of telling Jake that he has bladder cancer or honoring his family's request to keep the matter secret. "Whatever you do," John asks, "don't mention cancer to my father. He's terribly anxious and frightened by that word." To John's dismay, Dr. Santana, following his professional obligation, decides to tell Jake the truth, sending Jake into a state of painful shock, confusion, and withdrawal. The situation prompts many questions about the roles and responsibilities of physicians, patients, and other caregivers. What rights do family members have to conceal information about a patient's illness, even if that concealment is in the patient's best interest? Who within a family has the right to know about the health condition of another? Who has the right to make decisions based on that information?[18] In a moving scene, John wraps Jake up in a bed sheet and carries him out of the hospital, vowing to care for Jake himself rather than consign him to a hospital bed or a nursing home.

Iris (2001) is a biopic about the philosopher Iris Murdoch (played by Judy Dench), who suffers from Alzheimer's disease, and her husband and caregiver, writer John Bayley. We see Iris through John's feeling and memories, which oscillate between his youth, when the couple met and fell in love at Oxford, and the late-life plot in which John decides whether to institutionalize Iris or care for her at home.[19] As a caregiver, John must cope with his wife's incontinence, her wandering, her repetitive behavior, and her vacant stares. In an especially difficult moment, John lashes out at her: "I hate you! All your friends are finished with you now! I've got you now! Nobody else has you anymore! I've got you now, and I don't want you!" How does a caregiver deal with his or her own frustration or anger? When do the responsibilities of a caregiver become more than he or she can bear? John grapples with these questions as Iris's condition worsens, culminating when she flees from their home in a fit of panic and confusion. John decides to call the police and place her in a nursing home, where she soon dies.

In *Away from Her* (2003), Fiona and her husband, Grant Anderson, have enjoyed a long and fulfilling marriage. After a series of memory lapses and mishaps indicates that Fiona is becoming a risk to herself, she enters a long-term care facility. After a thirty-day waiting period, Grant goes to visit her only to find that she has forgotten him and turned her affections to Aubrey, a mute man in a wheelchair. She treats Grant with detached civility, as if he were a determined suitor – "my, but you're persistent," she remarks when he brings flowers – rather than her husband of more than forty years. Grant responds with both anger and guilt. We learn that many years ago, when he was a university professor, Grant cheated on Fiona with one of his students. Is her sudden affinity with Aubrey a manifestation of her disease, or a backhanded form of punishment for Grant's infidelity? When Aubrey leaves the home because of financial troubles, Grant visits Aubrey's wife in an effort to allow Fiona to see Aubrey again, preferring to see his wife happy with another man rather than miserable by herself. In a final scene, Fiona briefly remembers Grant and the long life that they shared together. The film ends as they embrace.

Amour (2012), Michael Henke's highly acclaimed French-language film, offers a harrowing portrait of late-life dementia that is both unflinching and compassionate. Georges and Anne, both retired piano players in their eighties, are an accomplished, loving, and active Parisian couple whose lives revolve around music and each other. They are quirky, willful, and fiercely independent people, ill-suited to accommodating the ravages of aging. A series of strokes leaves Anne demented. Georges watches the person whom he loves vanish before his eyes. Is their love also beginning to disappear? Having promised Anne that he will not take her back to the hospital, Georges becomes his wife's hospice caregiver. He sings to her. At times, when she is fiercely defiant at dinner, Georges must pry open her mouth in order to feed her. Despite the challenges, Georges remains devoted in his love for Anne, writing letters that she will never be able to read and recounting stories of their courtship. One day, as he is telling Anne a story, Georges picks up a pillow and smothers her. Viewers are left to ponder: is this mercy killing a final act of love and promise keeping? Is it murder? Or is it a terribly misguided act of desperation by a heartbroken old man?

The Iron Lady (2011) explores the experience of aging in the life of one of England's most powerful and polarizing recent figures, Margaret Thatcher. The film's portrait of Thatcher (played by Meryl Streep) is intimate and personal rather than purely political. We first see her frail and confused, as she slips out of her apartment to buy a carton of milk in a small, cluttered convenience store. A series of flashbacks explores her life as a teenager in Grantham, England; her entry into politics; her first meeting with her future husband, the successful businessman Sir Denis Thatcher; and the years of her political ascendancy as Britain's Conservative Party leader and prime minister, when she reigned for fifteen years as "the Iron Lady." All of these images contrast sharply with the film's present day scenes of Thatcher's growing dementia, her struggle with feelings of impotence and isolation, and her increasing reliance on her daughter.

Dad, Iris, The Iron Lady, and *Amour* contain a complexity and an existential realism that, for the most part, are absent in the films discussed in previous sections. While these films also focus on families and the crises of caregiving, they are less idyllic and more somber in tone. Instead of ending with the feelings of serenity or reconciliation that Norman finds in *On Golden Pond, Dad* ends with Jack's relapse and death. Rather than growing closer with her son, as Old Mrs. Watts does in *The Trip to Bountiful*, in *The Iron Lady* Margaret Thatcher's relationship with her daughter, Carol, remains strained.

AGING SEXUALITIES IN CONTEMPORARY FILM

Recent films have also begun to move beyond the cultural taboo imposed on sex in old age, but they often reinforce popular views of its repulsiveness. *About Schmidt* (2003), for example, offers a sad revision of the elder journey and a glimpse into late-life sexuality. We quickly learn that Warren Schmidt's problems are not with physical disease – he is a healthy, if flabby, older man – but with emotional and existential confusion. Schmidt (played by Jack Nicholson) is unsure whether he has lived a meaningful life. At his retirement party, Warren listens stoically to a colleague who praises his unique life and contributions. But Schmidt knows that, in truth, his life is not the one just described. Upon retiring, he is effortlessly replaced by a younger man. His marriage is joyless, empty, and marked by infidelity: his wife Helen has actually cheated with the very man who delivers Schmidt's retirement speech! In an effort to find meaning in his life, Schmidt "adopts" a Tanzanian orphan named Ndugu and writes him letters.

Helen abruptly dies, leaving Schmidt alone. Without a job, spouse, family, or community, he sets out on the open road in his Winnebago. While the conditions of his journey are not unlike Harry's in *Harry and Tonto*, Schmidt's experiences are marked by loneliness and failure. His childhood home has been demolished and replaced by an auto repair shop. At an RV campground, he makes a failed pass at an acquaintance's young wife and flees the scene. The final destination of his trip, his daughter's wedding, is filled with riotous scenes of drunken in-laws and unsuccessful attempts to talk his daughter out her engagement. At the reception dinner, Schmidt delivers the father-of-the-bride speech. It is a moving, eloquent speech given by a man who doesn't believe a word of what he is saying. A deep sense of resignation pervades the film. In the final scene, however, Schmidt receives a drawing from Ndugu (who cannot read or write) of a tall stick person holding a smaller stick person's hand under a blazing sun. He sees in that drawing the image of a better life of human connection and experiences a rare outpouring of emotion. Rather than concluding with a sense of reconciliation or regeneration, the film ends on a note of poignant ambiguity.

About Schmidt is also noteworthy for its portrait of late-life sexuality. Perhaps the most well-known scene (because it flaunts taboos and appeared in promotional trailers) is Schmidt's hot-tub encounter with the licentious Roberta, played by Kathy Bates. The scene occurs when Schmidt wakes from an uncomfortable night with a stiff neck and slips into the hot tub for some relief. Roberta's frank sexual advances in the hot tub, which are accentuated by her brash manner and corporeality, prompt Schmidt to flee the scene. The unapologetic presentation of aging female sexuality – exemplified by Roberta's flabby female flesh – is too much for Schmidt, and perhaps the viewer, to bear. This exchange between Nicholson and Bates is typical in Hollywood cinema. In *Iris* and elsewhere, films often juxtapose youthful scenes of lovemaking with current scenes of decline and disability, suggesting that older people's bodies are repulsive or incapable of desire and sexual activity.[20]

Beginners (2011) stands as an exception to Hollywood's reluctance to explore passion in late-life sexuality. The film follows the intergenerational relationship between Oliver, a thirty-eight-year-old graphic designer, and his father Hal, a seventy-eight-year-old retired art historian. After his wife's death, Hal comes out of the closet after forty-four years of marriage, a revelation that discomfits Oliver even as he tries to accept his father's new lifestyle. Hal decides to live openly as a gay man just as he learns that he is dying of cancer. He is thus faced with another dilemma: should he "come out of the closet" *and* tell others about his disease? Hal decides to come out as gay but to keep the news of his cancer a secret from everyone except Oliver. The news of Hal's cancer does not stop him from enjoying life and searching for a new partner, as he details in a candid personal ad:

> I'm looking for sex, with the hope it turns into friendship or a relationship, but I don't insist on monogamy. I'm an old senior [gay] guy, 78, but I'm attractive and horny. I'm an art historian, now retired. In addition to art, I like houses, gardens, parties, and walking with my Jack Russell. I'm 5'11, 160 pounds. I'm trim, gray hair, blue eyes, hairy chest.... If you are willing to try an older guy, let's meet and see what happens.

Even though he is pushing eighty with only a few years to live, Hal continues looking for love – and eventually finds it with a man nearly half his age. Like *Wild Strawberries*, *Harry and Tonto*, and *The Trip to Bountiful*, *Beginners* emphasizes that the lessons learned in old age are relevant to subsequent generations. When Hal's son Oliver reflects upon his father's life and its significance for his relationship with his girlfriend Anna, he learns that the journey toward love is a difficult one that does not end with marriage, old age, or even the onset of terminal disease. Oliver and Anna still have much to learn. They, like Hal, are "beginners."

"YES WE STILL CAN": THE AGING COWBOY IN AMERICAN CINEMA

In the early twenty-first century, as some of American cinema's most beloved male actors grew older, Hollywood gave birth to a new kind of hero, an aging hero whose waning physicality and strength become the stimulus for the reassertion of masculinity in later life. A number of films, from Harrison Ford's *Indiana Jones and the Kingdom of the Crystal Skull* (2008) to Sylvester Stallone's *The Expendables* (2010), imply that in spite of real signs of physical decline, aging men needn't relinquish any of their power or their dominance. This kind of exaggerated and compensatory masculinity is especially prominent within the genre of the western. Beyond the rolling plains, bawdy saloons, hostile Indians, and other iconic images of the genre, perhaps the most distinctive feature of the classic western film is the model of masculinity that lies at its core.[21] As Sally Chivers puts it, "enormous effort is made to shore up each male star's increasingly fragile sense of virility at the expense of others, usually women dismissively treated as potential or rejected sexual objects and racialized men easily killed off."[22] In many contemporary westerns, as Chivers notes, the role of the older male figure is recast from a man whose masculinity is thought to be fading to a man whose masculinity is exaggerated and compensatory.

Unforgiven (1992), which stars Clint Eastwood in his early sixties, presents a model of masculinity in which aging physicality is offset by means of "astonishing yet apparently justified violence."[23] Eastwood's character William Munny is a legendary, murderous villain who has become a family man and mended his ways thanks to his loving wife who is recently deceased. As a lonely pig farmer mired in poverty with his two children, Munny's body is beginning to fail him. He is first seen rolling around in the mud chasing his pigs, consistently unable to catch them. Munny fails to hit the mark a single time during target practice; he has even more trouble mounting his horse.[24] At the start, Munny seems resigned to his fate as an ex-outlaw, widower, father of two, pigpen owner, and over-the-hill cowboy. Soon enough, however, Munny is drawn against his will to avenge his friend Ned Logan (played by Morgan Freedman) who has been brutally whipped to death by the sheriff, Little Bill. As the reluctant, wifeless hero thrust back into the fray, Munny embarks on a flurry of retributive violent acts that reinforce his masculinity. The violence culminates in a gripping climax in which Munny guns down the inhabitants of the local saloon, including the corrupt sheriff Little Bill.

No Country for Old Men (2007) features an alternative conception of masculinity in old age. In this western, Sheriff Ed Tom Bell (played by Tommy Lee Jones) represents a unique character: an aging, ineffectual cowboy whose renunciation of violence leaves him uncertain about his identity as a man. Bell is the kind of officer who helps people coax their cats down from treetops and cares about his horses in a personal way. During his thirty-year tenure as the lawman of Terrell County, Texas, he's never had to kill anyone and has never failed to solve a murder case. The plot of *No Country for Old Men* is driven by two other characters, Anton Chigurh and Llewellyn Moss. Moss is a young welder who, on a hunting trip in the desert, stumbles upon a botched drug deal and a briefcase filled with just over two million dollars. Chigurh is a mysterious psychopath who has been hired to retrieve the money at all costs. Within a couple of weeks, there are eight drug-related murders and Bell is helplessly trailing the action in each of them. By the end of the film, Bell is overwhelmed. Chigurh has escaped with the money. Moss and his wife are dead. The peace in Terrell County has been shattered. Bitter, defeated, and bewildered, Bell retires from his job as a sheriff, no longer certain of who he is or where he fits in the world.

What is significant about Bell is how he differs from William Munny. In *No Country for Old Men,* there are no rejected women or racialized men who are sacrificed in order to reaffirm Bell's status as a patriarchal, strong sexy white man. Bell has lived in a long (if imperfect) marriage with his wife, Loretta, and he goes home to an uncertain renewal. Unlike Munny, who is motivated by revenge, Bell is developed through renunciation of violence. Bell makes a critical decision: he will not "*put his soul at hazard*" by pursuing Chigurh, who is a virtual killing machine.[25] Instead, he retires from his post as sheriff and admits that he no longer has easy answers or even confidence in his own views. By refusing to confront Chigurh, Bell stands apart from the violence characterized by typical heroes of the American western. In departing from traditional scripts of youthful aging, Bell takes an important step toward personal authenticity and intimacy, thereby offering an alternative, if uncertain, model of aging masculinity.

CONCLUSION

As we have seen, cinema over the last century reflects the difficulty of making sense of aging in modern culture. From the inception of Hollywood to contemporary film, old people on the silver screen have largely been either absent or viewed through the distorting lens of ageism. While some contemporary films defy negative stereotypes and images of old age, traces of ageism and fears of old age are alive and well. Although the plots have changed, the idea that age is physically demeaning has not.[26] Women, in particular, are cinematically represented as devalued, disabled, and undesirable. At the same time, the history of aging in film reveals a halting and uneven movement from ageist images and representations to portraits of heightened sensitivity and complexity. Despite the distorting lenses of ageism and sexism, some films do indicate paths to the realization of moral and spiritual possibilities in later life.

SUMMATION

This chapter explored portraits of old age in film. Beginning with a discussion of early Hollywood's cult of youth, it examined the slow emergence of aging characters in the 1950s and 60s; the themes of intergeneration and regeneration that frequently drove the plots of films depicting old age in the 70s and 80s; and the variable and complex images of aging presented in more recent age-related films. Then, with a focus on issues such as late-life sexuality and the trope of the "aging cowboy," it considered some of the ways that contemporary film has challenged negative stereotypes and images of old age. Overall, this chapter emphasized that most films present old age as physically and emotionally demeaning, and that a greater awareness of ageism can help us to move toward more nuanced and complex conceptions of old age.

EXERCISES FOR CRITICAL THINKING AND CHARACTER FORMATION

QUESTIONS FOR DISCUSSION

1. Think of the last older character you saw in a movie. How was he or she portrayed? How did you feel about him or her?
2. How did early Hollywood culture contribute to the "pathologizing" of age?
3. Distinguish between male and female representations of aging on the screen. How does the portrait of aging change across gender lines?
4. What's your favorite movie about an older person? What is it that you like about him or her?

WRITING EXERCISE

Watch the movie *About Schmidt*. Notice how the character struggles and how you feel about him. Write an additional scene in which Schmidt responds to Ndugu.

What would he say in this final letter? Would he use words or images to express himself? Write for five to ten minutes.

SUGGESTED VIEWING

Aging in America (2002)
All is Lost (2013)
The Expendables (2010)

Last Vegas (2013)
Red (2010)
The Wrestler (2008)

ADVANCED READING

Robert Butler, "The Life Review: An Interpretation of Reminiscence in the Aged." *Psychiatry* 26 (1963): 65–76.
Sally Chivers, *The Silvering Screen: Old Age and Disability in Cinema*

Thomas R. Cole, *The Journey of Life: A Cultural History of Aging in America*
Robert Yahnke, "The Experience of Aging in Feature-Length Films: A Selected and Annotated Filmography," in *A Guide to Humanistic Studies in Aging*

WEBSITES

Literature, Arts, and Medicine Database
http://litmed.med.nyu.edu/ European Network of Aging Studies (ENAS)
"http://www.agingstudies.eu/" www.agingstudies.eu/
"https://www.google.com/url?sa=t&rct=j&q=&esrc=s&source=web&cd=1&cad=rja&uact=8&sqi=2&ved=0CB0QFjAA&url=http%3A%2F%2Fwww.agingstudies.o

rg%2F&ei=imTaU82MB8mj8QGp9IHwDw&usg=AFQjCNEu-XrI27OizAFzeuuOgIpoO3Tw3Q&sig2=Hh7ayQ1_r1rOlHkQgnf6LQ" North American Network in Aging Studies (NANAS)
"http://www.agingstudies.org" www.agingstudies.org

JOURNALS

Age, Culture, Humanities
The Gerontologist (see, especially, the section on "Film and Digital Media")
Journal of Aging Studies

ORGANIZATIONS AND GROUPS

Gerontological Society of America
http://www.geron.org/

9 Medicine and Media

Although neither the medicine nor the bioethics of these TV dramas is real, both are often so compellingly portrayed as to provide us with extraordinary opportunities to use them to encourage more in depth discussion, and to make bioethics itself more accessible and democratic.

– George Annas[1]

ABSTRACT

This chapter explores how doctors have been depicted on American television. Beginning with a discussion of existing scholarly literature, it examines the origins of the doctor show formula on programs such as *Medic* and *Ben Casey*; the shift toward shows, like *M*A*S*H*, that focused on the lives and problems of physicians rather than patients; the new emphasis on the doctor's family life on programs like *The Cosby Show*; the growing sense of disillusionment presented on shows such as *ER*; and the representation of the doctor as anti-hero on shows like *House, M.D.* Then, with a focus on *The Mindy Project*, it considers some recent developments in the doctor show formula.

INTRODUCTION

Police shows and doctor shows have been a staple of American television for well over fifty years. It is striking that while police shows tend to focus on the taking of life (i.e., murder) doctor shows tend to focus on procedures for saving life (e.g., surgery). The ongoing popularity of both genres seems to indicate that the American public never seems to grow weary of watching the extremities of life.

This chapter introduces the reader to major themes in the history of doctor shows. A key source for this chapter is Joseph Turow's (1950–) *Playing Doctor.*[2] This book is regarded as the most substantial monograph on the topic. The chapter also includes critical scholarship in medical humanities as well as discussions of particular doctor shows. We begin by discussing medical humanities literature on medicine and media.

LITERATURE REVIEW

Types of Literature in Medicine and Media

There are a number of types of literature in medicine and media: edited volumes that compile scholarly perspectives, books that focus on particular doctor shows and other topics, scholarly monographs, and journal articles. Sampling this literature is one way to get some sense of the field.

The most significant book in the area of medicine and media in terms of scholarly rigor as well as representativeness of major scholars doing this work is Lester Friedman's (1945–) *Cultural Sutures*.[3] This edited volume is comprised of chapters from high profile writers in medical humanities and bioethics, including Jonathan Metzl, Arthur Caplan (1950–), Kirsten Ostherr, Therese Jones, and Tod Chambers, and includes essays by other major humanities scholars such as Sander Gilman (1944–). The book addresses journalistic treatment of mental illness, managed care ads on billboards, "medical monsters" in horror films, the depiction of empathy in doctor films, content analyses of doctor television shows, and other topics. In terms of being introduced to medicine and media, the actual topics that the book covers is less important than being introduced to these authors.

Another significant volume is Leslie Reagan, Nancy Tomes, and Paula Treichler's (1943–) *Medicine's Moving Pictures*.[4] This volume's focus, like Friedman's volume, is broader than television; it includes, for example, chapters on popular films as well as health films. This book also demonstrates a high level of scholarly rigor. Yet another significant book in this area is Sandra Shapshay's *Bioethics at the Movies*.[5] This edited volume, as the title intimates, explores bioethics issues as represented in film. It has chapters on movies such as *Gattaca*, *Eternal Sunshine of the Spotless Mind*, and *Million Dollar Baby*. This book, unlike the previous volumes, is content-driven and is important because of its sustained focus on films that are useful for teaching.

In addition to edited volumes, there are monographs and coauthored books that focus on particular doctor shows; Andrew Holtz's *House, M.D. vs. Reality*,[6] for example, focuses on *House*, and Alan Ross and Harlan Gibbs's *The Medicine of ER*[7] focuses on *ER*. There are, too, books that explore particular specialties (e.g., emergency medicine) in a number of doctor shows – e.g., Jason Jacob's *Body Trauma TV*.[8]

There are also rigorous scholarly monographs that focus on medicine and media such as Clive Seale's *Media and Health*[9] and Kirsten Ostherr's *Cinematic Prophylaxis* as well as her *Medical Visions*.[10] These scholarly books often focus on issues of representation, discourse, and power. And yet another kind of literature in the area involves journal articles. Some of these articles are brief commentaries published in major medical journals,[11] and others are full-length journal articles published in bioethics journals.[12] This literature is vast; this discussion is simply meant to give readers a sense of the kind of literature that exists in medicine and media as well as some of the key authors.[13]

Sample Topics in Medicine and Media: Representations of Disability and Pedagogical Debates

Another way of introducing medicine and media is by exploring sample topics; we introduce two here: representations of disability and pedagogical debates. The first topic concerns representations of disability. In *Media and Health*, Seale discusses literature from disability studies as it applies to media with an emphasis on television. He notes that two tropes tend to appear in a variety of forms. One set of images tends to idealize disability (e.g., when persons with a certain disability are portrayed as "supercrips," as when they are shown competing in the Paralympics), and another set of images tends to stigmatize disability (e.g., when persons with a certain disability are portrayed as victims, as when telethons portray persons with a disability as passive victims of charity). Seale also points out that a number of studies in the late 1970s and the early 1980s found that persons with a disability did not tend to appear as major characters on television shows, and that, when persons with a disability are represented at all, they are often misrepresented. A 1992 study, for example, found that representations of the wheelchair, in contrast to other forms of disability, were *over*represented, and that:

> Disabled people were less likely to be portrayed as having jobs, being sexually attractive, or involved in relationships, and more likely to be shown as loners, moody, violent or victims. They were also three times more likely to die than non-disabled people on television.[14]

Seale also noted that persons with a disability were often represented as "disabled persons," in contrast to "persons with disability" – that is, disability was featured as the main component of their character rather than being incidental to it. Seale reports findings from one focus group comprised of persons with disability: persons with disability "would like to see more disabled actors playing as disabled people, and ... that they liked it when disability is shown as a normal background feature of life, rather than a character's overriding focus."[15]

The second topic that we would like to introduce concerns the pedagogical use of doctor shows: To what extent are doctor shows useful as teaching tools? Matthew Czarny and his colleagues report data they collected from an online survey distributed to medical students and nursing students. The study found that most medical students and nursing students do watch doctor shows, and the study also reported other findings relating to ethical issues. While the study was not designed to ascertain whether television viewing habits actually influence the attitudes and the behaviors of medical students and nursing students, the authors suggest that "these television programs are of concern to the extent

that they *might* … influence the attitudes and behaviors of young professionals."[16] The authors also suggest that such viewing might be considered a part
of the "informal curriculum" in that health professional students might learn
bad behavior by watching bad role models on television. In a commentary on
this article, Mark Wicclair (1944–) suggests that these concerns are overblown
because "viewers of television programs and movies are able to recognize that
the behavior of characters who lie, cheat, abuse drugs, steal, rape, kill, and so
forth is not to be emulated in real life."[17]

In contrast to being worried about the potential negative messages sent to
health professional students via television, clinical ethicist Jeffrey Spike makes
a positive case for the educational value of doctor shows.[18] He notes that while
the medicine and the science may be inaccurate on these shows they nevertheless
capture ethical complexity better than the one-paragraph cases that are so often
used in medical education. Why? Television shows, especially if they develop a
character over the course of multiple episodes, are able to portray a person's
personality and their context. Spike also notes that there is much about communication that is nonverbal and cannot be captured with the written word but can
be captured by professional actors who are skilled in representing such subtleties
of conversation. Spike also notes that ethical and professional issues appear in
every episode of each doctor show because drama, by necessity, entails conflict.
Spike also points out that doctor shows often explore a wide range of professionalism issues that are usually overlooked in most bioethics courses.

Howard Trachtman provides a different view. He argues against the use of
doctor shows in medical education because (1) doctor shows need to compete
for ratings and thus tend to show extreme bioethical outliers to generate interest;
(2) television tends to "airbrush" out important details about socioeconomic
location; and (3) bioethical deliberations are often long and drawn-out processes
that require multiple meetings with family members and hospital administrators, and these are rarely depicted on television. While Trachtman's criticisms
are valid, it seems that they could be answered by producing better television.
Crime-related shows like *The Sopranos*, *The Wire*, and *Breaking Bad* have ushered in a new era of television that takes context and character development to a
new level – perhaps the same will happen with doctor shows.

THE HISTORY OF DOCTOR SHOWS: SNAPSHOTS

We now want to turn to a discussion of the history of doctor shows on American
television. During the last sixty years, many doctor shows have been featured
on American primetime television, such as *Medic* and *The Doctor* in the 1950s;
Dr. Kildare, *Ben Casey*, and *Marcus Welby, M.D.* in the 1960s; *The Interns* and
M*A*S*H in the 1970s; *The Cosby Show*, *Growing Pains*, and *Doogie Howser,
M.D.* in the 1980s; *Chicago Hope* and *Dr. Quinn, Medicine Woman* in the 1990s;

and *Grey's Anatomy, Scrubs, House, M.D.* in the 2000s; and *The Mindy Project* in the 2010s. Of particular importance is *ER*, which ran from 1994–2009, making it the longest-running doctor show. This list, far from being exhaustive, is some of the most prominent.

While there have been many doctor shows since the 1950s, it has been argued that these shows do not differ significantly. In a book chapter in *Medicine's Moving Pictures*, Joseph Turow and Rachel Gans-Boriskin provide a brief history of what they call the doctor show formula.[19] The basis for their formula – and its continuities and changes over time – is derived primarily from (1) interviews with producers, directors, writers, actors, and others involved with the creation of doctor shows; (2) viewing and analyzing doctor shows; and (3) engagement with scholarly literature about doctor shows. They argue that the doctor show formula emerged in the years following World War II when medicine was making great advances. Medicine then seemed to be the new "frontier" and doctors were the new "cowboys." In this context, the emerging formula centered on physician-specialists in hospitals with high-tech machines, drugs, and procedures, with no concern for cost. Shows tended to focus on patients who would present them with a problem, and, by the end of the episode, the patient was, more often than not, cured. There was also an emphasis on "realism" – defined as "a portrayal [that] reproduces as faithfully as possible certain aspects of the reality of what practitioners in the institution (lawyers, doctors, police) do and how they do it"[20] – from the beginning, though some shows emphasized realism more than others. A major change to the formula occurred during the 1970s when doctor shows began to focus on the lives and problems of physicians rather than on the lives and problems of patients. The evolution of this formula will be explored in more detail below.

But why did the doctor show formula emerge in the first place? Why is there a need for a formula? Turow suggests that formulas are one way to manage marketing uncertainty. Since there is much at stake with the launching of any television show, parties involved often want some way to minimize risk, and one way of doing so is by holding onto a tried and true formula.[21] In what follows, we focus on seven influential doctor shows, one for each of the decades from the 1950s to the 2010s.

The 1950s: *Medic* and the Origins of the Doctor Show Formula

Medic was the first doctor show to procure a spot on primetime television, created by James Moser. In preparation for creating his show, Moser went to the Los Angeles County Hospital to see what medicine was like. He "shadowed" there for two and a half years. His goal was to gain enough material to enable him to create a show that mixed the human side of medicine with science and technology. It worked. The idea for the pilot episode was derived from an actual experience that he had witnessed in the hospital: a young pregnant woman, diagnosed with leukemia, dies right before her baby is born.

This show established a new paradigm for doctor shows. The show was advertised with phrases such as "No compromise with the truth!" Previous doctor shows – such as programs and films based on CBS Radio's Dr. Christian (who served as the town cupid, philosopher, and detective *in addition to* his role as town physician!) – tended to dramatize the *lives* rather than the *work* of doctors. Moser shifted the drama to clinical experience and set the plot in the hospital. Moser's "realism," however, did not mean complete accuracy, and he was well aware of his limitations, particularly the limitation imposed by the twenty-two minute per episode constraint. Indeed, he realized that his show was not accurate in a number of ways: (1) his plots were physician-centric; (2) a cure almost always occurred; and (3) chronic diseases were rarely depicted. Despite these flaws – flaws that, as we will see, continue to this day – this show took important strides in the creation of a genre.[22]

The 1960s: *Ben Casey* and the Tried and True Methods of Television

Ben Casey was an important doctor show in the early 1960s. Strikingly, it was also created by Moser. After *Medic* had ended in 1956, Moser took leftover material from *Medic* and put a new medical twist on it by focusing on neurosurgery. Television episodes were also increasingly becoming an hour long, thus giving Moser more plot flexibility. To prepare for his new show, he again spent time shadowing in the hospital, this time spending ten months on a neurosurgery ward in L.A. County Hospital. Max Warner, a neurosurgeon, also helped with the accuracy of the show.

Moser created this show around the stereotype of the nasty attitudes of surgeons, linking this stereotype to the popular antiheroes of the 1950s such as James Dean. He also employed the tried and true conventions of television: he gave Casey a sidekick as well as a love interest, and he inserted an older-doctor/younger-doctor tension. Such relationships became key to the plot.

This photograph reveals a few elements of the contrivance behind a single shot in the series *Mercy*, which aired on NBC from 2009 to 2010. The bulky camera occupies a third of the frame; three crew members occupy a third, leaving roughly a third for the actor, the patient in the hospital bed.

What we don't see, farther back, could include more crew members – the photographer, the camera operator, the director, the script supervisor, a lighting crew, the sound crew, the props and set design team, electricians, and more equipment such as light stands and fixtures, cables, microphone booms and a recording console, video monitors, speakers, and miscellaneous carts, chairs, and equipment cases. The crew we see appear to be costumers and makeup artists.

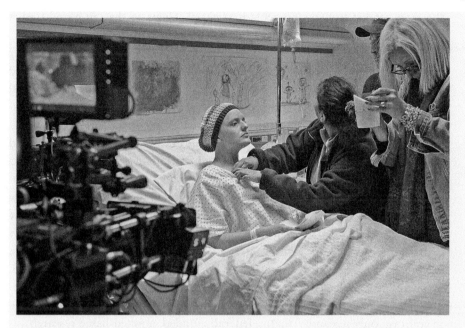

Figure 9. Television series *Mercy* production photo, 2009–10, NBC, NBCUniversal/Getty Images.

The frame of the shot to be recorded appears on the camera's viewfinder. The image is out of focus, but you can see that the camera position is low, relative to the patient's head. The framing leaves room for the doctor to stand in the area occupied by the crew.

What about the patient's cap, the patient's gown, the IV stand and bag, and what appear to be a child's drawings on the wall? We should assume that each item was selected and deliberately placed in the scene to support the story. Only the cap and drawings are unusual; the cap stands out because of its color and texture, while the drawings, at the distance they're seen in this shot, are generic. In an institutional setting such as a hospital, only a few elements like the hat and drawings can add texture to a scene. Doctor shows are usually fast paced with rapid cutting and camera movement, focused on exchanges between the actors or medical procedures.

One goal of this chapter is to help you become an informed consumer of popular media. To exercise what you've learned, compare a doctor show with an historical drama, which depends on elaborate costumes and settings, over which the camera lingers to convey a very different quality of life.

The series was filmed as a dramatic documentary. To preserve tension and mystery, the hospital was never named and details were withheld about Casey so that he would be portrayed as "raw," "puzzling," and "intriguing." The primary focus in each episode was on a guest star; thus, new plot devices could be introduced while also preserving Casey as a mystery. This also meant, however, that the show tended to focus on acute medical problems so that, in general, each episode had to result in either a cure or a death.

The show was a hit. The press loved *Ben Casey*. The combination of safety and adventure embodied in Casey especially appealed to women. People would write to Vince Edwards (who played the role of Casey), asking him for medical advice. Real doctors, too, wanted to discuss cases with Edwards. And even hospital schedules were changed to accommodate viewing of the show.

Yet not everyone was a fan of the show. Some health professionals complained that the show was teaching bad habits and inaccurate concepts of medicine. However, the American Medical Association, while sympathetic to these criticisms, believed that the show, on the whole, was good for the profession's image (and the AMA enjoyed its influence in determining what was portrayed in the show). The *Wall Street Journal* suggested that *Ben Casey* and other such shows constituted a good public relations strategy. Others, while not attacking the show, used it to criticize medical education. In an article published in *JAMA* in 1978, William Regelson laments the fact that a generation or two prior to 1978 teaching and patient care was valued in departments of medicine, but now (i.e., 1978), in contrast, only research – that is, federally funded, granted-based research – is valued, and that medicine is becoming controlled by economic forces, leading to "Ben Casey medicine."[23] The fact that Regelson could use the phrase "Ben Casey medicine" without any further explanation demonstrates the influence of the show. And his 1978 critique seems to be as true today as it was then.

With *Ben Casey*, the doctor show formula was now set. The doctor show formula mixes the tried and true dramatic elements of television with: (1) medical "realism," (2) a hospital-based focus, (3) a character selection that is physician-centric (with an emphasis on specialists), (4) a plot that is technologically driven, (5) representations of acute illnesses, and (6) a disregard for the costs of health care.[24]

The 1970s: *M*A*S*H* and the Existential Turn

No discussion of doctor shows is complete without *M*A*S*H*. During a time when there was skepticism about the viability of doctor shows in general – some television executives felt that there was only so much that could be depicted in hospitals and that doctor shows had run their course – *M*A*S*H*, which ran from 1972–1983, altered the doctor show formula in two significant ways: by shifting the existential focus from patients to physicians and by introducing comedy in a unique way.

M*A*S*H was set during the Korean War (1950–1953), but it was also indirectly about the Vietnam War (1955–1975). The show followed a mobile army surgical hospital (M.A.S.H.) unit. The show's theme song was an instrumental version of "Suicide is Painless," an indication of the dark comedy of the show. This thirty-minute show was based on a film with the same title, which had done well, and the movie, in turn, also was based on a novel with the same title.[25]

$M*A*S*H$, unlike previous doctor shows, was able to communicate the absurdity of medicine with doses of comedy to make the truth of inevitable death palatable. By locating medicine in a war zone – that is, by depicting doctors treating people who would then go back out on the battlefield to die – invited the viewer to consider his or her own mortality as well as the meaning of life: What is the point of life (and medicine) if we are just going to die anyway? What is striking about $M*A*S*H$ in contrast to other doctor shows is that the doctor is *not* in complete control. Just as the doctor is not the highest ranking military official (and therefore does not have ultimate authority), the doctor in $M*A*S*H$ does not have ultimate power over death; patients die. $M*A*S*H$, in other words, treated doctors as "reluctant draftees" and *not* as superhuman heroes.

EXERCISE: PREPARING A CLASS PRESENTATION

Pick a doctor show. Write a brief synopsis of the premise of the show. Describe the setting and the main characters. Next, pick a particular episode. Watch the episode once to become (re)acquainted with the basic narrative. Re-watch the episode, this time taking notes on ethical issues that are presented in the show. Now pick one ethical issue from the show on which to present. Next read ethics literature about the issue. Watch the episode a third time, and pick a scene to show in class for your presentation. Finally, prepare a presentation that includes the following elements: (1) background information about the show; (2) a synopsis of a particular episode; (3) a viewing from the show that presents the ethical issue; and (4) questions for discussion.

The show's key themes involved the emotional toll of operating on an ongoing stream of wounded soldiers; the difficulties of working with people whose personalities are quite different from one's own; and the pestering interference of military bureaucracy and hierarchy. The show would make political points, too. Some critics felt that the show did so effectively without moralizing. In any case, the original contribution of $M*A*S*H$ was that it dealt with these medical, political, and personal tensions with dark comedy that was not heavy handed. There was, to be sure, comedy about medicine before $M*A*S*H$, such as the "Doctor Kronkhite" sketch in the mid-twentieth century where the patient says, "It hurts when I do this," and the doctor replies, "Don't do this." This kind of comedy is referred to as "buffoonery." But the image of the doctor as a buffoon did not really last because, Turow suggests, organized medicine gained power and prestige during the 1950s. In other words, doctor shows were beginning to take off at precisely the time when organized medicine was concerned about its image, so buffoonery was out. *M*A*S*H*, in contrast to buffoonery pure and simple, provided a kind of comedy that humanized doctors without demeaning them.[26]

The 1980s: *The Cosby Show* and the Domesticated Doctor

The Cosby Show was a major – perhaps *the* major – television program of the 1980s. Bill Cosby, an African American comedian, played Dr. Cliff Huxtable, the central character of the show. *The Cosby Show* focused not only on the physician's life but also – straying significantly from the doctor show formula – on the physician's *home* life, thus bringing the existential turn from *M*A*S*H* back to American soil with domestic concerns. It is striking that *Growing Pains*, another major show during the 1980s, was also about a doctor. *Growing Pains* featured Dr. Jason Seaver as a psychiatrist, and this show, like *The Cosby Show*, used medicine as a backdrop.

Dr. Huxtable was an obstetrician/gynecologist who had an office in his home. The choice to make Dr. Huxtable an obstetrician/gynecologist was intentional on Cosby's part (he was a creator of the show and its lead actor), as he wanted to teach important lessons about family life, and he felt that this specialty especially lent itself to intimate conversations about birth and growth – the stuff of families.[27]

The show was more about family life than medical life. But the fact that medicine was in the background rather than the foreground did not deter doctors from praising *The Cosby Show*. In a 1985 commentary in *JAMA*, Roselyn Epps writes: "Dr. Huxtable is liked by physicians who hope they're a little like him, and by patients who appreciate that kind of doctor."[28] Perhaps another way of saying this is that doctors appreciated seeing a physician with a good work-life balance when they had difficulty maintaining their own.

It is worth pointing out that, in scholarly literature, *The Cosby Show* has been examined more along the lines of race than along the lines of medicine. Leslie Inniss and Joe Feagin build on research reported in Sut Jhally and Justin Lewis's *Enlightened Racism: The Cosby Show, Audiences, and the Myth of the American Dream*.[29] Inniss and Feagin draw on interviews that they conducted and found a genuinely mixed response to the show. On the one hand, some interviewees felt that the show was unrealistic in that there was an absence of the unique struggles that African Americans face and that the show more or less portrayed a white family with "black faces." On the other hand, other interviewees felt that it is not the job of television to be "realistic" and that fantasy images can be inspirational – that is, they can offer a picture of what life *should* be like, not what it *is* like, and that the Huxtables can be seen as role models in this regard. Discussions of race have been undeveloped in medical humanities and bioethics, so contributions such as these are much needed.[30]

The 1990s: *ER*, Diversity, and Cultural Pessimism

The longest-running doctor show in television history is *ER*, running, as noted, from 1994–2009; it also achieved 122 Emmy Award nominations. The show is noteworthy for these numbers alone. In addition to achieving these numbers, the show also blazed new trails (such as portraying doctors in racially, ethnically, and sexually diverse ways). Subsequent shows, such as *Scrubs* and *Grey's Anatomy*, as well as more recent female-centric shows such as *The Mindy Project* and *Emily Owens, M.D.*, benefited from the paths cleared by *ER*. Indeed, it was *ER* (arguably building on the success of *The Cosby Show*'s depiction of an African American doctor) that sculpted a new "mosaic" of American doctors, one that was in line with actual practice. Doctors in *ER* were male, female, white, black, South Asian, straight, gay, U.S. born, immigrant, and so forth.

A new sense of medical realism was also cultivated in *ER*. The show was fast-paced, high-tech, and quasi-documentary. It depicted weaker relationships with patients, more angst-ridden health professionals, and more bodily gore. In *Body Trauma TV*, Jacobs notes that Michael Crichton (1942–2008), the creator of *ER*, wrote the script for the show in 1974 but was unable to procure a pilot for a series until he teamed up with Steven Spielberg. Jacobs also notes that John Wells, executive producer of *China Beach*, felt that the script for *ER* was off-putting to many. He writes:

> [Y]ou didn't know who you were supposed to care about [and] ... there wasn't a beginning, middle and end .... *ER* was almost like a pointillist painting ... looking closely at the bits and pieces of scenes, they seemed not to make sense. But when you stepped back, they added up to an emotional tapestry that was very moving.[31]

Jacobs also notes that the tone of *ER* was different from previous doctor shows. The show often offered a spirit of disillusionment rather than reassurance. This, to Crichton, was a part of his take on "medical realism." Jacobs adds that this spirit of disillusionment could be a reflection of a growing cultural pessimism in American society.[32]

In any case, this new dark sense of realism was appreciated by viewers. One reviewer wrote, "There are few miracles, and stories don't always have happy endings. People do die."[33] The reviewer also noted that the days when health professional groups controlled the content of doctor shows (to portray health professionals in a favorable light) are over, as *ER* depicts some health professionals in a less than favorable light (such as residents sleeping on duty and a nurse over-dosing on drugs). The show also portrayed residents working for eighty hours a week and making only $36,000 a year – a truth that was not widely known among the general public. But the show was unrealistic in other ways. Medical students, for example, do not spend an entire year in the emergency room, as was depicted on the show. Turow observes that the show still contained the traditional problems of doctor shows: it dealt primarily with acute incidents; health care was depicted as hierarchical and physician-centric; and top-of-the-line care was provided without a sense of the costs. Despite these shortcomings, the show was a huge success and was important for the development of the genre.[34]

The 2000s: *House* as a New Kind of (Anti)hero?

The most significant doctor show of the 2000s, at least during the latter half of the decade, was *House, M.D.*, which ran from 2004–2012. *House* is about Dr. Gregory House (or simply "House"), whose specialty is infectious disease. He is portrayed as a kind of Sherlock Holmes figure, able to figure out bizarre medical cases with flashes of insight. He is also depicted as a brash diagnostician who has questionable personal and professional ethics (e.g., he often speaks uncaringly to patients and suffers from an addiction to pain medication).

In *House, M.D. vs. Reality*, Andrew Holtz offers a broad look at the show and its context. Many of the criticisms of doctor shows previously noted still apply to *House, M.D.* – the show, for example, tends to focus on sensational issues and cost is not taken into account sufficiently. However, one study found, strikingly, that *House, M.D.* as well as other recent medical dramas actually display *worse* than actual health outcomes in hospitals.[35] This is counterintuitive, because doctor shows historically have *overrepresented* cures. Some media scholars think that this is because networks like HBO have pushed the boundaries of television, enabling a number of shows to emerge that can yield "a darker, grittier portrayal of life – and more frequently death."[36]

Bioethicists and medical humanists have displayed a recent interest in *House, M.D.*[37] One thoughtful analysis by Elena Strauman and Bethany Goodier published in *The Journal of Medical Humanities* analyzed the first two seasons of the show. They found that:

> *House* is at once similar to, and different from, the classic medical drama. On the one hand, *House* repeats a familiar formula – a central physician-hero who cures patients with the help of a supporting team. However, while early doctor shows focused on the all-knowing, all-caring physician hero and later generic iterations focused on a caring but infallible physician-hero, *House* challenges audiences by offering a physician who, on [the] one hand, is the heroic, maverick scientist who always finds the answer in time to cure the patient, and on the other, a wholly flawed and often unlikable character who lacks empathy and decency toward patients and co-workers.[38]

Strauman and Goodier also observe that the show, as a whole, *does* recreate the early physician hero who is both scientifically competent and empathetically attuned by complementing House with other physicians and health care professionals who *do* attend to the non-biomedical aspects of healing even while he does not. As they put it: "It literally 'takes a village' to produce 'ideal' medicine."[39] The show, in any case, does privilege the science (i.e., the biomedical aspects) over the art (i.e., the patient care aspects) of medicine. In the words of House: "Treating illness is why we became doctors. Treating patients is actually what makes most doctors miserable."[40]

The 2010s and Beyond: *The Mindy Project* and Future Directions for Doctor Shows

The Mindy Project premiered on Fox in 2012. The show centers on Mindy Kaling (the stage name of Vera Mindy Chokalingam), who is well known for her roles in producing, directing, writing for, and acting in the comedy *The Office*. In *The Mindy Project*, Kaling plays the role of Mindy Lahiri, an obstetrician/gynecologist. While *The Mindy Project* is not the first doctor show to feature a woman as the series lead – *Dr. Quinn, Medicine Woman* was a prominent precursor – it is the first American television series to feature a South Asian American as the lead actor. Kaling also writes for the show. Time will tell how influential this show will prove to be; it very well could alter the doctor show formula in unprecedented ways, perhaps by being informed by the experience and epistemologies of women.

CONCLUSION

"Although neither the medicine nor the bioethics of these TV dramas is real," influential bioethicist George Annas (1945–) writes, "both are often so compellingly portrayed as to provide us with extraordinary opportunities to use them to encourage more in depth discussion, and to make bioethics itself more accessible and democratic."[41] This chapter intimated pedagogical, pragmatic, and political reasons for medical humanists and bioethicists to pay attention to doctor shows while tracing the evolution of the doctor show formula through seven notable doctor shows. We noted that the doctor shows produced to date have had their limits: what counts as "realism" has changed over time and is never neutrally or objectively determined; visual technologies and time constraints have often determined how disease is represented; plot concerns have sometimes worked against the virtues and values often promoted by medical humanities and bioethics (especially when doctor shows encourage the illusion that costs do not have to be controlled and when diseases have been depicted as acute rather than chronic); and these shows have tended to be physician-centric and patriarchal. But these limits, in any case, do not weaken Annas's point; they strengthen it. Indeed, these weaknesses are all the more reason for bioethicists and medical humanists to engage, critically, these shows, exploring the opportunities identified by Annas that television, as a unique form of media, has to offer.

SUMMATION

This chapter explored how doctors have been depicted on American television. Beginning with a discussion of the existing literature, it examined the origins of the doctor show formula on programs like *Medic* and *Ben Casey*; the shift toward shows, like *M*A*S*H*, that focused on the lives and problems of physicians rather than patients; the emphasis on the doctor's family life on programs like *The Cosby Show*; the growing sense of disillusionment presented on shows like *ER*; and the representation of the doctor as antihero on shows like *House, M.D.* Then, with a focus on *The Mindy Project*, it considered some recent developments in the doctor show formula. Overall, though, this chapter attempted to emphasize that, while these TV dramas do not depict "reality," they can still provide us with extraordinary opportunities for discussion and reflection.

EXERCISES FOR CRITICAL THINKING AND CHARACTER FORMATION

QUESTIONS FOR DISCUSSION

1. Do you watch doctor shows? Which show or shows do you watch, and why?
2. To what extent should doctor shows be based in "reality"?
3. To what extent should doctor shows attempt to educate the public about matters of health and disease?
4. To what extent should doctor shows engage social issues?

SUGGESTED VIEWING: POPULAR AND IMPORTANT DOCTOR SHOWS

Ben Casey
Chicago Hope
China Beach
The Cosby Show
Dr. Kildare
Dr. Quinn, Medicine Woman
Emily Owens, M.D.
ER

Grey's Anatomy
House, M.D.
M*A*S*H
Marcus Welby, M.D.
Medic
The Mindy Project
Nip/Tuck
Scrubs

ADVANCED READING

Virginia Berridge and Kelly Loughlin, eds., *Medicine, the Market and the Mass Media*
Lester Friedman, ed., *Cultural Sutures: Medicine and Media*
Kirsten Ostherr, *Medical Visions: Producing the Patient through Film, Television, and Imaging Technologies*

Leslie Reagan, Nancy Tomes, and Paula Treichler, eds., *Medicine's Moving Pictures: Medicine, Health, and Bodies in American Film and Television*
Clive Seale, *Media and Health*
Sandra Shapshay, ed., *Bioethics at the Movies*
Joseph Turow, *Playing Doctor: Television, Storytelling, and Medical Power*

JOURNALS

Continuum: Journal of Media and Cultural Studies
Feminist Media Studies
Historical Journal of Film, Radio and Television

Journal of Popular Film and Television
Media, Culture, Society
Television and New Media

PROGRAMS

Berkeley
http://ugis.ls.berkeley.edu/mediastudies/
The New School

http://www.newschool.edu/public-engagement/
ma-media-studies/

ONLINE RESOURCES

Bioethics in Television Entertainment
http://bioethicsmedia.org/about/
The Medical Futures Lab

http://www.medicalfutureslab.org/
The Museum of Broadcast Communications
http://www.museum.tv/

10 Poetry and Moral Imagination

I don't see any reason why doctors shouldn't read a little poetry as a part of their training.[1]

– Anatole Broyard

ABSTRACT

This chapter explores how poetry can contribute to medical humanities. Beginning with a discussion of how poetry deals with the raw material of human experience – including experiences of illness and injury, healing and grief, love and death – it examines five poems that are particularly relevant to students of medical humanities: Alan Shapiro's "Someone Else," James Dickey's "The Scarred Girl," Robert Cooperman's "What They Don't Know," Stephen Knight's "FROM *The Fascinating Room*," and Sharon Olds's "The Learner." Then, with a focus on how poetry "makes language care," it considers how these poems – experienced vicariously but intimately – animate our moral imagination and transport us into the lives of others in ways that enhance our empathetic understanding.

INTRODUCTION

Medical people are taught to read for facts and data, an undeniably useful skill. But there is so much more to the written (and spoken) word than information. We read for pleasure and inspiration as well as edification. We read because we want to learn and to be informed. And we read to deepen our knowledge and expand our horizons. Reading can broaden our experience and enrich our lives; it can enchant us, quicken our spirits, and shape our sentiments. To read for meaning yields sympathetic understanding; to read for inspiration yields hope, and possibly transformation. We filter our self-understanding and the way we see others through experiences encountered vicariously in our reading of imaginative literature. But poetry? Why poetry?

Marianne Moore (1887–1972) had this to say about it:

"I, too, dislike it: there are things that are important beyond all this fiddle.
Reading it, however, with a perfect contempt for it, one discovers in
it after all, a place for the genuine.
      Hands that can grasp, eyes
        that can dilate, hair that can rise
            if it must, these things are important not because a

high-sounding interpretation can be put upon them but because they are useful...
      if you demand on the one hand
the raw material of poetry in
      in all its rawness and
      that which is on the other hand
            genuine, then you are interested in poetry."[2]

The raw material of human experience – including experiences of illness and injury, healing and grief, love and death – *and* that which is genuine, honest, and authentic will serve our purposes here as a good enough answer to the question: why poetry? To be sure, "Poetry belongs to the *strange*," as Cynthia Ozick (1928) once put it. "But when we say that poetry is strange, we mean not that it is less than intelligible, but exactly the opposite: poetry is intelligibility heightened, strengthened, distilled; and also made manifold .... A poet has the same access to the language pool as a tailor, an archaeologist, or a felon. How strange that, scooping up words from the selfsame pool as everyone else, a poet will reconfigure, startle, and restart those words!"[3]

But what to make of Moore's idea that poetry can be *useful*? Useful in what way? The conventional view is that a poem is what it is, stands on its own, and is therefore not "usable" instrumentally toward some extrinsic end. W. H. Auden's (1907–1973) claim that poetry makes nothing happen seems plausible in a strict sense: "Poetry is not concerned with telling people what to do, but with extending our knowledge of good and evil, perhaps making the necessity for action more urgent and its nature more clear, but only leading us to the point where it is possible for us to make a rational and moral choice."[4]

Particularly pertinent to our consideration of poetry and moral imagination, Auden says elsewhere, "Poetry is speech at its most personal, the most intimate of dialogues. A poem does not come to life until a reader makes his response to the words written by the poet .... Poetry must either be 'read,' that is to say, entered into by a personal encounter, or it must be left alone."[5]

This chapter explores the idea that poetry must be entered into by an active reader, one who engages in what Ozick calls "the labor of human imagination,"[6] the readerly endeavor to move from words to meaning, from letter to spirit. It will do this by offering interpretations of a selection of contemporary poems that bear in various ways on experiences of illness and injury in the context of modern medical practice.[7]

Poetry may seem forbidding at first but on closer acquaintance it can be seen to be just another language. And fortunately, as Kenneth Koch (1925–2002) observes, "Like other languages, the poetic language can be picked up starting anywhere. One can study it or just begin reading."[8]

So let's begin.

Someone Else

When she had come to live with them, by then
vanity was all her stroke had left her.
Yet it became another kind of health,
a way to get through days when she would wake
in her wet bed, a child again, afraid
she might be found before the sheets were clean;
or showering, when she would have to see her body
like someone else resisting her, so stiff
it only let her turn enough to reach,
not wash the bitter smell that clung like shame.

So she would spend the mornings struggling
with her silk slip and dress, and work her stockings
up her legs till they seemed agile with shimmering.
the rouged cheek, the hair done up, the nails polished till the brightness made her hands
(if only they'd keep still) less like a stranger's –
these enabled her to leave her room
and face them, and believe the care she needed was what they owed her,
what she permitted them to give. They were,
she would tell herself, tottering her great
weight down the stairs, no better than her husbands,
those first betrayers: the sullen courtesy
her grandchild showed, the irritation hiding
in her daughter's pity, she could at least ignore them
(at least there would be power there), and wait
till they went out, wanting them out,
so she could feel finally at home,
the tv on, just her and her celebrities.

She could anticipate each set response,
each misery. Nothing could surprise her.
And with a kind of joy she could be certain
that even if some star walked from the screen
the mirror, always at hand, would show her hair
in place, her face powdered; she could feel
the aftertaste of mouthwash, could even savor
the bitter cleanness of her mouth, and know,
nearly invincible, that she was ready,
should anybody come to take her out.

– Alan Shapiro[9]

The subject of this poem is a mother and grandmother who, betrayed by her body, has come to live with her daughter's family. It is an arrangement dictated by necessity. She needs their care but resents it. They pity her and tolerate her, all the while wishing it weren't so. She maintains a kind of control over a life unexpectedly thrust upon her by putting necessity to work for her, in *allowing* her family to provide the care she needs. In a body grown strange and recalcitrant, it is vanity that lets her come out at all and settle down to watch the reassuringly predictable television soaps. Her vanity is "another kind of health" that gets her through days of shame and bitterness. More than this, there, is "a kind of joy" in the certainty that if a celebrity were to step from the screen (or if death were to announce itself?), she would be composed, well groomed, ready to "go out."

Poetry persuades not by argumentation or exhortation but by evocation. Poems are often not immediately transparent to meaning but require studied attentiveness accompanied by an openness to possibility. The search for sense is sought by sorting and weighing evidence available in or alluded to in the text. In this process, insights take form in the reader's (or listener's) imagination. As a plausible rendering of Shapiro's poem begins to dawn, we are able to imagine: so this is how it can feel to live with the aftereffects of a stroke.

CASE STUDY: ALAN SHAPIRO AND EVOCATION

With the idea that poetry persuades not by argumentation or exhortation but by evocation in mind, go back and read Alan Shapiro's "Someone Else" again, paying close attention to the details he uses to help you imagine what it might be like to live with the aftereffects of a stroke.

1. While humans tend to privilege the sense of sight, there is more to experience than vision alone. What senses does Shapiro engage in "Someone Else"? How do these details give you a better understanding of the woman's experience of illness?
2. The third and fourth stanzas of "Someone Else" indicate that the woman looks forward to time away from her family, time when she can be alone with television and her mirror. Why might the woman feel like this? What evidence is there for your position?
3. Consider the title of the poem: "Someone Else." How does this title relate to the rest of the poem?

The Scarred Girl

All glass may yet be whole
She thinks, it may be put together
From the deep inner flashing of her face.
One moment the windshield held

The countryside, the green
Level fields and the animals,
And these must be restored
To what they were when her brow

Broke into them for nothing, and began
Its sparkling under the gauze.
Though the still, small war for her beauty
Is stitched out of sight and lost,
It is not this field that she thinks of.
It is that her face, buried
And held up inside the slow scars,
Knows how the bright, fractured world

Burns and pulls and weeps
To come together again.
The green meadow lying in fragments
Under the splintered sunlight,

The cattle broken in pieces
By her useless, painful intrusion
Know that her visage contains
The process and hurt of their healing,

The hidden wounds that can
Restore anything, bringing the glass
Of the world together once more,
All as it was then she struck,

All except her. The shattered field
Where they dragged the telescoped car
Off to be pounded to scrap
Waits for her to get up,

For her calm, unimagined face
To emerge from the yards of its wrapping,
Red, raw, mixed-looking but entire,
A new face, an old life,

To confront the pale glass it has dreamed
Made whole and backed with wise silver,
Held in other hands brittle with dread,
A doctor's, a lip-biting nurse's,

Who do not see what she sees
Behind her odd face in the mirror:
The pastures of earth and of heaven
Restored and undamaged, the cattle

Risen out of their jagged graves
To walk in the seamless sunlight
And a newborn countenance
Put upon everything.

Her beauty gone, but to hover
Near for the rest of her life
And good no nearer, but plainly
In sight, and the only way.

– James Dickey[10]

In James Dickey's (1923–1997) poem, we encounter a girl who lies hugely bandaged ("her face, buried") as the result of an accident that threw her face first into the windshield of the car in which she was riding. Just prior to the accident, "the windshield held" – it was intact, it shielded her in the vehicle, and it framed a bucolic scene. In a flash, at the moment of impact, this pastoral scene, this peaceful life, was needlessly, painfully broken. The poet metaphorically conflates the girl's face and the car's windshield. They splinter simultaneously. We know that a shattered windshield cannot be repaired. We infer from the poem's title that the girl's face cannot be restored to seamlessness. But in spite of the brute facticity of brokenness here, this poem speaks, finally, of restoration and reconciliation.

The poet imagines what the girl may be thinking as she waits for her wounds to heal: "All glass may yet be whole." This is more than a mere thought; it is a yearning and a dawning. As she thinks of the field as she last saw it, and all that it signified of beauty and wholeness, it comes to the girl that the countryside and the animals that splintered on impact can be restored. The restoration will depend on her; the fate of the fragmented meadow and the broken cattle lies in her way of seeing. The girl can recall the view through the windshield prior to the crash, thereby resurrecting the pastures and cattle from their "jagged graves."

But there is another field here, one the girl does not (yet) think of. It is a battlefield whereon a war for her beauty is already lost. Her face is not only buried under gauze; it is gone for good. Although she knows that her face will not be as before, she cannot imagine how it will look when the wrappings come off. We – doctor, nurse, reader – transported by the poet into the girl's presence, dread the girl's reaction when she confronts her scarred face. But our anxious anticipation is misplaced. What the girl sees in the mirror is an "odd face," but that is not all. Looking past the face to the surrounding background, she sees all glass made whole – the pastures and the cattle, once in pieces, now restored and undamaged, the splintered sunlight seamless again, and "a newborn countenance put upon everything." What is this countenance? The girl's outlook, perhaps, her way of seeing herself and the world, now changed. She will live with the memory of her former beauty, which must be kept at arm's length for the rest of her life, and she will come to terms with the hard fact of her new face. Though her face is scarred, she and her world are intact. The scarred girl is reconciled. It is "the only way."

What They Don't Know

Big companies figure out all sorts of stuff about us we don't even know ourselves – from how many headaches we get to how much dust we vacuum up. They know how many times we change the babies' diapers, how often we lose the cap to our toothpaste and what we think of our local car dealer.

– The Wall Street Journal

But they haven't figured out his last headache
began to build when the specialist
told them his wife had cancer,
and he had to listen, her hand trembling in his,
his head buzzing as if his next door neighbor
had once again gone berserk

with his chainsaw and dwindling stand of trees.
Afterward, he escorted his wife to the car,
feeling her feather-light on his arm, no, more like a rag filthy
from cleaning toilets and furnaces.
He felt ashamed of his fear of touching her,
and knew she sensed his terror,
when her fingers withdrew
as he opened the car door
and they drove home silent as the sky
minutes following the freight train of tornadoes.

After he took the babysitter home
he fumbled for the aspirins,
considered taking them all
while his wife changed the baby's diaper,
clucking too casually that the girl
had conveniently forgotten that chore.

That night, as he lay on his back in bed,
the bottle of aspirins on the night table,
he still heard the world buzz
in the doctor's words; his wife
touched his arm that felt made
of wood petrified a million years ago.
"What about me?" she whispered,
the first words she had spoken in hours,
her voice dry as trees
about to burst into forest fires,
her tears trembling echoes
of hot film enveloping the whole forest.

– Robert Cooperman[11]

The mood of this poem is one of dread. The voice speaking from the poem is that of a husband terrified, "petrified," by his wife's cancer diagnosis. He treats her as if she were contagious. His head is buzzing, the world is buzzing, and he harbors thoughts of suicide. The poem is full of foreboding and menace. Only hours later, when she reaches out to him, does he hear in her voice and see in her tears *her* fear of the coming conflagration.

Poems are schools of feeling; they go straight to the heart – the heart of the matter, and the reader's heart. But if we readers are to be edified as well as touched or moved, our emotions must be schooled. It is not a question of either/or, but of both/and. Cooperman's poem arouses our emotions *and* challenges our intellect. We feel the husband's head buzzing, his shame at feeling that his wife is tainted, and his inability to reach out to her. And we feel his wife's despair and deep sadness at having been left so utterly alone. We feel all this with an immediacy that, if left at that, might come to nothing more than a fleeting upsurge of emotion. As a *school* of feeling, the poem also challenges us to *think* about the meaning of what we have felt.

But are thinking and feeling two distinct activities? Might it be that the long-honored distinction between intellect and emotion fails to illuminate what is happening when we readers try to plausibly account for the abundance of emotion evoked by Cooperman's poem? Maybe the perceived divide between heart and head is a distinction without a difference. Perhaps, instead, it is the faculty of imagination, conceived as what Northup Frye (1912–1991) calls "the *combination* of emotion and intellect," [emphasis added] that is at work here.[12] Or perhaps, as Mary Warnock (1924–) has argued, it is best thought of as a *capacity*, a "capacity to look beyond the immediate and the present,"[13] "a power in the human mind which is at work in our everyday perception of the world and is also at work in our thoughts about what is absent; which enables us to see the world, whether present or absent as significant, and also to present this vision to others, for them to share or reject. And this power ... is not only intellectual. Its impetus comes from the emotions as much as from the reason, from the heart as much as from the head."[14]

We are taught to distinguish poetry from prose by the form it takes on the printed page, most commonly the use of stanzas, which are groups of two or more short lines, as you see in this picture. The form of poetry on a printed page also highlights the qualities of the art of typography.

Compare the letters in the title of the poem *Musée Des Beaux Arts* to the letters in the first stanza. How are they different in height, width, letter style, use of upper and lower case, spacing between letters, and spacing between lines? Examine the paper. Imagine rubbing the page between your thumb and forefinger. Would it feel smooth or textured? How does the paper of this book feel between your fingers?

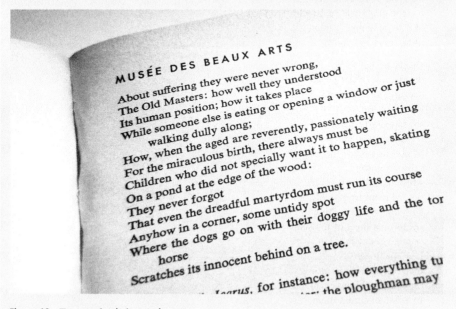

Figure 10. *Typography,* designer unknown.

Compare the typography of this poem with any other printed form you have near you – this book, other books, a business card, the label on a bottle of prescription medicine. How is the typography of the poem different from other typography around you, even on your computer screen? Why might the typography of a roadside billboard be different from the typography of the *Physicians' Desk Reference*?

Does your handwriting approach art in the way you shape letters? Can you imagine drawing each of the letters in this poem by hand and trying to put into each letter something of the poem itself? That was the goal of the printers and type designers who revolutionized intellectual life after 1450. They not only made millions of books widely available for the first time in history; they also made beautiful books that are treasures in form and content.

To pursue these ideas, search the web for the history of printing, Johannes Gutenberg, Aldus, Manutius, and typography. For terms to describe typography, search for "white space," "serif and sans-serif," and "monospace or proportional type."

FROM *The Fascinating Room*
Her bedroom hardening
to a small museum:
stilts of light
breaking the clouds,
freckled with dust
and quietly
rusting the wallpaper;
the mattress and the sheets
rippling with her shape;
the burning bedside lamp. . .
I log these observations
by repeating them to myself
like the nine times table
or learning quotations.

On the desk,
the shadow of her pencil
deepens, minute by minute,
like a bruise –
she has sharpened it
to within three inches
of nothing. Now, I watch
saliva evaporate
where teeth have cracked
the red paint irreparably.
Her plump handwriting
swims on a sheet of foolscap
capable of cutting skin.
I cut my finger
then run my tongue along
the thin and bloodless crack.
In a dish of liquid sugar,
five dead honey bees

have folded their wings
like hairy full stops.
In the corner, her lemonade
is going flat:
bubbles rise
from the side of the tumbler
to vanish on the surface.
I count them for a while
then turn to her essay.
Floral curtains,

she begins,
frame the window
where six crystal birds
stand on the window-sill.
There, the rays
of the morning sun
make them flash
with an iridescent light.
A family of china rabbits
lives on my bedside table,
under the shelter of the lamp.
Tucked in an alcove
on his bed of moss on the shelf,
my horse's skull grins at me.

Brick on brick, her paragraphs
Crumble down the page:
everything her room contains
is falling into place.
And with a tact
her father would admire,
she doesn't mention the tree
pushing up to her –
from the foundations,
through the dining-room –
spreading branches
on her ceiling,
leaning against the sill.
Her carpet peels back from the trunk.

In the undergrowth
of scribbles, *I remember,*
she has written,
the warm summer afternoon,
when we all went
into the countryside
looking for a sheep's skull
to put with my books.
My brothers have one in their room
and I was envious
for I collect things too.
Instead, I discovered
The horse's skull
Now they are the envious ones!

And still
not a word of the tree –
how it widens
the hole in her floor
year after year; how branches
twist round the legs of her desk;
how still it is,
being so excluded
from every breeze...
As the sun
fades from the runnels of the trunk,
I rise and listen to the thunder:
like the Twenty-Third Psalm
mumbled in assembly.

– Stephen Knight[15]

In Stephen Knight's poem, we find ourselves in a bedroom, whose we do not know except that it is "Her bedroom." Only gradually is it revealed that she is a child: she has sharpened her pencil to the quick and chewed on the stub as children are wont to do; her handwriting is plump; and her essay bears childlike characteristics of composition and tone. But before we get to the essay, central as it is to the poem, as announced in the poem's title, we learn that the bedroom is museum-like, small and quiet. And the words used to describe the setting are dust and rust and bruise. There are, as yet inscrutable, hints of irreparability and finality – honey bees that have given up the ghost, lemonade bubbles rising in a glass and vanishing. And yet, the bed bears the shape of its occupant, the bed-side lamp is burning, saliva is still evaporating from her pencil, and her lemonade is only now going flat. All these observations are being made by a witness who is never explicitly identified. I log, I watch, I cut, I count – not unlike chart dictation. Let's imagine this "I" to be the girl's doctor who attended her in her dying.

The doctor's attention turns from the girl's room to her essay. As he reads, he conjures what she must have been feeling toward the end. Her paragraphs do not build up brick by brick, but "crumble down the page." And yet, though the end is near, everything in her room begins to make sense from the girl's point of view. Her essay is about floral curtains, crystal birds, morning sun, and iridescent light. What she thinks of when contemplating her coveted horse head is not its death grin but the warm summer afternoon outing on which she trumped her brothers' treasured sheep's skull with her more impressive discovery. The mood of her essay is contentment. She describes the family of china rabbits sheltered by a lamp, and the horse's skull comfortably tucked away on a bed of moss in an alcove. And never a mention of the "tree," ominous and invasive, overtaking her body. While cancer was sapping her life, everything in the girl's room spoke to her of satisfaction, protection, and comfort. Her room, to her, was fascinating.

The observer who records this experience is meticulous, even reverentially attentive, allowing us to see what the girl sees and what she has written, and to "overhear" what he imagines her state of mind to have been near the end. The

observer rises in response to having witnessed something profound and hears in
the thunder the words of the Psalmist, "Yea, though I walk through the valley
of the shadow of death, I will fear no ill, for thou art with me ...." The entire
experience is imbued with a sense of wonder.

The Learner

When my mother tells me she has found her late husband's
flag in the attic, and put it up,
over the front door, for her party,
her voice on the phone is steady with the truth
of yearning, she sounds like a soldier who has known
no other life. For a moment I forget
the fierce one who raised me. We talk about her sweetheart,
how she took such perfect care of him
after his strokes. *And when the cancer came*
it was BLACK, she says, and then it was WHITE.
–What? What do you mean? –It was BLACK, it was
cancer, it was terrible,
but he did not know to be afraid, and then it
took him mercifully, it was WHITE.
– Mom, I say, breaking a cold
sweat. *Could I say something and you not*
get mad? Silence. I have never said anything
to question her. I'm shaking so the phone
is beating on my jaw. *Yes... – Mom,*
people have kind of stopped saying that, BLACK for bad,
WHITE for good. – Well, I'M not a racist,
she says, with some of the rich, almost sly
pride I have heard in myself. *Well I think*
everyone is, Mom, but that's not
the point – if someone Black heard you,
how would they feel? – But no one Black
is here! she cries, and I say *Well then think of me*
as Black. It's quiet, then I say *It's like some of the*
things the kids tell me now,
"Mom, nobody says that any
more." And my mother says, in a soft
voice, with the timing of a dream, *I'll never*
say that anymore. And then a little
anguished, *I PROMISE you that I'll never*
say it again. – Oh, Mom, I say, *don't*
promise me, who am I,
you're doing so well, you're an amazing learner
and that is when, from inside my mother,
the mother of my heart speaks to me,
the one under the coloratura,
the alto, the woman under the child – who lay
under, waiting, all my life,
to speak – her low voice, slowly
undulating, like the flag of her love,
she says, *Before, I, die, I am, learning,*
things, I never, thought, I'd know, I am so

fortunate. And then, *They are things*
I would not, have learned, if he, had lived,
but I cannot, be glad, he died, and then
the sound of quiet crying, as if
I hear, near a clearing, a spirit of mourning
bathing herself, and singing.

– Sharon Olds (1942–)[16]

Who is the learner here? The mother, certainly, but also the daughter. Here is a woman looking through her deceased husband's things, stored in the attic, and finding a flag, a keepsake perhaps from his stint in the military. She has displayed it over the front door in preparation for "her party." It could be Memorial Day or the Fourth of July. The poet encourages us also to imagine it to be the widow's first attempt to come out following her husband's death. The daughter is talking with her mother on the phone. The cadence is conversational, though intense – call and response, parry and thrust – ultimately yielding sympathetic understanding.

The mother's voice is "steady with the truth of yearning, she sounds like a soldier who has known no other life." The truth of yearning. What truth is this? The life the widow has known has been that of taking good care of her husband following his stroke, then caring for him when cancer came, and yearning for it to end, and – hesitantly, tentatively – also yearning for a life of her own beyond that of a soldier "who has known no other life." Yearning also for him. As a result of his stroke, the mother's husband was unaware that cancer was killing him, but to her it was "terrible," and to her his death was a relief.

Then the mother-daughter quarrel, tinged with anger and anguish, pride and shame, about racism and respect, but also about long suffering, language, love, and guilt. Not until the daughter catches herself and shifts from disapprobation and instruction to comfort and reassurance – "you're doing so well, you're an amazing learner" – does she hear the mother of her heart speak the truth in mature, measured tones – not now the calm truth of yearning but the conflicted truth of knowing that she could not have come into her own as long as her husband lived and needed her care, but that "I cannot, be glad, he died." At the utterance of this sad truth from deep within her and the weeping brought on by its recognition, the mother's spirit of mourning emerges, in the poet's imagination, into a place where she is bathing, not her child nor her sick husband but herself – "and singing."

"The Learner" temporarily transports us out of our own experience into the life of another in such a way that empathy is evoked. To empathize is to simultaneously feel one's way into another person's situation while holding to the awareness that the other person's experience exists independent of us. In "The Learner," the widow's experience is brought within the range of something we can imagine. It remains the widow's experience, not ours. And yet, through the poet's labor of imagination, and ours as readers, we can come to know what it's like to be in such a situation, to undergo such an experience, to suffer like that.

CONCLUSION

"Poetry makes language care," writes John Berger (1926–), "because it renders everything intimate. This intimacy is the result of the poem's labor."[17] Berger's insight has been borne out by our reading of the poems in this chapter. Thanks to the poems' labor, we have been present as the scarred girl begins the process of coming to terms with a life-changing injury. We have been within earshot of a married couple reeling from the wife's disturbing diagnosis. We have taken in the girl's fascinating room and read the essay she wrote shortly before she died. And we have overheard a tense conversation between a mother and her daughter occasioned by shame and deep grief. The experiences vicariously but intimately encountered in these poems animate our moral imagination and transport us into the lives of others in ways that enhance sympathetic understanding.

SUMMATION

This chapter explored how poetry can contribute to medical humanities. Beginning with a discussion of how poetry deals with the raw material of human experience – including experiences of illness and injury, healing and grief, love and death – it examined five poems that are particularly relevant to students of medical humanities: Alan Shapiro's "Someone Else," James Dickey's "The Scarred Girl," Robert Cooperman's "What They Don't Know," Stephen Knight's "FROM *The Fascinating Room*," and Sharon Olds's "The Learner." Then, with a focus on how poetry 'makes language care,' it considered ways in which these poems can enhance our empathic understanding. Overall, it emphasized that poetry must be entered into by an active reader who engages in "the labor of human imagination," and that this activity can help us to learn how we move from words to meaning.

EXERCISES FOR CRITICAL THINKING AND CHARACTER FORMATION

QUESTIONS FOR DISCUSSION

1. Do you like poetry? Why or why not?
2. How do you think the language of poetry might be different from an essay or a short story?
3. What do you think it means to have "moral imagination"?
4. Are you convinced by Marianne Moore's claim that poetry can be useful? Why or why not?

SUGGESTED WRITING EXERCISE

Go back through the chapter and select a poem that you find interesting. Spend a few minutes "close reading" the poem – that is, reading with an attention to the poem's style, language, and tone. Write, for about ten minutes, on *why* you find the poem interesting. Does your interest stem from what the poem is "about"? Or does it come from another place – from a specific word, image, or metaphor?

FURTHER READING

Dannie Abse, *The Yellow Bird*
Rafael Campo, *Alternative Medicine*
Alice Jones, *The Knot*
Jane Kenyon, *Otherwise: New and Selected Poems*

Sharon Olds, *The Unswept Room*
John Stone, *Music From Apartment 8: New and Selected Poems*

ADVANCED READING

Angela Belli and Jack Coulehan, eds., *Primary Care: More Poems by Physicians*
Gillie Bolton, *Reflective Practice: Writing and Professional Development*
Rafael Campo, *The Healing Arts: A Doctor's Black Bag of Poetry*

Marilyn Chandler McEntyre, *Patient Poets: Illness from Inside Out*
Robert Coles, *The Call of Stories and Teaching the Moral Imagination*
Donald Hall, *Without*

ONLINE RESOURCES

American Literature Association
http://www.calstatela.edu/academic/english/ala2/
The Institute for Poetic Medicine
http://www.poeticmedicine.com/

Modern American Poetry
http://www.english.illinois.edu/maps/

11 Doctor-Writers

I want a doctor with a sensibility.[1]

– Anatole Broyard

ABSTRACT

This chapter explores some of the many doctor-writers who have reflected on the practice of medicine and the qualities of a good doctor. Beginning with a discussion of the merged scientific and humanistic sensibilities of these writers, it examines the work of five prominent figures: William Carlos Williams, Richard Selzer, Kate Scannell, Danielle Ofri, and Pauline Chen. Then, with a focus on their pleas that we attend to the patient's illness and life world as well as to the patient's ailing body, it considers how their work helps us to think about what it means to practice purposefully.

WILLIAM CARLOS WILLIAMS

William Carlos Williams (1883–1963) is best remembered today as a revolutionary modernist who wrote poetry in the American idiom – poetry that reflected the distinctive way Americans speak the English language. He was also a prolific writer of prose – novels and essays – and a playwright. But Williams's day job was as a doctor who practiced general medicine and pediatrics for four decades and composed stories emanating from his practice experience. Williams's "doctor-stories" reveal a physician seeing patients during office hours in his home clinic and making house calls in and around Rutherford, New Jersey, especially among the often immigrant poor. The physician is genuinely interested in his patients ("fascinated" would not be too strong a word), intrigued by their lives, touched by their humanity, and struck by their authenticity. The narrator speaks in the story, "Ancient Gentility": "In those days I was about the only doctor they would have on Guinea Hill. Nowadays some of the kids I delivered then may be practicing medicine in the neighborhood. But in those days I had them all. I got to love those people, they were all right. Italian peasants from the region just south of Naples, most of them, living in small jerry-built houses – doing whatever they could find to do for a living and getting by, somehow."[2]

In this story, a neighbor asks the doctor to look in on the couple next door. An old man opens the door of the small house – one room downstairs, another above – and, speaking no English, smiles and bows his head several times "out of respect for a physician." "He was wonderful. A gentle, kindly creature, big as the house itself, almost, with long pure white hair and big white moustache. Every movement he made showed a sort of ancient gentility."[3] The man points to a ladder leading to the upstairs room, and the doctor climbs up to find the woman he had been sent to see. "Her face was dry and seamed with wrinkles, as old peasant faces will finally become, but it had the same patient smile upon it as shone from that of her old husband. White hair framing her face with silvery abundance, she didn't look at all sick to me."[4] The woman says something in Italian, which the doctor took to mean that she didn't feel so bad and didn't think she needed a doctor. After listening to her heart and palpating her abdomen, he assured her that she was fine, said goodbye, and backed down the ladder.

The old man, waiting by the door, seemed to be trying to thank the doctor for coming and apologizing for not being able to pay him. He then pulled a small silver box from his vest pocket and handed it to the doctor, who was at a loss as to what to do with it. Seeing this, the old man opened the box and took a small amount of what appeared to be brown powder between his thumb and forefinger and placed it on the other thumb. The doctor marveled, "Why snuff! Of course. I was delighted. As he whiffed the powder generously into one nostril and then the other, he handed the box back to me – in all, one of the most gracious, kindly proceedings I had ever taken part in." Desiring to show his gratitude but unaware that a pinch of snuff goes a long way, the doctor overdoes it and bursts into a sneezing frenzy. "Finally with tears in my eyes, I felt the old man standing there, smiling, an experience the like of which I shall never, in all probability, have again in my life on the mundane sphere."[5]

Beyond his deep interest in and admiration for his patients, Williams's doctor is also unsparingly honest and unforgiving of his own moral lapses and missteps that occur in the course of his daily rounds.

In "The Use of Force," there is Mathilda Olsen, a very sick little girl whose worried parents contacted the doctor after three days of home remedies had failed to bring down her fever. The mother led the doctor to the kitchen, the only warm room, where Mathilda was sitting on her father's lap. "Has she had a sore throat? Both parents answered me together. No ... No, she says her throat don't hurt her .... Have you looked? I tried to, said the mother, but I couldn't see."[6]

Concerned that the girl might have diphtheria (a number of cases had recently been diagnosed in other schoolchildren), the doctor assumed his best professional manner and proposed to take a look at her throat. Mathilda refused to open her mouth. Taking his time but persisting, he coaxed the girl to let him look. Despite his entreaties, Mathilda remained defiant. Suddenly, she took a swipe at the doctor's face, knocking his eyeglasses to the floor. Retrieving his glasses, the doctor issued an ultimatum. "Look here, I said to the child, we're going to look at your throat. You're old enough to understand what I'm saying. Will you open it now by yourself or shall we have to open it for you?"[7] Thereupon, a struggle ensued, escalating into a battle that ended with the doctor overpowering the girl and forcing a kitchen spoon into her mouth until she gagged, revealing both tonsils covered with membrane.

Thinking back remorsefully on this experience, the doctor confesses his shame at having entered the fury with the child despite getting a successful diagnosis: "the worst of it was that I too had got beyond reason .... The damned little brat must be protected against her own idiocy, one says to one's self at such times. Others must be protected against her. It is a social necessity. And all these things are true. But a blind fury, a feeling of adult shame, bred of a longing for muscular release are the operatives. One goes on to the end."[8]

By means of aesthetic appreciation and moral reflection, these two stories convey a sense of what Joanne Trautmann (1941–2007) described as Williams's "merged sensibility." "In him," she wrote, "we cannot easily discern separate medical and humanistic sensibilities."[9] In his autobiography, Williams had this to say about what might be thought of as the source of this "merger": "We catch a glimpse of something, from time to time, which shows us that a presence has just brushed past us, some rare thing .... [T]he physician, listening from day to day, catches a hint of it.... Humbly, he presents himself before it and by long practice he strives as best he can to interpret the manner of its speech. In that the secret lies. This, in the end, comes perhaps to be the occupation of the physician after a lifetime of careful listening."[10]

This is the doctor who wrote about overpowering a little girl and forcing a kitchen spoon into her mouth in order to confirm that she had tonsillitis. Does anything in this portrait of William Carlos Williams indicate that he was capable of "a blind fury," as he put it? Does the picture display his ability to merge medical and humanistic sensibilities in the stories that he published about his patients? Is there any indication that the subject is both a writer and a physician?

The goal of the portrait artist, in painting or photography, is to reveal something of the character of his or her subject. In the frame, the artist may position the whole figure from head to toe, half the figure (as in this portrait of Williams), or perhaps only the subject's face. In the space that remains, the artist often includes objects that relate to the subject in some way.

How did Williams's photographer allocate space within the frame? Williams himself occupies the entire left half of the image. Why do you think the photographer positioned his camera so that shelves of books frame Williams's head? How did the artist use the rest of the space, and to what purpose?

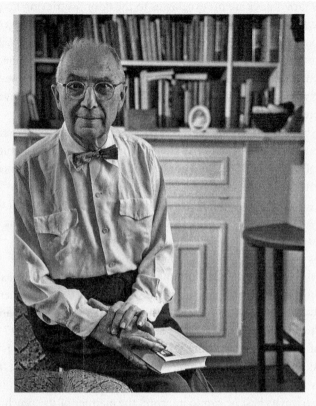

Figure 11. *American Poet* (William Carlos Williams), 1955, Hulton Archive/Getty Images.

Williams presented himself to be photographed in a shirt with two pockets, buttoned, a bow tie, and eyeglasses with large, light-colored frames. What does each of these choices contribute to your overall impression of him as a physician and an artist? Would you want to meet Williams? How might you start a conversation with him?

Portraits of physicians, nurses, and other health care specialists are often displayed in the public spaces, corridors, and meeting rooms of medical schools, hospitals, and clinics. When you encounter them, even in passing, examine your first impression. What is the setting? How is the person dressed, and what might a suit or a lab coat signify? Does the person appear distant or accessible?

RICHARD SELZER

Richard Selzer's (1928–) stories are peopled with the ill and injured, damaged survivors of close calls, and casualties of the surgical theater. But for all their suffering, these patients are not pitiable. They are estimable. What is endlessly fascinating to this doctor-writer is a sacredness that pervades and envelopes the space of suffering that they occupy. For Selzer, surgery is a sacred art, redolent with ritual. Surgery is sacred not in a sectarian, but rather a spiritual sense. Acknowledging "a strong note of spirituality" in his work, Selzer remarks, "This is only natural for a writer who sees flesh as the spirit thickened."[11]

Selzer's *surgeon* is expertly knowledgeable and highly accomplished technically. Beyond these necessary attributes of competence, his work is informed and enlivened by a certain sensibility, a refined responsiveness to pathos. This surgeon has attended many a patient over the years. There was Joe Riker, the short-order cook with a cancer that had eaten a hole through scalp and skull, who refused surgery and healed himself with holy water from Lourdes. And Pete, the hospital mailman with acute abdominal pain: "Narcotized, he nods and takes my fingers in his own, pressing. Thus has he given me all of his trust .... 'Go to sleep, Pete,' I say into his ear, my lips so close it is almost a kiss" – the trust received.[12]

Another of Selzer's characters is a young man, back from an excavation of ancient Guatemalan ruins who presented with an abscessed wound in his upper arm out of which emerged a menacing-looking gray worm with black pincers. With deftness (and even greater self-satisfaction), the surgeon stood poised, hemostat at the ready, and extracted the offender, only to learn from the pathologist that the organism was the larva of a botfly that was burrowing its way out, whereupon it would have dropped to the ground and died without the dramatic intervention of the surgeon. These patients have taught the surgeon humility in the face of the inexplicable, the necessity of fellow feeling and the boon of comfort, and modesty.

Selzer, the *writer*, is a parablist. A parable is a story with meaning beyond the literal. This second meaning is not buried beneath the words of the story to be excavated and analyzed, but is there in plain view although only obliquely discernible – perceptible at a slant.

Selzer's story, "A Parable," opens with a doctor discreetly witnessing an early morning scene in a hospital room where a man lies, inert and near death, breathing erratically in rapid bursts followed by the suspension of breathing, then more rapid bursts. "It is called Cheyne-Stokes respiration. When they start that, you know it won't be long."[13] An elderly physician in surgical scrubs, stooped and seemingly somewhat worn down, enters the room. With a moistened tissue, he wipes pus from around the man's eyes and says something to him that the witness cannot hear. The patient then twice tries to speak but cannot. "When the doctor turns his head to bend an ear to the lips of his patient, I can see the deep furrow that divides his brow, extending from the bridge of the nose almost to the hairline. It gives his face a pained expression. It is a line of pain. Had he been born with it? No, I think he had not. Rather, it had appeared on the day that he treated his first patient. At first, it was merely a shadow on his forehead, then a slight indentation that, over the years, has deepened into this dark cleft that is the mark of all the suffering he has witnessed over a lifetime as a doctor. It resembles a wound that might have been made with an ax."[14]

As he palpates the patient's abdomen, the doctor asks, ""Am I hurting you?" whereupon the patient shakes his head and, astonishingly, stretches a trembling hand toward the doctor's head. "The sick man finds the furrow with his finger, touches, then strokes it from one end to the other, a look of wonder upon his face, as though he were just waking from a deep sleep. As he does so, a spicule of light appears to emanate from the doctor's forehead. It is a warm light that grows to engulf the two men and the bed. From this touching, the doctor does not withdraw, but smiles down at the patient with his sapphiric gaze .... From the doorway, the two men appear to be luminous .... It is as if I were witnessing a feast .... The two men are dining together, each the nourishment of the other."[15]

The doctor returns the following morning to find the man lying perfectly still. After unsuccessfully trying to find a pulse, he observes the man's body before placing a hand over his heart and closing his eyes. "As he leaves the room, it seems the furrow is not quite so deep and dark as on the day before."[16]

W. H. Auden (1907–1973) said, "You cannot tell people what to do, you can only tell them parables; and that is what art really is, particular stories of particular people and experiences, from which each according to his immediate and peculiar needs may draw his own conclusions."[17] Parables are narratives that disclose moral quandaries and illuminate spiritual relations. Instead of leading listener or reader toward a robust conclusion, as was perhaps possible at times when matters of the spirit were less unsettled than they are today, modern parables often simply raise a question for pondering or persuade by intimation and indirection. What all parables, ancient and modern, have in common is an impatience with the obvious and a search for significance that come together in moments of insight. Parables have an arresting quality that etches them in memory. Because they engage imagination, they penetrate deeply into experience. They possess the power to do more than provoke curiosity. They arouse something within by calling up what the hearer, or the reader, vaguely senses but now can fully see.

In his essay, "Religion, Poetry, and the 'Dilemma' of the Modern Writer," David Daiches (1912–2005) observed that literary and religious answers to questions about suffering tend to be responses rather than solutions. "The answers have force and meaning in virtue of their poetic expression, of the place they take in the myth or fable or situation presented, and of the effectiveness with which they project a mood."[18] The projection of a mood does not solve anything, but, if it is persuasive, it may make life more tolerable, more interesting, even. Moreover, if life is made more tolerable by the telling of stories and the artful use of imagery, patients and doctors alike may thereby be enabled to return to the daily round in the face of experiences that would otherwise threaten to become unbearable.

KATE SCANNELL

In her memoir, *Death of the Good Doctor: Lessons from the Heart of the AIDS Epidemic*, Kate Scannell recalls the challenges she faced and the rewards she reaped while caring for patients dying from AIDS at the height of the epidemic in the 1980s. Soon after completing a three-year fellowship, Scannell assumed responsibility for a newly established AIDS ward in a large county hospital and was quickly overwhelmed by the depth of suffering and the ubiquity of death she encountered there. These patients were suffering with occult fevers, exotic infections, disfiguring cancers, and they were dying miserably. Scannell had been trained to aggressively attack AIDS with the most up-to-date knowledge medicine had to offer. And fight she did. "I stalked the AIDS ward like a weary but seasoned gunfighter, ready for medical challenges to present themselves. I would shoot them down with my skills and pills." Maintaining this sharpshooter mentality came to seem increasingly futile in the face of such mass agony. More fundamentally, Scannell had to admit to herself that she was even "incapable of understanding and articulating my own experiences."[19]

Then one day, Manuel, a twenty-two-year-old man with advanced Kaposi's sarcoma was admitted to the ward. "He arrived as a huge, bloated, violaceous, knobby mass with eyelids so swollen that he could no longer see. His dense purple tumors had infiltrated multiple lymph nodes throughout his body, and two had perforated the roof of his mouth. One imposing mass extended from the bottom of his foot so that he could no longer walk. Massive amounts of fluids surrounded and compressed his lungs, making his breathing laborious. Tears literally squeezed through the slits between his puffy eyelids. One of the first things Manuel said to me was, 'Doctor, please help me.'" Scannell sprang into action, bringing her finely honed diagnostic skills and every appropriate assessment measure and treatment modality to bear on Manuel's case – laboratory tests, supplemental oxygen, intravenous fluids with potassium, blood transfusion, and so on. Checking on Manuel before leaving that first evening to satisfy herself that she had left no stone unturned, Manuel said again, "Doctor, please help me," and Scannell, though shaken by his suffering, assured him that his medical problems were being evaluated and treated and that she would discuss next steps with him once he was stabilized.

Upon her arrival on the ward the following morning, Scannell learned from a night nurse that Manuel had died. He had asked the evening duty doctor to help him and the physician, after familiarizing himself with the case, responded by withdrawing futile treatments that would only prolong dying and administering additional morphine for comfort. "The nurse said that Manuel smiled and thanked the doctor for helping him." Scannell writes, "My entire body cringed and my soul clenched as I imagined Manuel's agony sustained through my unconscious denial of his dying . . . . Years later I continue to think of Manuel often, and I ask him to forgive me. I tell him that I have never practiced medicine in the same way since his death .... I began learning – how to recognize the sound of my own voice, listen to my patients, validate the insistent stirrings of my compassionate sensibilities."[20] And, as these lessons from the heart of the AIDS epidemic convey, Scannell was also learning how to cultivate a humane professional self-understanding.

DANIELLE OFRI

In *Incidental Findings: Lessons from My Patients in the Art of Medicine*, internist Danielle Ofri recalls and recounts from her early years in practice a shameful encounter with patient Nazma Uddin and her eleven-year-old daughter, Azina. Mrs. Uddin is what doctors sometimes call a "difficult patient." At this appointment, as on previous visits, with Azina translating from Bengali, Mrs. Uddin complained of "abdominal pain and headache, diarrhea and insomnia, back pain and aching arches, a rash and gas pains, itchy ears and a cough, no appetite. And more headaches."[21] While listening to the litany of complaints, Ofri saw on the computer screen that in the five weeks since her last visit, the patient had been to several specialty clinics, to no avail.

Ofri recalls her own mounting frustration with Mrs. Uddin, to the point where she desperately wanted the woman out of her clinic office. She had talked to the patient about stress and depression and their somatic symptoms, but Mrs. Uddin refused to take antidepressant medications and did not follow through with psychiatry referrals. Getting nowhere, "I start to resent her, to hate her, to hate everything about her .... I hate that she routinely keeps her daughter out of school to facilitate her wild overuse of the medical system. And I hate how she makes me feel so utterly useless."[22]

Now no longer able to mask her anger, she instructed Azina to tell her mother in no uncertain terms that she was healthy, that most of her symptoms were related to depression, and that she needed to see a psychiatrist. Azina dutifully translated the doctor's orders, then asked, "Are you almost finished?" Ofri, still seething, nearly failed to notice that Azina, for the first time ever, was speaking directly to her. The child explained that she had to take her mother home on the bus, then catch another bus to school, and she was afraid that if they didn't leave soon she'd miss a whole day of school. Ofri wondered aloud why Mrs. Uddin didn't come to the clinic by herself – "We do have interpreters available." Azina: "My mother is afraid to go out by herself .... My brother is in college, and my father works ...." Realizing that she had, until this moment, paid no heed to Azina in her own right, Ofri turned to her and quietly asked, "What is it like at home?" As tears began to flow, Azina mumbled, "She doesn't *do* anything .... She just sits there .... She doesn't say anything to us. She doesn't cook dinner anymore. She doesn't go anywhere." Hearing Azina's anguished confession, Ofri saw in her mind's eye "a little girl cut off from her mother, reeling in the wretched vacuum that depression creates – a child conscripted to be the fulcrum of cultures, illnesses, and torments, all the while trying to complete the fifth grade."[23]

As Ofri's perspective shifted from herself and her frustrating inability to make any headway with this patient, she understood: "Mrs. Uddin ... is truly suffering. Her daughter is truly suffering." Moreover (here is the insight that prompts the reawakening of compassion), "*I* am not suffering. *I* am actually the complainer."[24] Chagrined and humbled, Ofri took the hands of both Azina and her mother, "for they are both my patients now," and acknowledged that "Depression is a painful illness .... Broken souls hurt as much as broken bones, and the pain spreads to everyone around them." And she patiently explained, once again, why it is important to take antidepressants and see a psychiatrist. Mrs. Uddin agreed to do so. Ofri admitted to herself that she wouldn't be surprised if it didn't happen. "But I think, or at least hope, that I will no longer view Nazma Uddin as a personal torment. Azina has cured me of that."[25]

Among the aspirations of those who choose a career in medicine is the desire to care for the ill and injured. Because medicine in our society is generally thought of in heroic terms, it should come as no surprise that for medical students and trainees the prevailing image of what it means to care for the sick should be that of curing disease, saving lives, rescuing patients. It is a noble sentiment but one that is out of sync with the typical trajectory of illness in modern societies where *chronic* illness is the norm.

CASE STUDY: DANIELLE OFRI'S *INCIDENTAL FINDINGS*

In the following passage, Danielle Ofri recounts her thoughts upon leaving the hospital with her husband after giving birth to her first child. The trip to the hospital has already been more confusing than Ofri, a doctor herself, could have imagined, and, on top of that, she has been informed that her child is missing an artery. She has been told that this is "a normal anatomical variant," an "incidental finding"; but as she reflects on her experience, she finds herself thinking differently.

"We walk out into the sunlight, stepping gingerly since I'm a little sore. But I'm more shaken than sore. I reflect back on how discombobulated I'd become from the simple act of getting lost this morning. How many patients do I send for procedures, many of whom have little education or command of English? How many have wandered the hallways, holding up their referral forms to strangers, hoping someone will have the knowledge and the patience to help them out? How many of my patients give up in frustration and simply go home? I'd never thought about how hard it could be just to *get* there.

And how do we convey mildly bad news? We obviously try to be careful about the big bad news – cancer, HIV, Alzheimer's disease – with sensitive, empathic discussions. But what about the incidental findings – the bit of gastritis seen during an endoscopy, the benign calcification noted on a mammogram, the simple ovarian cyst picked up on a sonogram. For us in the medical profession, these are small potatoes, hardly worth much thought given the more serious issues we must face with our sicker patients. But as I learned today, there is no such thing as incidental to a patient. Nothing is incidental. The location of the room is not incidental. The "normal anatomical variant" is not incidental. The "little pinch and a tiny bit of pressure" is not incidental. The frigid room and skimpy gowns are not incidental. I want to announce it to the receptionists and the radiologist and the obstetrician and the gray-brained designers of this infernal building. "I am not incidental!" – I want to enunciate every syllable. I want it to echo down the sterile carpeted corridors.

I am *not* incidental.

But I am now wiser."[26]

1. What does Ofri mean when she says that "there is no such thing as incidental to a patient"? Come up with a list of things that might seem "incidental" to a patient, but that, on closer inspection, turn out to be quite significant.
2. How does Ofri's own experience as a patient make her wiser? Have you had any experiences as a patient or caregiver that have made you wiser?
3. Anatole Broyard has said that he wants a doctor with "sensibility." What sort of "sensibility" does Ofri seem to have? What sort of "sensibility" do you want your doctor to have?

PAULINE CHEN

Looking back from mid-career at her initiation into the medical profession, transplant surgeon Pauline Chen writes, "From the moment I had begun to contemplate this career path some fifteen years earlier, I knew that I would want to use my profession to help people. Most of my classmates were no different ... we were for the most part determined to learn how to save lives. What many of us did not realize was that despite those dreams, our profession would require us to live among the dying. Death, more than life, would become the constant in our lives."[27] Setting out from this insight, Chen begins to reflect on her experience with this "constant" and on the ways she learned to deal with it.

Beginning one's formal medical education with the dissection of a human cadaver has long been recognized as an emotionally fraught experience. Chen remembers it as the "first lesson in disengaging from the personal ... suppressing the fundamental and very human fear of death."[28] For her, this first phase of disengagement was facilitated by her fascination with all there was to learn about the intricacies of the human body, and by the rigors of memorizing anatomic principles and Latin terms, and practicing proper dissection technique. The process of disengagement accelerates during third-year clerkships as students are inducted into the culture of clinical medicine with its distinctive attitudes and behaviors, including attitudes about death and behaviors in encounters with dying patients and their families.

Experiences with patients dying or lingering near death commonly elicit the seemingly paradoxical clinical response of arm's-length solicitude, for which sociologist Renée Fox coined the term "detached concern."[29] Try as she might to adopt such a posture, Chen found it impossible to treat death as only a clinical event. "In my mind, dying had as much to do with fate as with biology .... That great passing of life was too sacred; it was nearly magical. Death was an immutable moment in time, locked up as much in our particular destiny as in the time and date of our birth."[30]

Throughout her years of clinical education, from medical school through residency and fellowship training, Chen assiduously strove to become an ever-more superbly skilled surgeon. But beyond that, without guidance or support, she felt unschooled in how to care for patients near the end of their lives. What she had were her own experiences – some painful, others instructive – and it was to these experiences and the perceptions and insights they evoked that she began to pay close attention.

Max was only a few months old when Chen met him during her transplantation and liver surgery fellowship. Max had developed a life-threatening condition in utero that left his intestines twisted and starved of blood supply. Immediately following his delivery by cesarean section, pediatric surgeons operated, removing most of his bowel. Of necessity, Max was fed intravenously, which led to numerous complications, including liver failure. At ten months of age, Max received a liver and small bowel transplant. Two months later, he was back in the pediatric intensive care unit teetering between life-threatening infections and organ rejection.

With the attending surgeon, who was relentlessly dedicated to sustaining the transplant and saving Max, Chen became deeply involved in the team's all-out effort to rescue the child. A month later, after almost a dozen additional surgeries, Max died of a raging fungal infection. Having experienced firsthand the damage can be done by heroic efforts and fear of failure, Chen adopts a tempered view of a single-minded commitment to cure.

There comes a point in complex cases such as Max's when additional interventions may cause more harm than good ... or only prolong dying. Discerning when that point has been reached is difficult but is nonetheless a key component in sophisticated clinical judgment. It involves a forthright, humane conversation with patients and, where appropriate, with loved ones, about when enough is enough. When is the flame no longer worth the candle, the suffering to be endured too burdensome to bear? Certainly, addressing this question requires medical expertise. But it is fundamentally an existential question, one that draws on fundamental beliefs about life and death, and meaning and suffering, and that therefore can appropriately be answered only by those who will live with, or bear up under, or die from, whatever decision is made.

By the time Chen met Alfred, a sixty-five-year-old businessman who had been diagnosed with bile duct cancer who wanted a second opinion about the feasibility of a curative operation, his tumor had spread beyond his liver and was inoperable. During his brief hospital stay, Alfred told Chen about a dream he had had in which he was being enclosed in a brick-like box from which he could not escape. "I'm going to try chemotherapy," he told Chen. "When the time comes, I want to be at home and be comfortable and with my family .... but right now, I don't want to be passive in my box."[31]

Following six months of chemotherapy at a different hospital, Alfred's wife, Judy, brought her husband back to Chen. Alfred's condition had worsened dramatically. He was confused. His face was wasted, his belly bloated with fluid, and his jaundice unresolved. "Looking at Alfred, I knew that we could transfer him into the intensive care unit; put tubes into his mouth, nose, bladder, and rectum; hook him up to a ventilator; and probably cure his confusion. But he was dying and any remedy would be temporary."[32] Alfred appeared moribund, occasionally rousing to make nonsensical mumbling sounds before dropping off again. With Judy at her side, Chen knelt at Alfred's bedside, "so that my face was close to his," and said, "Mr. Lipstein ... we can either take you to the intensive care unit or we can let you go home. I'm not sure how much longer we have, but I want to know what you want." Not expecting Alfred to respond, Chen was startled when he opened his eyes, looked straight at her and said in a deep, lucid voice, "Dr. Chen ... Let me go home," and lapsed back into semi-consciousness.[32]

Chen contacted hospice and arranged for Alfred to be taken to his home where he died one week later. She learned of his death in a phone call from Alfred's brother-in-law. Chen recalls feeling the wave of helplessness rising in her chest that she always experienced upon hearing of the death of one of her patients. "I wondered silently why I still could not save my patient despite all the knowledge and training and technology. I began to speak, saying what I always did with grieving loved ones. I wish I could have cured him. I wish I could have done more." But then she heard Alfred's brother-in-law thanking her for helping Alfred die at home surrounded by his family. "'You know, Dr. Chen,' he said, 'it was just as he had wished.' It was then I realized that I *had* done more. I had comforted my patient and his family. I had eased their suffering. I had been present for them during life and despite death. I had caught a glimpse of the doctor I could become."[33]

In listening for patients' yearnings beyond their chief complaints, Kate Scannell came to an appreciation of the deeper meaning of "help me, doctor." With the dawning of the insight that, no matter how occasionally frustrating a doctor-patient encounter might be, the patient is the one in need, Danielle Ofri learned humility. And in realizing that "doing more" need not always mean more medical interventions, Pauline Chen discovered the power of comfort and care.

CONCLUSION

In "The Patient Examines the Doctor," an essay composed in the months between his prostate cancer diagnosis and his death, literary critic Anatole Broyard (1920–1990) made this intriguing claim: "I want a doctor with a sensibility. And that seems almost like an oxymoron, a contradiction in terms. A doctor is a man of science." But Broyard was disinclined to accept as necessary the supposed contradiction inherent in using "sensibility" and "science" in the same breath. He goes on to say, "Imagine having Chekhov, who was a doctor, for your doctor. Imagine having William Carlos Williams, who was a poet, or Walker Percy, who's a novelist, for your doctor. Imagine having Rabelais, who was a doctor, as your physician."[34]

These doctor-writers were men of science *and* sensibility. Today, in English and American parlance, we tend to associate the term "sensibility" solely with aesthetics. But it was not always so. Predating what T. S. Eliot (1888–1965) dubbed a dissociation of sensibility, a supposed disjunction between reason and emotion, sensibility signified a *general* perceptiveness and responsiveness irreducible to either thought or feeling but combining them in a single way of being. It is this way of being, now transposed into the realm of doctoring, to which the physicians whose work we have sampled seem to be aspiring – attentiveness to the patient's illness experience and life world as well as the patient's ailing body.

Underlying the soul-searching evident in the writings of these physicians is a desire to rethink what it takes to practice purposefully. Dissatisfied with a description of doctoring limited to the acquisition of specialized scientific knowledge and technical expertise, they seek a more capacious conception of their craft.[35] In caring for their patients, and then reflecting upon and writing about their experience, they have discovered that humanistic medical practice requires both a feeling intellect and personal engagement – in a word, a sensibility.

SUMMATION

This chapter explored some of the many doctor-writers who have reflected on the practice of medicine and the qualities of a good doctor. Beginning with a discussion of the merged scientific and humanistic sensibilities of these writers, it examined the work of five prominent figures: William Carlos Williams, Richard Selzer, Kate Scannell, Danielle Ofri, and Pauline Chen. Then, with a focus on their plea that we attend to the patient's illness experience and life world as well as to the patient's ailing body, it considered how their work helps us to think about what it means to practice purposefully. Overall, this chapter has emphasized that a greater attention to the work of doctor-writers helps us not because it provides solutions to difficult problems but because it illuminates those problems in vivid and unique ways.

EXERCISES FOR CRITICAL THINKING AND CHARACTER FORMATION

QUESTIONS FOR DISCUSSION

1. Think about your favorite doctor. What combination of his or her attributes makes you feel most taken care of?
2. Anatole Broyard declared that he wants a doctor with a "sensibility." What is distinctive, in your opinion, about doctors who practice with both science *and* "sensibility"?
3. Why do you think that these doctors wrote about their experiences? What value might the act of writing have had for these doctors?
4. What recurring themes do you notice among the doctor-writers in this chapter?

SUGGESTED WRITING EXERCISE

Write a short essay on what Richard Selzer considers sacred about the doctor's vocation.

FURTHER READING

Anton Chekhov, *Ward Number 6 and Other Stories*
Oliver Sacks, *The Man Who Mistook His Wife for a Hat: And Other Clinical Tales*
Richard Selzer, *The Doctor Stories* and *Letters to A Young Doctor*

Abraham Verghese, *My Own Country: A Doctor's Story of a Town and its People in the Age of AIDS*
William Carlos Williams, *The Doctor Stories*

ADVANCED READING

Rafael Campo, *The Poetry of Healing: A Doctor's Education in Empathy, Identity, and Desire*
Carol Donley and Martin Kohn, eds., *Recognitions: Doctors and Their Stories*
Michael La Combe, ed., *On Being a Doctor 2: Voices of Physicians and Patients*

Danielle Ofri, *Incidental Findings: Lessons from My Patients in the Art of Medicine*
John Stone, *In the Country of Hearts: Journeys in the Art of Medicine*

JOURNALS

Literature and Medicine

ORGANIZATIONS AND GROUPS

William Carlos Williams Society Online
http://wcwsociety.wordpress.com/

12 Studying Medicine

As medicine becomes increasingly sophisticated, its technical sides and human sides seem to be growing ever farther apart.[1]

– Ellen Fox

ABSTRACT

This chapter provides an "insider's view" of medical education since the 1960s. Relying on the voices and writings of students and reformers, it examines student protests against injustice and against a dehumanizing education as well as a growing skepticism about an emphasis on biomedical science and technology as adequate preparation for clinical practice. Then, with a focus on the recent rise in humanities courses and full-fledged medical humanities programs in many medical schools, it considers how medical education is adapting to meet the challenges of the twenty-first century.

INTRODUCTION

Chapter 3 provided a historical sketch of the contours of medical education from antiquity through the twentieth century. Chapter 12 provides an "insider's view" of how studying medicine has been experienced by students and trainees and viewed by reform minded educators in an era dominated by a bioscience and technology ethos.

In the decades following the publication of the Flexner Report in 1910,[2] medical educators aspired to make medicine scientifically sound, and virtually all medical curricula conformed to the Flexner model – two years of basic science study followed by two years of clinical training – which remained dominant for decades, and whose fundamental framework was not seriously challenged for a century.

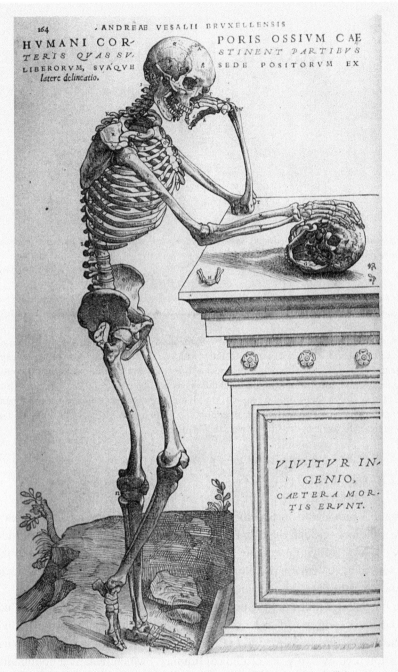

Figure 12. Full-length side view of a skeleton contemplating a skull (Skeleton with Skull) from '*De Humani Corporis Fabrica*', page 164 (Liber I), 1534, Courtesy National Library of Medicine.

If this were a person rather than a skeleton, with one hand resting on a human skull, what might he or she be thinking? What if the image depicted a health care professional resting his or her hand on the head of a patient? Rest your cheek on one hand, as the skeleton does. If you then lay your other hand on any object within reach, what do you feel?

If you replaced the skull with a plant or a rock, how would the skeleton's relationship with the object in hand be different? Because the skull is part of the skeleton, the image could be seen as a visual representation of the Greek aphorism "Know thyself."

Vesalius was concerned with improving the education of physicians, as was Abraham Flexner, whose modern reforms are summarized in this chapter. By including this image, how might Vesalius have been suggesting that knowledge of medicine involves more than the study of anatomy?

BIOSCIENCE EDUCATION AND ITS LIMITS

By the 1950s, social scientists had begun to document some unintended consequences of a single-minded focus on bioscience education. Their studies revealed evidence of feelings of anxiety among many medical students who agonized about what medical education was doing to their capacity for fellow feeling, and who often coped by adopting cynical attitudes about their medical school experience.[3] Moreover, the bioscience ethos of the post-Flexner years, when coupled with a technological imperative that equated every technical advance with progress, came at the expense of cultural learning about the human condition, existential experiences of illness and injury, and the social contexts of sickness.[4]

In the 1960s, students across the country were restive and rebellious. Medical students were no exception. Many of them found the medical school regimen inattentive to and complicit in the injustices of the health care delivery system in which care was considered a commodity rather than a right. They were offended by the unspoken messages conveyed in the informal, or "hidden curriculum," which condoned attitudes and behaviors of disregard, disdain, and callousness toward patients made doubly vulnerable by sickness and poverty. These concerns persist to this day.[5]

The sense of moral unease resulting from such experiences is captured in a poem penned by a medical student in Philadelphia at the time.

On Being Poor
Being poor is watching all the residents practice passing a laryngoscope down your dead baby's throat.
Being poor is being told in front of 115 people that you are a "veritable museum of pathology."
Being poor is coming to the emergency room at 10:30 a.m. with severe pain and not being seen until 1:30 p.m. in the clinic.
Being poor is having four young men put their fingers in your vagina and only one of them has his name end in M.D.
Being poor is having a med student stick your arm seven times unsuccessfully while a staff physician stands by and watches.

Being poor is being called "stupid" because you do not have the sense to feed your five kids
more protein when you get only $3,100 a year.
Being poor is being afraid to go to the hospital because you do not want to die.

– L. Kron[6]

Reflecting on a lacuna in his medical education, activist physician H. Jack
Geiger (1925–) recounted an incident that occurred in 1965 in Alabama where
he was working at a first-aid station during the civil rights confrontations in
Selma. An eleven-year-old girl was brought to the station with a hot, swollen,
and painful knee after having been caught up in a white mob attack on black
protesters. "Training and routine carried me through the process of history and
examination, treatment, and bandaging," Geiger recalled, "but as I worked I
was seized with the most intense feeling that these technical skills were deeply
irrelevant to the real damage .... There was little in my professional medical
training, or within the usual *professional* behaviors, that pointed the way toward
being human in this situation, that is, toward giving full recognition to the girl's
humanity .... Both the girl and her knee needed care. My training to deal with
the knee was excellent; my training to deal with the interpersonal dynamics was
fair. But my preparation for understanding the social, racial, and political context – which were not context but the very core of the pathology afflicting this
girl – had to come entirely from sources outside my professional training."[7]

In the preface to the 2006 edition of his 1976 memoir of medical education,
White Coat, Clenched Fist: The Political Education of an American Physician,
pediatrician Fitzhugh Mullan (1942–) recalls how the world of medicine looked
when he went to medical school in the sixties. "One in ten students in my medical school class was a woman. One in seventy-two was black – and he came
from Nigeria. The main functions of the Student American Medical Association
(SAMA) on campus was social, and the American Medical Association was
engaged in a last ditch effort to prevent the enactment of Medicare to provide
health insurance for the nation's elderly. A student did not have to arrive in medicine as a radical to be troubled by the moral posture of the profession in the
1960s."[8]

Mullan's experience was emblematic of that of a cadre of likeminded and similarly conscientious students in this era who committed themselves to reform –
who insisted that human values are a critical part of doctors' ability to care for
patients, and that physicians have a responsibility to make the health care system
fairer and to contribute generally to the betterment of society. A 1974 survey
of physicians who had been student activists in medical schools in the 1960s
revealed that, to a great extent, these former students continued to pursue their
idealistic goals in their later practice.[9]

The 1970s marked the advent of more widespread concern about the shape
and direction of medical education. A growing number of medical educators
became critical of an education system that was evidently better at training

"disease technicians" than educating "thinking doctors."[10] By the 1980s a veritable chorus of voices, within medicine and without, was expressing skepticism about the sufficiency of a continuing emphasis on bioscience and technology alone as adequate preparation for the practice of humanistic medicine, and calling for the integration of cultural learning into premedical and medical education and for explicit attention to moral conduct in residency programs.[11]

Residency training came under special scrutiny in the early 1980s on the heels of the publication of *The House of God*, a satirical novel by Samuel Shem (1944–) based on his experience as an intern at a Harvard Medical School hospital. The novel exposed the inhumane conditions of residency training programs and the bad medical behaviors they engendered. It soon achieved the status of a cult classic among medical students and residents, a status it continues to enjoy.[12]

Jack Coulehan (1943–) and Peter C. Williams (1946–) observe that medical students and young physicians struggle with the challenge of reconciling medicine's espousal of the importance of such virtues as empathy and compassion with its tacit commitment to an ethic of objectivity and detachment. They note that some students deal with this challenge by limiting their professional identity to the notion of technical competence. Others develop a broader conception encompassing a commitment to humane values and to habits of moral introspection and reflection, which they strive to appropriate and internalize in their attitudes and actions. It is this latter form of professional self-understanding that the humanities aim to conceptualize and cultivate.[13]

THE HUMANITIES AND EXPERIENTIAL LEARNING

From the time that the first department of humanities in an American medical school was established (at the Pennsylvania State University School of Medicine at Hershey in 1969), humanistic studies began to be programmatically introduced at selected medical schools around the country. In addition, many individual faculty positions were created in medical schools that lacked full-fledged humanities or ethics programs, so that by the early 1980s the humanities had, in the words of Edmund D. Pellegrino (1920–2013), one of the principal leaders of this movement, "established a beachhead in an unpromising place, the medical school curriculum."[14]

Related reforms and curricular innovations in recent decades have included the development of special programs aimed at encouraging active, small-group problem-based learning,[15] improving cultural competence,[16] encouraging moral growth and promoting professional behaviors,[17] and attending more carefully to what Renée C. Fox (1928–) aptly called "the human condition of health professionals."[18] Many of these initiatives evolved in response to perceived omissions and deficiencies: a lecture-based curriculum glutted with ever-expanding quantities of scientific information, substandard competence in relating to and communicating with patients and colleagues, and unprofessional attitudes and behavior.

Interpersonal skills can be taught and learned, and attitudes may be changed by raising awareness, but human values – personal values, moral values – take shape slowly, over time, in response to one's life experiences. As noted earlier in this chapter, in medical school such indirect learning experiences are a part of the hidden or informal curriculum wherein both good behavior and bad are on display,[19] examples of which are typified in the following vignettes.

Medical school graduate Melanie M. Watkins recalls an experience she had as an applicant visiting a medical school for an interview in the late 1990s. One of the doctors giving a hospital tour remarked, "I really miss the days of deliveries when a happy husband and wife looked forward to seeing their baby. Now all we have are single women on Medicaid with four and five children." Watkins, a single black mother, remembers thinking, "Doesn't he know that single women may need even more support? Does he think that none of them look forward to having their baby? Does he think that because they cannot afford a camcorder to record the birth that it is any less important?"[20]

No sooner had Karen C. Kim been admitted to medical school than she began to entertain doubts about her decision because it seemed to her "that many of the concerns that originally led me to medicine are simply not valued by the medical establishment." She was made to feel out of line when she drew attention to the paucity of class time devoted to such issues as gun violence, poverty, and racial disparities in health care, and the ethics of the pharmaceutical industry. "With thirty hours a week of class time spent sitting in a lecture hall looking at PowerPoint slides, who has the time? [W]ho wants to spend extra time and energy caring about stuff we aren't tested on?"[21]

From the vantage of her residency, Tista Ghosh remembers being anxious and agitated on the first day of her surgery rotation with "Dr. Snead," whose reputation for gruffness and volatile temper had preceded him. When he appeared that day, Dr. Snead sized up the students from head to toe, barked an order at each of the three male students on the rotation, then turned to Ghosh. "'What's the matter, honey? You nervous?' A sarcastic smile on his lips. 'The rest of you, follow your resident to the wards. But you, sweetheart, you're coming with me. We're going to the OR.'" Snead's misogyny knew no bounds. His browbeating was relentless, and his patronizing remarks were humiliating and demeaning. When it was Ghosh's turn to answer a question, Snead would often pass over her and ask one of the male students because the question "might be too hard for you, sweetheart." Looking back on her third year, Ghosh found that she "had become hardened and jaded by the so-called learning experience of clinical rotations. Did fear, discomfort, and intimidation really enhance a student's educational environment? Apparently they're supposed to, I often thought cynically."[22]

David Hellerstein recalls an experience from his third year in medical school that left him feeling embarrassed, disturbed, and disappointed. A young woman had come to the gynecology clinic complaining of chronic pelvic pain. After listening to the information the student had gathered during the patient interview, Hellerstein's teacher Dr. Snarr (not his real name) dismissed it as nonsense and said, "She couldn't possibly be feeling that kind of pain." The novice and the senior physician then entered the examining room to do a pelvic exam. Though a novice, Hellerstein considered himself reasonably good technically, having spent the past month working on his ob-gyn rotation. When he began the manual exam, the patient screamed and slid up on the table. Hellerstein desisted and, sweating now, promised to try again, more gently. This time the patient didn't scream, only breathed deeply, but the student was unable to feel anything. When Dr. Snarr took over, the woman screamed and writhed. Snarr withdrew and said, "All right, hon …. Wipe yourself off; we'll come back and see you in a minute." Once outside, Snarr told Hellerstein, "I don't know why the heck she hurts …. Give her some estrogen cream." As the two debriefed before seeing the next patient, Hellerstein, when asked what he thought the woman's problem was, mentioned a couple of possibilities but stopped short of saying what he really thought, that his would-be teacher was insensitive and obtuse, "that he has no sense of what he put her through …. I'm disappointed, too, but I'm not sure why. Perhaps it's that I wished he was a better doctor, a better role model …. [What] I needed to know was how to be with patients, how to deal with the feelings they evoked, how to make them feel at ease."[23]

Physician-poet John Stone (1936–) recalls an experience of a different sort from his student clinical rotation with the chairman of the department of internal medicine. "One young woman, about my age and terribly ill with cystic fibrosis, a respiratory ailment sure to be fatal, stands out in my memory of rounds with Dr. Moore. He took a careful history from the girl, performed an exemplary physical examination, all the while keeping the patient completely at ease." Afterwards, as the small retinue of students and their teacher turned to go, Dr. Moore called their attention to a vase of flowers on the patient's bedside table. "Someone must love you very much,' he said to the young woman, 'to send you those beautiful flowers." "I realized, in that instant," Stone recalls, "that such a sensitive comment from a physician can be an absolutely vital part of whatever healing there is to be done." Such small acts of thoughtfulness and comfort are at risk of becoming vanishingly rare in the increasingly hustle-and-haste academic hospital environment where teaching is seldom highly regarded or rewarded. In addition to Dr. Moore's parting gesture being one of profound courteousness and generosity of spirit, student Stone remembered it years later as an absolutely vital part of "what clinical skill really means, how to handle difficult moments with a patient; in short, how it *should* be done."[24]

As Stone's experience attests, sometimes learning happens serendipitously, as is also the case in a short story by nurse practitioner and writer Cortney Davis

(1945–).[25] The story's narrator sets the scene in the hospital room of James Harris, an eighty-four-year-old dying man who is receiving comfort measures. Shortly before midnight, Mr. Harris's private duty nurse, Irene McNamara, pages medical intern Peter Locke because she is concerned that the patient's pain is not being adequately controlled. We learn that, in addition to being sleep deprived and in a foul mood, Locke "hated being among the dying."[26] As Locke turns to leave after increasing Mr. Harris's morphine, the nurse asks him to help her scoot the patient up in bed. Peter seemed unsure how to respond. "Just go around to the other side and we'll hoist him up a bit. He's sliding." This they do together, "their heads almost touching."[27] Before leaving, Peter asks Irene if she thinks Mr. Harris will die this night, adding "I've never pronounced anyone before."[28]

When Peter returns a couple of hours later, he finds Irene washing and massaging Mr. Harris's back and wonders why she bothers. "Massage helps. Even if it doesn't, it lets Mr. Harris know I'm here," she explains.[29] Peter sits down and the two begin to talk about Mr. Harris's family and what he did for a living. In the course of this conversation, Peter mentions his grandfather who died when he was Mr. Harris's age. Irene asks Peter if he has ever seen anyone die. "Not really," he replies.[30] Irene continues to busy herself with making sure Mr. Harris is comfortable. Raising her voice, she says, "Jim, your doctor, Peter, is here with us again. He called his grandfather Poppy." Then "She looked at Peter as if to say, your turn." Peter begins haltingly, looking to Irene for cues, "Hello, Mr. Harris ... I've been working with your internist for the last few weeks. I admitted you to the hospital." Stroking Mr. Harris's hand, Irene says "You're doing great, Jim ......Don't worry. We're here with you."[31]

Peter looks in once more as day breaks following another sleepless night and sees Irene sitting on the bed next to Mr. Harris, holding his hand, and chanting "ahhh" with each of his labored exhalations. "It sounded to him as if they were singing together, or praying."[32] Peter asks Irene about the sound she is making. She explains, "It's called breathing with the patient .... It's like going part of the way them, a way of letting your life and their death overlap."[33] Irene asks Peter if he'd like to try it. He is speechless. She assures him that all he has to do is follow Jim's lead. And before he can give it a second thought, he begins. When Irene whispers, "this is it," Peter becomes anxious. "But as Mr. Harris let go a final, slow moan of air, Peter found himself joining in, his deeper *ah* blending with Mr. Harris's and Irene's, the three notes braiding around one another. Mr. Harris's lips paled, his eyes darkened, and together their three breaths rose into the room, fading out in unison."[34]

An experience such as this is likely to make a profound impression on a novice physician. Nevertheless, without some context for *understanding* what was learned, the impression risks becoming fleeting. The perverse practice of disvaluing experience in medical training has long been recognized.[35] In addition to teaching practice skills, clinical education at all levels is a moral apprenticeship. And experience is central to learning appropriate behavior. Moral formation occurs in the process of observing an exemplary role model such as Dr. Moore or Nurse McNamara in action, imitating the observed behavior, appropriating it and internalizing it until it becomes second nature. In order for student Stone and intern Locke to fully appreciate the importance, for their patients *and* for themselves, of what they have experienced, it must be brought to their awareness and legitimated. This is best accomplished in small group humanities discussions in which participants share meaningful clinical experiences and analyze what made them so.

Pediatrician Perri Klass writes of an exercise that is part of a course on learning to do a proper patient interview. She takes a group of four first-year students to the threshold of what she calls "the zone of the patient's story." "Clinical medicine," Klass wants these novices to appreciate, "is all about stories."[36] It's about "saying – and meaning – all over again that every hospital room, every life, is full of stories more complicated and more tangled than we can ever hope to tease out, but also making the commitment to learn to ask the questions and listen carefully to the answers that may help you understand, at least a little."[37]

On the occasion she recounts, Klass took her charges to meet the father of a two-year-old girl with a putative diagnosis of osteogenesis imperfecta, commonly called brittle bone disease. After admiring the little girl who was carefully positioned in a stroller with a cast on her broken leg – the seventh such fracture in her short life – the students began to ask the father questions. He willingly obliged, telling the students what it is like to be the parent of a child who has a serious illness, one she will likely have to learn to live with. He told them about a previous misdiagnosis at a different hospital. He told them that he and his wife had a new baby who was at home with its mother while he stayed at the hospital to keep his daughter company. As Klass observed her students interacting with this man, she realized that they were beginning to understand that they had "chosen a career which brings them into the room with what is truly important in people's lives, and sometimes what is truly important is difficult and sad and even tragic."[38]

Following the interview, the group went to a seminar room to reflect on what they had experienced. Klass asked the students to think about all the stories this father had told them – a genetic story, a biological story, a medical system story, a child development story, a family story, an immigration story, a day-by-day story, and "probably even a religious story, since the father clearly identifies his faith as the only thing that keeps him going, since he asked you over and over to pray for his family, and we should never forget to think about where patients get their strength."[39] As Klass listened to the students work through their encounter with this young father, their teacher for the day, she saw with satisfaction that they had stepped over the threshold into the zone of the patient's story.

Opportunities provided in medical humanities programs to reflect openly and think through such experiences as these can enhance what Suzanne Poirier calls "emotional honesty," a constructive alternative to the suppression of troubling emotions and the stunting of moral growth.[40]

Historian of medical education Kenneth M. Ludmerer (1947–) has observed that despite the fact that there are dedicated teachers on virtually every medical faculty, formidable obstacles to good teaching are pervasive. The incentive and reward structure in academic health systems favors research and "clinical productivity."[41] Studying medicine, as Perri Klass's students learned, is serious business. Consequently, teaching is a serious responsibility, in the humanities as in the sciences. Just as competent, humane medical care depends significantly on the quality of patient-physician relationships, so also does good teaching turn importantly on meaningful interactions between teachers and students – around humanistic ideas as well as scientific concepts. The concepts count, the ideas matter, and discerning their appropriate use in practice has consequences in the lives of the ill and injured. The success or failure of teaching and doctoring revolves around human relationships – teacher and student, doctor with patient.[42]

CONCLUSION

Toward the end of Abraham Flexner's (1866–1959) seminal report on American medical education a century ago is this prescient and largely overlooked passage: "[T]he practitioner deals with facts of two categories. Chemistry, physics, biology enable him to apprehend one set; he needs a different apperceptive and appreciative apparatus to deal with other, more subtle elements. Specific preparation is in this direction much more difficult; one must rely for the requisite insight and sympathy on a varied and enlarging cultural experience. Such enlargement of the physician's horizon is otherwise important, for scientific progress has greatly modified his ethical responsibility."[43]

As we learned in Chapter 3, a new Carnegie Foundation Report on Medical Education published its findings in 2010, a century after Flexner's Report. Not surprisingly, it confirmed what students and educational reformers had been saying for decades. Medical training was not oriented toward student learning and professional identity formation; it was too long and inflexible; book learning and clinical learning were poorly coordinated; students had little opportunity for holistic learning about patients' experiences; and an overly commercialized health care system undermined the broader responsibilities for advocacy and civic engagement.

Medical humanities is designed to attack many of these problems. It contributes to the study of medicine by encouraging a self-reflective disposition. It teaches clarity of thinking and skill in reasoning about aspects of life that elude quantification. It teaches elements of the arts of dialogue – attending to patients, listening respectfully and responding appropriately. It shapes medical sensibility so that doctors are better able to imagine what patients are going through, what their illnesses mean to them, and what their futures may hold. In sum, the humanities help stimulate the development of professional identity. They contribute, in Flexner's words, to the "enlargement of the physician's horizon" by cultivating personality, intellectual curiosity, emotional honesty, social awareness, and the exercise of sound judgment and moral imagination – virtues and skills indispensable to good doctoring.

SUMMATION

This chapter provided an "insider's view" of medical education since the 1960s. Relying on the voices and writings of students and reformers, it examined student protests against injustice and against a dehumanizing education as well as a growing skepticism about an exclusive emphasis on biomedical science and technology as adequate preparation for clinical practice. Then, with a focus on the recent rise in humanities courses and full-fledged medical humanities programs in many medical schools, it considered how medical education is adapting to meet the challenges of the twenty-first century. Overall, this chapter emphasized how, in an effort to counteract trends of depersonalization, biological determinism, and mechanistic medicine, medical education is evolving to help future physicians cultivate social awareness and responsibility, personality, intellectual curiosity, emotional honesty, and the exercise of sound judgment and moral imagination.

EXERCISES FOR CRITICAL THINKING AND CHARACTER FORMATION

QUESTIONS FOR DISCUSSION

1. What are some of the benefits to studying medicine today?
2. What are some of the disadvantages to studying medicine today?
3. In "On Being Poor," how does the author redefine poverty? What is he trying to say about the state of medical education? Why do you think that he chooses a poem to express these themes?
4. If you are a medical student, are there parts of your medical education that you find unnecessary? Are there parts of your medical education that you wish you could explore further? If you are an undergraduate, what elements of your education are needed to prepare you for an active life in the professional and/or public world?

SUGGESTED WRITING EXERCISES

Write, in as much concrete detail as you can, about your worst experience studying medicine. Write for about fifteen minutes. Now write, for ten minutes, about how it might shape your experiences in the future. If you are an undergraduate, write about your best and worst experiences in college. What changes might strengthen your education?

SUGGESTED VIEWING

Gross Anatomy (1989)
The Interns (1962)

Scrubs (television show, 2001–2010)

FURTHER READING

Lee Gutkind, ed., *Becoming a Doctor: From Student to Specialist, Doctor-Writers Share Their Experiences*
Melvin Konner, *Becoming a Doctor: A Journey of Initiation in Medical School*
Suzanne Poirier, *Doctors in the Making: Memoirs and Medical Education*

Kevin M. Takakuwa, Nick Rubashkin, and Karen E. Herzig, *What I Learned in Medical School: Personal Stories of Young Doctors*

ADVANCED READING

Kenneth M. Ludmerer, *Learning to Heal: The Development of America Medical Education*

Kenneth M. Ludmerer, *Time to Heal: American Medical Education from the Turn of the Twentieth Century to the Era of Managed Care*

JOURNALS

International Journal of Medical Education
Journal of Continuing Education in the Health Professions
Medical Education

ORGANIZATIONS AND GROUPS

The American Medical Student Association
http://www.amsa.org/AMSA/Homepage.aspx

PART III
Philosophy and Medicine

PART OVERVIEW
Philosophy and Medicine

Part 3 of this book deals with philosophy. What is philosophy? Philosophy, or *philosophia* in Greek, literally means love of wisdom. One could say that philosophy is the search for truth and that it seeks to explore ultimate and fundamental questions: How do we know? What is reality? What is good? How should we live? What does it mean to be human?

As an academic discipline, philosophy can be divided into several branches: epistemology (the study of knowledge), logic (the study of reasoning), metaphysics/ontology (the study of reality), ethics (the study of values), and aesthetics (the study of beauty). There are various intellectual traditions of philosophy. For example, there are regionally and historically based traditions such as Greek stoicism, German idealism, American pragmatism, and French existentialism. And within twentieth century philosophy there is a great divide between continental and analytic philosophy. This list is not exhaustive. Indeed, there are many other schools of thought and methodological approaches, such as phenomenological, structuralist, poststructuralist, materialist, feminist, and race-critical. And there are major specialized subfields within philosophy, such as philosophy of religion, philosophy of science, philosophy of language, and philosophy of mind. Philosophy of medicine is another such subfield.

What is philosophy of medicine? Philosophy of medicine engages traditional questions of philosophy in light of medical practice. In other words, it examines medicine in light of epistemology, logic, metaphysics, ethics, and aesthetics and in doing so asks questions such as:

- What is health? What is disease?
- What is death?
- What are the goals of medicine?
- How does one make clinical judgments? What counts as evidence in the production of medical knowledge?
- What is it like to be a doctor? What is it like to be a patient?

- In what ways does medical knowledge assume and (re)produce certain power relationships?
- How can one resolve ethical dilemmas in clinical practice?
- To what extent is health care a right?

The chapters following in this section address, sometimes explicitly and other times implicitly, these questions and more. It is worth noting that each of these questions engage, in one way or another, what it means to flourish as a human being, and how debate within philosophy of medicine follows from one's own core understanding of human flourishing.

"Any physician who goes beyond technique to contemplate the human object of his ministrations," Edmund Pellegrino writes, "must turn to the humanities for those meanings which medical science alone cannot give."[1] Pellegrino (1920–2013) is the single most important person in the subfield of philosophy of medicine. "Bioethics and the medical humanities, especially their emergence in the latter part of the twentieth century," H. Tristram Engelhardt Jr. (1941–) and Fabrice Jotterand note, "cannot be understood apart from Edmund D. Pellegrino."[2] Engelhardt and Jotterand suggest that he, more than any other person, was able to connect the humanities to the teaching and the practice of medicine in a substantive way. While others, such as Abraham Flexner (1866–1959), were able to pay lip service to this ideal in the early twentieth century, they were not able to articulate a robust connection. But Pellegrino's work, they observe, demonstrated that "bioethics cannot be understood outside the context of the medical humanities, and that the medical humanities cannot be understood outside the context of the philosophy of medicine."[3] Pellegrino, in other words, expanded the scope of bioethics beyond traditional moral questions in bioethics (questions concerning, for example, abortion, end-of-life care, and resource allocation) by arguing that (1) various disciplines and fields of the humanities are needed to provide a concrete vision of human flourishing; and (2) the discipline of philosophy provides an essential critical self-awareness that directs humanistic inquiry.

No book on medical humanities would be complete without addressing philosophy of medicine, and so we dedicate an entire section to the topic. As with history and medicine and literature and medicine, there has been a substantial amount of writing on philosophy and medicine during the latter part of the twentieth century and the early decades of the twenty-first century. This section introduces the reader to some of the most important topics and influential thinkers.

13 Ways of Knowing

To speak of clinical medicine as human *medicine is no mere gloss: it calls less for the ingenious conceptual grasp of* episteme ... *than for a kind of discernment (*phronesis*) characteristic of the knowledge that human beings have of other human beings – rooted in long experience, cultivated in years of practice.*

– Stephen Toulmin[1]

ABSTRACT

This chapter explores the principal theories of knowledge that are at work, and sometimes at odds, in the practice of medicine. Beginning with a discussion of Cartesian rationalism and the ideal of objective and dispassionate observation, it examines how theories of interpretive, imaginative, empathic, and narrative knowledge can supplement the knowledge derived from biomedical science. Then, with a focus on clinical practice, it considers two vignettes in which doctors move past the model of detached objectivity and instrumentality toward a dialogical and collaborative attempt to discern the elusive sources of patient suffering.

INTRODUCTION

What do we know and how do we know it? How can we be certain that what we know is true? These are epistemological questions about the sources and validity of knowledge. Two principal theories of knowledge, or ways of knowing, are at work, and sometimes at odds, in medicine: the way of biomedical science, and that of clinical practice.

A medical scientist wants to know *about* the human body, how it functions and why it fails. For the scientist, the ideal is to study the body, its organs, tissues, cells, and genes *objectively* and dispassionately and to make the knowledge gained thereby available for use in the prevention and treatment of disease. Medical knowledge derived from the biological sciences, although indisputably indispensable, is insufficient for the practice of clinical medicine. Something more is called for.[2]

Practicing medicine is inadequately understood when limited to selectively applying the validated results of laboratory studies and clinical trials in diagnosing and treating disease. It also involves engaging patients, one at a time, in discerning what ails them and deciding what course of action is most likely to lead to their betterment. In this process, the patient is not an object but a fellow *subject*, and the way to understanding and healing is intersubjective[3] – relational, person to person, a joint venture. An exploration of this latter way of knowing will be the focus of this chapter.

RATIONALISM

As we noted in Chapter 2, major changes began to occur at the dawn of the modern era in the way European thinkers viewed human nature and the human condition. Rene Descartes (1596–1650), commonly considered the father of modern philosophy, derived his rationalist ideal of true knowledge from geometry. Enlightenment thinkers of the eighteenth century further advanced the idea that reason was the primary source of knowledge. Particularly in science, the path to sure knowledge was believed to be through reason's objective gaze. The ideal of the scientist or scholar as disengaged and rational – unencumbered by preconceptions and free from mere opinion – and of mathematical certainty as the epitome of knowledge, came to seem unquestionable.[4] This Cartesianism became thoroughly integrated into mainstream Western thought over the course of three centuries until it came under critical scrutiny beginning in the mid-nineteenth century.[5]

INTERPRETIVE UNDERSTANDING

Competing conceptions of knowledge were evolving as early as the seventeenth century. Particularly notable were the views of rhetorician and historian Giambattista Vico (1668–1744) for whom adopting mathematics as a model for *all* knowledge was to restrict knowledge to the abstract and the analytical, making it thus unsuited to understanding *human* life, which is imbued with imagination, intuition, memory and feeling. According to Isaiah Berlin (1909–1997), "Vico uncovered a species of knowing not previously clearly discriminated – the idea of empathetic insight or intuitive sympathy, a sense of knowing that is basic to all humane studies, the sense in which I know what it is to be poor, to fight for a cause, to belong to a nation, to join or abandon a church or a party, to feel nostalgia, terror, the omnipresence of a god, to understand a gesture, a work of art, a joke, a man's character .... It is not a matter of 'knowing that'. Nor is it like knowing how to ride a bicycle, or to win a battle, or what to do in case of fire, or knowing a man's name, or a poem by heart .... [It] is the sort of knowing which participants in an activity claim to possess as against mere observers."[6]

This capacity for imagining what it may have been like to live in a bygone place or time, or to appreciate what it may be like to walk in another person's shoes, yields understanding unlike the knowledge gained by empirical observation or abstraction and analysis. Vico's alternative epistemology (called acquaintance-knowledge by some later scholars), was a mode of perception best suited to understanding cultures and persons, ways of thought and feeling and expression. Though obscured by the Cartesianism of his time, it was taken up anew in modern humanistic and social scientific thought when interest in the ancient practice of hermeneutics reemerged in the wake of the demise of philosophic and scientific positivisms. Central to this "interpretive turn" was a reevaluation of the concept of *Verstehen,* or interpretive understanding, as it was developed by Wilhelm Dilthey (1833–1911), Max Weber (1846–1920), Hans Georg Gadamer (1900–2002), Jürgen Habermas (1929–), and Charles Taylor (1931–), among others.[7]

Knowledge in the form of interpretive understanding (also called, variously, by different authors, "imaginative insight" or "imaginative understanding," and "empathic insight" or "empathic understanding") is especially relevant to the practice of medicine. It is inherently dialogical and its principal focus is on seeing things from the perspective of another. In the practice of patient care, this means paying careful attention to patients' perceptions about what ails them. It entails not only observing patients from a bioscientific perspective but also engaging them in order to discover how things seem to them, and the significance, to them, of various metaphoric and symbolic meanings attaching to their experience of illness.

Although modern medicine is generally unreflectively considered "scientific," it is so in no obvious way. Kathryn Montgomery (1939–) observes that "The assumption that medicine is a science – a positivist what-you-see-is-what-there-is representation of the physical world – passes almost unexamined by physicians, patients, and society as a whole." Curiously, medicine continues to idealize this antiquated view of science as providing incontrovertible facts and explanations of how things really work. Montgomery calls this "medicine's epistemological *scotoma,* a blindness of which the knower is unaware."[8] In practice, however, medical practitioners make selective use of generalized biomedical knowledge in the diagnosis and treatment of individual instances of malady guided by narratively constructed and conventionally agreed upon experiential knowledge.[9]

Whether interviewing a patient or making a chart entry, consulting a colleague or presenting on hospital rounds, physicians practice according to narrative conventions of the plot, taking prescribed steps from chief complaint to diagnosis to prognosis and formulation of a plan of care, and arrive at clinical judgments case by case informed by the collective wisdom of the practice community and their own professional experience. Clinicians use the findings of modern biomedical research in a *practice* that is fundamentally experiential and interpretive. Clinical medicine's epistemology is not hypothetical and theoretical, as the term "scientific" suggests, but engaged and practical.

As we learned in Chapter 12, medical students are taught to this day that mastery of the rudiments of science, with adherence to principles of objectivity, regularity, and certainty is the *sine qua non* of competence in medicine. But when these students move from the study of the basic sciences to hospital and clinic, the regularities and certainties of lecture hall and laboratory are challenged by the variability and uncertainties of patient care. Here, on the threshold of practice, a different way of knowing is called for, the way of sympathetic insight, available by means of dialogue and discernment, eventuating in human understanding and sound clinical judgment, the raison d'être of *clinical* medicine.[10]

Isaiah Berlin writes, echoing Giambattisa Vico (1668–1744), "A medical chart or diagram is not the equivalent of a portrait such as a gifted novelist or human being endowed with adequate insight – understanding – could form; not equivalent *not at all* because it needs less *skill* or is less *valuable* for its own purposes, but, because if it confines itself to publicly recordable facts and generalizations attested by them, it must necessarily leave out of account that vast number of small, constantly altering, evanescent colors, sense, sounds, and the psychical equivalent of these, the half noticed, half inferred, half gazed at, half unconsciously absorbed minutiae of behavior and thought and feeling which are at once too numerous, too complex, too fine and too indiscriminable from each other to be identified, named, ordered, recorded, set forth in neutral scientific language."

Moreover, Berlin observes, "there are among them pattern qualities ... habits of thought and emotion, ways of looking at, reacting to, talking about experiences which lie too close to us to be discriminated and classified – of which we are not strictly aware as such, but which, nevertheless, we absorb into our picture of what goes on, and the more sensitively and sharply aware of them we are the more understanding is the insight we are rightly said to possess. *This is what understanding human beings largely consists in.*"[11]

Berlin at times refers to such insight or understanding as a gift, suggesting that it is something with which one simply is or is not endowed. On other occasions, he speaks of it as an achievement, implying that it can be learned. Perhaps it is best thought of as a capacity that can be cultivated, say, by a physician, a capacity to imagine something of what it may be like to be a patient sitting in the examining room or lying in a hospital bed. Not to know for sure, of course, not to *identify* with another's experience but to come to some *sense* of what it may be *like* to be in that other person's shoes. As when Berlin writes, "When the Jews were enjoined in the Bible to protect strangers 'for ye know the heart of a stranger, seeing ye were strangers in the land of Egypt', this knowledge is neither deductive, nor inductive, nor founded on direct inspection, but akin to the 'I know' of 'I know what it is to be hungry and poor.'"[12] Knowledge of this sort is essential to the healing arts and is accessible through the cultivation of empathic insight.

NARRATIVE MEDICINE

When we or someone we love falls ill, we begin to think about what it is like compared to how it was and in relation to how we thought it was going to be, and might still turn out to be. Thus do we try to locate ourselves in our story as we understand it and seek the counsel of others to help us make sense of this unexpected turn of events. We size up the situation in which we newly find ourselves. We move through the situation guided by "readings" taken in transit. As things change, or cues become unclear, we make midcourse corrections in our evolving sense of what is going on. When messages seem mixed, or obstacles to understanding crop up and the fluid motion of our lives is seriously interrupted, we pause long enough to step back and figure out why. And often, we seek the counsel of others, including doctors.

What a doctor is often expected to do in such an encounter is not only to solve the problem posed by the patient's chief complaint, but to follow a story – about pain and discomfort, to be sure, but also about love, loss, loyalty and the like. Such encounters begin with patients and doctors talking with each other about what the hurt is like, why it hurts like that just now, and what it might mean. Meaning is not latent in the patient's symptoms waiting to be made manifest and deciphered. It is located contextually and articulated metaphorically in the give and take of dialogical discernment. Such a dialogue does not proceed logically from premises to conclusion. As with any story, one looks to the plausibility rather than the necessity of what transpires. The emphasis is on contingency – uncertainty and probability – and the interpretive task is to relate the current episode of illness to what has happened in the story thus far and to what might be anticipated by introducing a medical explanation of events or an unwelcome prognosis into the narrative. "Following the story" is not so much a matter of trailing along or keeping track but of becoming aware and getting the gist of the story as it evolves. Nor is the doctor the "reader" and the patient the "text."[13] Rather the two of them together are interpreters of the illness and joint authors of the illness narrative.

How many ways of knowing does this painting display? Is the scalpel, held by Dr. Samuel Gross, a way of knowing? How has the artist drawn our attention to it? What is the source of the light that strikes it?

What type of knowing do Gross's assistant surgeons demonstrate as they retract and explore the incision in the patient's left thigh and anesthetize and stabilize the patient on the table of the operating theater? If you could read the operative notes being recorded by the clerk who sits just beyond the surgeon's right shoulder, what might you learn, even today?

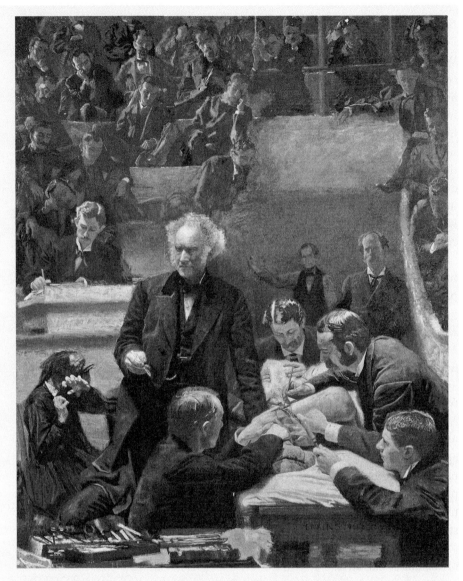

Figure 13. *Portrait of Dr. Samuel D. Gross* (The Gross Clinic), 1875, Thomas Eakins 1844–1916, Courtesy of the Pennsylvania Academy of the Fine Arts, Philadelphia. Gift of the Alumni Association to Jefferson Medical College in 1878 and purchased by the Pennsylvania Academy of the Fine Arts and the Philadelphia Museum of Art in 2007 with the generous support of more than 3,400 donors.

Which students appear to have the discipline and perception to turn the opportunity to see this operation into knowledge? How is their way of learning in 1875 different from students learning today? Finally, what sort of knowing did Eakins demonstrate in creating this work? Can you think of any elements of the actual scene that the artist was not able to capture? Which elements might suggest that Eakins knew what it was to be a surgeon, a student, a patient?

In order to develop a capacity for the type of human understanding described in this chapter, what can we learn from Thomas Eakins' ability to record, in Isaiah Berlin's words, "the minutiae of behavior and thought and feeling which are too numerous, too complex … to be set forth in neutral scientific language"?

For a detailed description and history of the painting, visit: http://www.jefferson.edu/about/eakins/grossclinic.html.

This Is the Child

In his searching narrative of his son's struggle with leukemia,[14] Terry Pringle (1947–) reflects, "As a child I always knew there were boundaries. A bully would chase me, but would stop at the front door. My father might beat me, but would stop short of killing me. We are subject to illness, but it can always be cured. We are safe within these boundaries. And when I see that the boundaries are imaginary, I feel sick … I want my son to live. I have never begged for anything in my adult life, but now I am begging."[15]

Pringle introduces the reader to Dr. Pope, the Abilene pediatrician who is to execute the medical treatment plan devised by Houston specialists. At first, Dr. Pope appears to Brenda Pringle to be insufficiently concerned about her son. When initial miscommunications between Houston and Abilene regarding drug dosages occur, it is Eric's mother, not the doctors, who sorts things out. However, Dr. Pope persists, staying in touch with Eric and his parents. "The words he speaks," recalls Eric's father, "aren't nearly so important as the effort he makes. We need at least one doctor to confirm that Eric is important to him, that he is thinking as well as acting, that he recognizes the treatment comes from a standardized schedule, but our son is not a compilation of statistics and probable responses."[16]

The relationship between Eric and Dr. Pope grows over time. Eric tells his parents that Dr. Pope is as skilled as the specialists at doing spinal taps. On another occasion, Eric objects to having to lie down to receive injections. "'Okay,' the doctor says, 'we'll do it your way.'"[17] When there is a choice of physicians, Eric always wants Dr. Pope.

As the Pringles begin to run out of therapeutic options and decide to try an experimental drug, they call their pediatrician. "He asks Brenda how we're doing. 'Fine,' she said. 'Now tell me how you're really doing.' A friend tells us later that the doctor had asked him if anyone had heard from us; he had thought about us all day."[18] When it becomes clear that cure will not come, Terry Pringle breaks down. "Once loosed, the sobs are unstoppable. I sit on the coffee table with my head in my hands; Dr. Pope crosses the room and pulls me up, embracing me. I understand instinctively the move he has made. We don't know each other well, he is as reserved as I am. And I know the steps across the room were long ones for him, not only to me, but out of a role that protects him. The doctor says, 'Lord, this hurts.'"[19]

While the Pringles decide about next steps, the doctor listens. Do they want Eric hospitalized? No, they wish to keep him home. From then until the end, Dr. Pope attends Eric at home. When Brenda and Terry are overwhelmed by the burden they bear, the doctor steps in, gently but steadily. It is a sad, beautiful dance, with one partner leading for a time, and then the other. Terry Pringle telephones Dr. Pope in the middle of an October night to tell him Eric has died. "He is there within a few minutes and sits beside Eric for a long time, sniffing and rubbing Eric's arm and head. Before he checks for a heartbeat, he performs the same ritual he always has – rubbing and blowing on the stethoscope to warm it before touching it to Eric's chest."[20]

Of the dynamic typical of a relationship in which conversation partners take each other seriously and hold each other in mutual regard, Martin Buber (1878–1965) wrote: "what is essential does not take place in each of the participants or in a neutral world which includes the two and all other things; it takes place between them in the most precise sense, as it were in a dimension which is accessible only to them."[21] This sense of connecting in the space "in-between" can accompany experiences ordinary or grave, as, in this story, in serious conversation between a sick child and his parents, and their doctor about how things are going, what to expect, what to do next, and how to hold up under the weight of the unthinkable. This hyphenated space of connecting is a place of moral and spiritual encounter, with parties in the relationship alternately speaking and listening, seeking mutually bearable meaning by means of which an illness that threatens to fray or even sever the storyline of this family's life may be woven into the fabric of that life.

The lived experience of illness may usefully be approached as a "text" requiring "reading," ideally by a patient and a doctor comparing notes. On this analogy, the patient-doctor relationship is collaborative, and the work of healing commences not when the doctor settles on a diagnosis but when text and readers converge in a common narrative. Thus construed, medical practice is seen to be a storied practice. In place of the stainless-steel apparatus and vital-sign monitors so central to rescue medicine, what is required of the doctor in patient encounters is less often swift judgment and deft action than a discerning reading of the situation at hand. What does the ailment portend for the life of the patient? Is the suffering to be relieved or endured, and in what measure? What can reasonably be expected to result from this or that intervention? Are there fates worse than death? Answers to such questions must be thought through and talked about case by case, person to person. In this process of reflection and conversation, courses of action evolve in which the right thing to do – the reasonable action to take – is not the result of discursive reasoning but is an "ingredient conclusion" that is embedded in and inseparable from the narrative as it unfolds.[22] Discerning an appropriate "fit" between selectively relevant generalized biomedical knowledge and the unique human story of a particular patient is the mark of sound clinical judgment.

A Vague Pain

Clinical care always begins with a patient's story, which is an invitation to a conversation – as in a case story recounted by gastroenterologist Richard Weinberg, of his encounter with a patient in her mid-twenties who arrived at his clinic with a complaint of chronic severe abdominal pain, a condition with which she had lived since her mid-teens.[23]

Her description of the pain was vague. She had been seen by several other gastroenterologists, had undergone all the appropriate tests, and tried virtually all the available medicines. What, Weinberg wondered, did she expect from him? "As I questioned her, I studied her with growing fascination. She was anxious and withdrawn, but nonetheless she projected a desperate courage, like a cornered animal making a defiant last stand. She kept her gaze directed downward, but every now and then I caught her staring at me intensely, as if searching for something."[24] Because she seemed uncomfortable talking about herself, Weinberg moved on to the family history. Her parents had emigrated from Italy. Her father was a baker who had worked and saved to buy his own shop, which she now managed. Her mother had died when she was a young girl, and primary responsibility for her five siblings had fallen to her. Following her mother's example, she went to mass every morning. "But I don't take communion," she volunteered.[25]

At a bit of a loss as to where the interview was headed, Weinberg responded to this last bit of information by saying that cooking was his hobby but that he was not much of a baker, which, he went on to say, was especially unfortunate because he was addicted to Napoleons which he purchased at the French Gourmet Bakery. "For the first time her eyes came alive. 'I wouldn't feed the French Gourmet to my cat ... the French learned all they know about baking from the Italians ....'"[26] Her outburst took Weinberg by surprise but disappeared as abruptly as it had appeared. The rest of the interview was yes or no. Her physical exam was normal. Weinberg conjectured that she probably was suffering from severe irritable bowel syndrome, which elicited no response from her. He prescribed a bland diet and an antispasmodic and asked her to come back in a month. Instead, she returned the following week but was curiously uncommunicative. So Weinberg switched back to Italian pastries, the one subject they so far had in common. As before, she became animated, and he discovered how knowledgeable she was. She made no mention of abdominal pain. He scheduled a return visit one month hence.

When, as before, she reappeared the following week, Weinberg noticed dark rings under her eyes. "'Are you sleeping well?' I inquired. 'No.' 'Why?' 'Because I have a nightmare.' 'A nightmare, the same nightmare every night?' 'Yes.' 'Can you tell me about it?'" With great effort, she describes a lurid dream that could have only one meaning. "Were you ever sexually assaulted? 'Yes ... when I was fourteen.'"[27] Whereupon she proceeded to recount the grim details of being raped by her sister's boyfriend, something she had before now told no one. Weinberg consoled her as best he could, and when she stopped sobbing, gently suggested that he refer her to a rape counselor. She would not hear of it and told him she would talk to no one else.

Despite feeling out of his depth, Weinberg scheduled weekly visits during which he mostly listened to her explain the lengths to which she had gone to try to expiate her guilt – giving up communion, giving up eating, then secretly bingeing on pastries, purging herself until her stomach ached, and so on, in a vicious cycle. Weinberg researched the link between rape and eating disorders. He consulted a psychiatrist colleague. Nothing seemed to help – except the visits themselves, which continued for several months. They talked about her pain, and when that became difficult, they talked about baking.

Over time, Weinberg noticed, subtle changes began to occur. She gained some weight and began taking communion again. Her visits came at longer intervals. Then, after a hiatus of three months, she reappeared, looking healthy and strong to announce to Weinberg that she was going to quit the bakery, spend the summer in Italy and, on her return, become a full-time college student. "'I wanted to see you before I left so I could bring you these,' she said, handing me a white cardboard box, carefully tied with a bright ribbon. 'Should I open it now?' I asked. She nodded. Inside the box, neatly resting on individual doilies, were six perfect Napoleons, the pastry puffed high, the fondant a smooth glassy sheet, the chocolate chevrons meticulously aligned. 'I made these myself just for you,' she said."[28] And took her leave.

In this story, the offending cause of the patient's complaint is not discoverable by objective means. But having ruled out every objectively plausible reason for the patient's abdominal pain, Dr. Weinberg eschews the subject-object mode of detached objectivity and instrumentality, shifting instead to mutuality and dialogue in a collaborative attempt to discern the elusive source of the patient's suffering. The kind of knowledge gained in the course of conversing with each other about what the ache in the abdomen is like, and what it may portend, is not a knowing that or a knowing how but a sympathetic sense of what it means to be in this vexing situation. This knowledge, this shared sense – this "communion" – is what human understanding largely consists of.

How did the physicians featured in the two vignettes presented herein acquire the knowledge to conduct themselves in the way they did? Where did Dr. Pope learn to be solicitous without being intrusive? How was he able to express his own grief over losing Eric while remaining a steady companion to Brenda and Terry Pringle in their grieving? What prompted Dr. Weinberg to entertain the possibility that the anxious but defiant patient who had sought him out might be "searching for something?" And how was he able to imagine that it might be the visits themselves and the open-ended conversations that went on there that were therapeutic?

We cannot know the answers to these questions regarding Dr. Pope and Dr. Weinberg in particular. What we can say is that, as characters in these stories, their responses to their patients contain clear evidence of humane knowledge – capacious human understanding. There are numerous ways to acquire such knowledge, such as emulating an admired person. However, one way recommends itself to students aspiring to become health professionals, namely, expansive exposure to, and deep dives into, works of imaginative literature, not only for the pleasure of engaging lifelike characters in fictional worlds (which is its own reward), but also for edification: for knowledge gained in experiencing, at one remove, the way the world turns and what makes people tick – acquainting oneself vicariously with the myriad ways people live their lives, cherish what they cherish, suffer, make up their minds, discover their desires, fill in the gaps, deal with adversity, and try to make sense of the sometimes apparently senseless; and, not least, for self-knowledge gained, as we readers see ourselves in others.

CONCLUSION

The meaning of malady emerges in a dialogue with the text of affliction. The analogy between textual interpretation and ordinary conversation between patients and doctors, though not exact, is suggestive. As the interpreter of a novel, poem, or play imaginatively places the text being read for the sense it makes in an illuminating context (a genre, say, or a parable), so also do interpreters of the text of a life event closely read its lines – and between the lines – searching for insight. In a therapeutic encounter, the doctor turns a trained ear to a patient's account of misfortune or malaise, places it in the company of similar accounts he or she has heard before, and then attends not only to what is said but also to what is unspoken, and to what may be unspeakable, all the while conversing with the patient to test the fit of the patient's experience with similar, potentially telling, experiences in the physician's repertoire. This requires a capacity to imagine the illness experience from the patient's perspective, and an awareness of the impossibility of finding a perfect fit. It is a kind of listening with a discerning ear for narrative possibility, a capacity for empathic insight that yields knowledge appropriate to understanding human experiences of illness.

SUMMATION

This chapter explored the principal theories of knowledge that are at work, and sometimes at odds, in the practice of medicine. Beginning with a discussion of Cartesian rationalism and the ideal of objective and dispassionate observation, it examined how theories of interpretive, imaginative, empathic, and narrative knowledge can supplement the knowledge derived from biomedical science. Then, with a focus on clinical practice, it considered two vignettes in which doctors move past the model of detached objectivity and instrumentality toward a dialogical, collaborative attempt to discern the elusive sources of the patient suffering. Overall, this chapter emphasized that meaning is not latent in the patient's symptoms waiting to be made manifest and deciphered, but is located contextually and articulated metaphorically in the give and take of dialogical discernment.

EXERCISES FOR CRITICAL THINKING AND CHARACTER FORMATION

QUESTIONS FOR DISCUSSION

1. Think about a time when you felt understood. What contributed to this feeling?
2. How do you try to understand others when you talk to them? How do you help them to understand you? What are the limits of understanding?
3. Think about your encounters with doctors. Was there ever a time when you thought your doctor didn't understand you? What did it feel like? What, in your opinion, caused the problem?
4. Now think about your encounters with doctors again. Was there ever a time when you felt particularly well understood? What did that feel like? What, in your opinion, made the encounter work?

SUGGESTED WRITING EXERCISES

The epigraph to this chapter refers to the concept of *phronesis*, a Greek term meaning "practical wisdom" or, to use Stephen Toulmin's words, knowledge "rooted in long experience" and "cultivated in years of practice." Think about something of which you have deep practical knowledge – a musical instrument, perhaps, or a sport or a hobby. Then spend fifteen to twenty minutes writing about how you put this knowledge into practice when you are engaged in the activity.

SUGGESTED VIEWING

Healing Words: Poetry and Medicine (2008)
Worlds Apart: A Four-Part Series on Cross-Cultural Health Care (2003)

ADVANCED READING

Isaiah Berlin, *The Hedgehog and the Fox*
Richard J. Bernstein, *Beyond Objectivism and Relativism: Science, Hermeneutics, and Praxis*
David R. Hiley, James F. Bohman, and Richard Shusterman, eds., *The Interpretive Turn: Philosophy, Science, Culture*
Kathryn Montgomery Hunter, *Doctors' Stories: The Narrative Structure of Medical Knowledge*
Kathryn Montgomery, *How Doctors Think: Clinical Judgment and the Practice of Medicine*
Richard Rorty, *Philosophy and the Mirror of Nature*
Charles Taylor, *Sources of the Self: The Making of Modern Identity*
Stephen Toulmin, *Cosmopolis: The Hidden Agenda of Modernity*
David Tracy, *Plurality and Ambiguity: Hermeneutics, Religion, and Hope*

14 Goals of Medicine

The relief of suffering is the fundamental goal of medicine.[1]

– Eric J. Cassell

ABSTRACT

This chapter addresses some ways of thinking about the goals of medicine. Beginning with a discussion of the two principal ways of specifying medicine's *raison d'être* – the social constructionist approach and the essentialist approach – it examines how these two seemingly incompatible approaches might be kept in balance. In particular, it discusses a mid-1990s study by the Hastings Center which found common ground between these two camps by pointing toward four broad notions that can serve as guideposts along the path toward determining modern medicine's goals and limits. Then, with a focus on enhancing human traits and end-of-life issues in America, it considers how our understanding of the goals of medicine has evolved in recent years.

INTRODUCTION

This chapter addresses the crisis of purpose occasioned by the proliferation of medicine's goals, beginning in the middle of the twentieth century. Two examples – enhancing human traits and end-of-life care – will illustrate the sorts of challenges faced by efforts to demarcate modern medicine's legitimate sphere of activity.

Until the late 1940s, medicine in economically developed countries consisted mostly of taking care of sick people using modest therapeutic means. As Robert Martensen (1947–2013) observed, preoccupation with medically managing the human body is of relatively recent origin. "Indeed, aside from vaccines and a few antibiotics and hormones to control infections and metabolic derangements like high blood sugar, the idea that anyone could control desperate *medical* conditions has only arisen since World War II .... When therapeutic modesty gave way to widespread new enthusiasm for technologies of bodily control that began with the mid-1960s and took off in the 1970s, the older way did not linger for long."[2]

In the twenty-first century, due to the great array of goals and activities of medicine, it is difficult to arrive at a coherent notion of its principal purposes. Medicine is about curing disease, discovering new knowledge, developing innovative technologies, defying death near the end of life, choosing children, rescuing premature newborns, enhancing human traits, preventive health maintenance, rehabilitation following accident or injury, and on and on. And the pursuit of each of these goals involves interaction among various institutions (hospitals, clinics, health science centers), government agencies (National Institutes of Health, the Centers for Disease Control and Prevention, Food and Drug Administration), and commercial enterprises (pharmaceutical companies, device manufacturers, insurance conglomerates) which often have competing goals of their own. It is an open question whether clarity of purpose can offer alternatives to what has become an unwieldy, expensive, and sometimes harmful "biomedical-industrial complex."[3] Many would argue, however, that as medicine's goals have multiplied, its core values seem to have eroded.

CONSTRUCTIVISM VERSUS ESSENTIALISM

There are two standard ways of specifying medicine's raison d'être – a social constructionist approach, and an essentialist approach. The social constructionist approach takes into account the diverse social factors and cultural values that shape healing practices. Social constructionists hold that medicine's ends and purposes are *externally* determined and thus culturally variable.[4] According to the essentialist view, the goals of medicine are derived *internally* from values inherent in the practice of medicine. The essentialist considers such values as preventing and curing disease, relieving pain, and mitigating suffering to be invariant or unchanging.[5]

Social constructivist and essentialist approaches to specifying medicine's goals are not necessarily incompatible. While advocates of one or the other view may joust theoretically over their relative merits, it is reasonable in practice to keep the two approaches in balance or otherwise in fruitful contention where possible. This was the position taken by participants in an international study project on the goals of medicine undertaken by the Hastings Center in the mid-1990s. The project's final report puts it this way: "A medicine that has no inner direction or core values will be too easily victimized and misused by society if it lacks the resources to resist encroachment upon it .... Yet it is also naïve to think that medical values can remain uninfluenced by society. Since doctors, health care personnel, and patients will be part of society, it will never be possible to find a sharp line between the institution of medicine and other social institutions."[6]

The report called for dialogue between adherents of these two ways of thinking about what medicine ought to be for – with one caveat: the risk to medicine's integrity and to patient well-being is greater when the balance of these views tips too far in the direction of social construction.

How might this drawing be interpreted to represent the opposing views of the goals of medicine summarized in this chapter? How might what appears to be a hole, on the left, represent the essentialist view that medicine's goals are derived internally from core values? Could the black disk on the opposite page represent the social constructionist view, that the goals of medicine are applied from the outside?

Notice the background. The pattern of dots is braille, the tactile writing system created for the blind. The artist, Michael Golden, took two pages from a braille book to use as his canvas. Why would a visual artist incorporate braille pages in his work, since most viewers could not be expected to read it?

On the other hand, a blind person who could read braille, running her fingers along the rows of dot patterns, might not detect the hole or the disk because the disk and the hole are superficial. Golden created the appearance of a hole by using powdered charcoal to shade the outer circumference of a circle and to add a dark crescent of to suggest depth. Likewise, the black disk on the opposite page is only powdered charcoal applied directly to the braille sheet. There's a French term for works like this, "trompe l'oeil," which is translated as "deceive the eye." There's an element of deception in most works of art, most commonly the appearance of three-dimensional space on the two-dimensional surface of a painting.

Now that you know the hole and disk are illusions, how might you use the drawing to clarify the two perspectives on the goals of medicine?

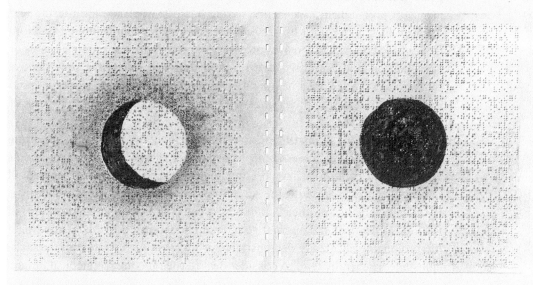

Figure 14. *Untitled* (Moons), No. 4, 1998, Michael G. Golden 1959–, (Braille text from work by James Baldwin, 1924–1987), Museum of Fine Arts, Houston, Bequest of Mary Pat Golden © Michael Golden 1998.

BALANCING APPROACHES

Over the course of four years of study and dialogue among essentialists and social constructionists, the Hastings group, comprised of individuals from humanities, biomedical sciences, clinical medicine, and social sciences, came to a consensus around four broad notions that may serve as guideposts along the path toward determining modern medicine's goals and limits: (1) disease prevention, and health maintenance and promotion; (2) relief of pain and mitigation of suffering caused by disease or injury; (3) care and cure of those with an ailment, and care for those who cannot be cured; and (4) avoidance of premature death, and pursuit of a peaceful death.

First, disease prevention and health maintenance are valuable for common-sense reasons. For example, as the public becomes knowledgeable about the dangerous health implications of tobacco use, a great deal of suffering and premature death is avoided. The same logic applies to maintaining a healthy diet, practicing safe sex, and so on.[7]

Second, avoidance of pain and suffering have long been among the main reasons people seek medical care. However, physicians generally are not prepared to respond adequately to pain of indeterminate physiological origin or to mental anguish.[8] Pain relief and the amelioration of suffering rank among traditional goals of medicine, but they merit special emphasis, especially in the United States, in view of continuing physician reluctance to prescribe adequate analgesic medication for pain, resulting in unnecessary suffering.[9]

Third, care and cure have figured historically among medicine's defining goals. But as scientific and technological methods of cure have risen to prominence in post-industrial societies, caring has often become an afterthought or given little more than lip service. This is an especially troubling development in societies where the lives of people contending with chronic diseases of aging can be made more livable with the aid of knowledgeable and attentive practitioners. To restore a healthy balance between curing and caring in modern social contexts requires a reassertion of the importance of the virtue of caring.[10]

Fourth, avoiding premature death is an obvious core goal, while supporting a peaceful death sometimes seems less so. Since the 1970s, emergency rooms and intensive care units have become highly successful in saving acutely ill patients from premature death. An unforeseen consequence of this success is that dying patients and their families have come increasingly to view rescue in the face of death as the optimal goal, even in circumstances where additional life-prolonging efforts are demonstrably of no avail. And doctors in these circumstances generally tend to consider death, when it comes, a medical failure.

These attitudes, and the practices engendered by them, are changing so slowly that it remains important to affirm humane care of the dying as a core value of modern medicine.

ENHANCING HUMAN TRAITS

The practice of medically enhancing human traits raises questions regarding the legitimate *limits* of medicine. To enhance is to make something better than it presently is, to improve it. But is it fair, say, for the parents of the runner up in last year's spelling bee to give their child a memory enhancing drug in preparation for this year's contest? The parents may see this simply as a means of enhancing their child's natural ability, ratcheting up her memory capacity, a matter of degree rather than an artificial alteration in consciousness. Questions of fairness aside, surely there is no harm in augmenting ordinary human traits, for example, by taking prescription medication to feel better if you only feel good most of the time. Or is there?[11] And if one believes that such decisions are matters of individual choice, the question remains: Does any of this appropriately belong within the purview of medicine?

Is enhancement a legitimate goal of medicine? A plastic surgeon is consulted by a person who has decided he wants to fly. Is it a legitimate medical goal for the surgeon, as long as he has the means and skill, to create "a marvel ... a person with animal parts – say, a tail or wings."[12] Why, or why not? To cite less frivolous examples, if you feel unhappy with your body, what would be wrong with asking a surgeon to change your appearance with breast augmentations or a facelift?[13] Are such enhancement techniques analogous to "working out" and staying in shape, ways of achieving the widely accepted goal of self-improvement? Does it matter that requests for such interventions are unrelated to remediation of pathology? How should surgeons respond?

To take an example other than pharmacological and surgical enhancement techniques, do doctors have a legitimate role in the practice of prenatal sex selection? As early as 1994, the ethics committee of the American Society for Reproductive Medicine said "no," arguing that medical involvement in sex selection would likely lead to gender discrimination, and would also likely eventuate in misuse of limited medical resources more appropriately utilized in the treatment of infertility. The committee also expressed concern regarding the likelihood that fertility specialists might be lured away from treating patients with infertility into this more lucrative business.[14] What the committee did not mention is that the high cost of infertility treatment puts it well beyond the reach of all but the affluent.[15]

CASE STUDY: SEX SELECTION

You are a gynecologist specializing in infertility. A married couple in their late thirties comes to you for help. Not long ago, you helped the couple conceive and the wife delivered a healthy baby girl, who is now four years old. This time they return asking for your help in conceiving and selecting a male. They argue that they are running out of time; that they desperately want a male child and their daughter wants a baby brother. They see no problem in selecting the sex of the child.

1. What is your answer to the couple?
2. What reasons do you give for agreeing or not agreeing to help them select a male baby?
3. Can you imagine a situation in which you would have responded differently?

What is medicine's role, if any, in activities such as these? Recalling the goals previously enumerated in this chapter, the relevant criteria are these: the relief of pain and suffering caused by an ailment or injury, and the care and cure of those with a malady. Using these criteria to distinguish "treatment" from "enhancement" is analogous to the distinction between efficacious treatment and futile measures in caring for gravely ill patients. When doctors reach the outer limits of medicine's ability to cure, they are, of course, expected to continue to care utilizing interventions responsive to pain and suffering. But they need not (*ought not?*) continue curative efforts. Analogizing from this "futility" distinction, Eric Juengst argues that the notion of enhancement functions similarly as a normative boundary concept. Once medicine moves beyond treatment of pathology to enhancement, it becomes just another service commodity in the commercial marketplace.[16] Moreover, as Michael J. Sandel argues, "eugenic parenting is objectionable because it expresses and entrenches a certain stance toward the world – a stance of mastery and domination that fails to appreciate the gifted character of human powers and achievements, and misses the part of freedom that consists in a persisting negotiation with the given."[17]

END-OF-LIFE CARE

Now we will turn our attention to the Hastings study group's third and fourth goals: care for those who cannot be cured, and the pursuit of a peaceful death – this latter being what the project report identifies as "perhaps [the] most humanly demanding responsibility of the physician."[18] What is the social context for this claim?

The 1960s and 1970s witnessed a growing public controversy over dissatisfaction with technologically managed rescue medicine for incurable and irreversibly dying patients. Public interest reached fever pitch during the long legal battle, journalistic coverage, and public debates culminating in the New Jersey Supreme Court ruling in the Quinlan case.[19] In the aftermath of *Quinlan,* lawyers, philosophers, physicians, and religious studies scholars concerned with questions of medical ethics, devoted special attention to relations between patients, families, and health care professionals in end-of-life care situations.

In 1978 Senator Edward Kennedy called for the establishment of "an interdisciplinary committee of professionals ... to work together to try to give the society guidance on some of the most difficult, complex, ethical and moral problems of our time,"[20] a call that led to the formation of the President's Commission for the Study of Ethical Problems in Medicine and Biomedical and Behavioral Research. Of several reports issued by the commission during its four-year tenure, *Deciding to Forego Life-Sustaining Treatment* (1983) was to become the most influential. As commissioner Albert R. Jonsen (1931–) observes, this report "endorses the patient as the most 'suitably qualified decisionmaker,' elaborates on various forms of proxy decision-making for the incompetent (stressing, for the first time, the value of 'durable power of attorney' arrangements), and sets out the considerations for resuscitation policy, for care of the permanently unconscious patient, and the ill newborn."[21]

In their influential 1979 book, *Principles of Biomedical Ethics,* Tom L. Beauchamp (1939–) and James F. Childress (1940–) advocated an approach to moral reasoning grounded in four principles, which they considered fundamental to ethically sound biomedical decision making – autonomy, nonmaleficence, beneficence, and justice [see Chapter 16].[22] The widespread adoption of the autonomy principle (the freedom to decide for oneself what course of action is most consistent with one's values and beliefs) and the informed consent requirement provided an effective antidote to physician paternalism ("doctor knows best"), prompted a fresh focus on patient prerogatives, and became the gold standard for ethical end-of-life decision making. However, although the affirmation of patient self-determination proved salutary in *decision making*, it was an insufficient guide to end-of-life *care*. There remained a need for thoughtful consideration of the existential (personal, social, and spiritual) dimensions of dying, and of the meaning of care near the end of life.[23]

DEATH AND THE SELF

In contemporary American culture, mortality has become an offensive fact and we are goaded into believing that there is nothing worse than death. Driven by this belief, we empower medicine to do whatever it takes to defeat death. Modern medicine – marvelously inventive and superbly equipped – takes us at our word and launches an all-out assault. But the enemy is unyielding and in the process of sustaining the attack, medicine neglects its other aims. In girding itself for ever-more challenging feats of death defiance, it often harms those it intends to help and squanders precious public and private resources. Ingenuity and the best materiel money can buy can keep death at bay only so long. Finally, medicine must fail, given the terms of the bargain.

Daniel Callahan (1930–) observes that these terms are not etched in stone.[24] Instead of fighting death on every front, he asks, might it be possible to pick our battles with a view not to defeating death but to shaping it to our own ends? Callahan prods us to ponder big questions about life's purposes in the hope that, with some serviceable answers in hand, we may be able to put death in perspective. "The relationship of death to the self, to the way we think about our individual fate, is the most central issue."[25]

What is this self that must die? In the culture of American individualism and autonomy, the self is a sovereign self, a maker of rational choices. The sovereign self sustains its identity through self-mastery and control of its destiny, up to and including the conditions of its dying. But as Callahan and others point out, at the end of life, the foolishness of this idea is revealed. It is I myself, an embodied, mortal self, who must die; it is I who must at some point relinquish control. If I have neglected to accommodate this important detail in my understanding of myself and have instead authorized medicine to fight death to the finish, my body is likely to become the scene of a doomed final assault, the site of death's dominion.

On the question of the right relation of death to the self, Callahan concludes that we must rethink the image of ourselves as sovereign. He invokes instead "an image of the self that is more flexible, less manipulative, more interdependent with others, more open to risk, a self appropriate to a peaceful death."[26] Instead of vainly trying to control death, Callahan recommends that we create conditions conducive to peaceful death, a death marked by an awareness that one is dying, by the relative absence of life-sustaining apparatus and, when possible, by the presence of family and friends.

In addition to the need to rethink the self and its relation to death, philosophers and theologians have reminded physicians of the moral imperative to care for the dying. In his landmark book *The Patient as Person* (1970), theologian Paul Ramsey (1913–1988) made a case for physicians' *obligation* to help patients and families prepare for a peaceful death.[27] "The patient," he argued, "has entered a covenant with the physician for his complete *care*, not for continuing useless efforts to *cure* ...."[28] He goes on, "Just as it would be negligence to the sick to treat them as if they were about to die, so it is another sort of 'negligence' to treat the dying as if they are going to get well."[29] Moreover, "What doctors should do in the presence of the process of dying is only a special case of what should be done to make a human presence felt to the dying. Desertion is more choking than death, and more feared. The chief problem of the dying is how not to die alone. To care, if only to care, for the dying is, therefore, a medical moral imperative."[30]

PREPARING FOR THE END OF LIFE

Dying in familiar surroundings in the presence of those who know us best is at the heart of the modern hospice movement, which originated in Britain,[31] got its start in America in the mid-1970s[32] and gained momentum from 1982 when hospice services became an entitlement under Medicare and the Joint Commission on Accreditation of Health Care Organizations initiated hospice accreditation (see Chapter 6). Over the ensuing twenty years, hospice care became a part of mainstream medical practice, although it remains an open question whether the hospice commitment to comfort care and attention to patients' values can be maintained in an era of cost cutting and profit making.[33]

Along with the proliferation of hospice programs came renewed attention to advance-care planning. Joan M. Teno and Joanne Lynn articulated a broad vision of such planning that reached well beyond a bare-bones determination of desired or declined life-prolonging interventions such as a do-not-resuscitate or do-not-intubate order. "Our emphasis is on advance planning as a means of communication and negotiation about the patient's life goals and the care that will be received in the final years of life .... Helping patients make the right choices for themselves is an important part of medical practice .... Physicians can't offer choices only when a patient is dying; rather a physician-patient relationship must be based on mutual understanding and shared decision making throughout the patent's clinical course."[34]

The 1990s witnessed a new professional interest in palliative care whose purpose is that of providing effective control of symptoms, especially pain management. Its major themes include: attention to the personal, social, and spiritual dimensions of dying; self-awareness on the part of caregivers regarding their own views and feelings about dying and death; and awareness of the relational nature of quality care in the final phase of life.[35] Particularly revealing of the need for better end-of-life care was a major multi-institutional study funded by the Robert Wood Johnson Foundation designed to improve end-of-life decision making and to reduce the frequency of medically supported, painful and prolonged dying.[36] The results were less than gratifying. Despite vigorous efforts to improve communication between doctors and patients, aggressive interventions aimed at prolonging life generally continued, even in the face of futility.

Over time, the drive to improve end-of-life care gained momentum within medicine. In 1997, the Institute of Medicine published a report calling for, among other measures, the creation of a new subspecialty of palliative medicine.[37] The American Board of Medical Specialties approved the creation of hospice and palliative care as a subspecialty in 2006, and in 2008, the Accreditation Council for Graduate Medical Education approved program requirements for fellowship training. An important related development was the stance taken by the Joint

Commission on Accreditation of Health Care Organizations on the need for standards for appropriate pain management.[38]

Meanwhile, informative educational resources such as *Handbook for Mortals: Guidance for People Facing Serious Illness*, and *Guidelines for Decisions on Life-Sustaining Treatment and Care Near the End of Life* were becoming available to the general public.[39] An excellent four-part Public Affairs Television series, "On Our Own Terms: Moyers on Dying," accompanied by a useful discussion guide, reached a sizable public audience when it aired in 2000.[40] And studies of the views of terminally ill patients and their families challenged long-held assumptions and professional practices.[41]

CONCLUSION

Our views about right and wrong, about what is permissible and what is impermissible, are acquired (socially constructed). To the extent that they embed themselves in our cultural habits and practices, they seem inherent and indispensable (essential). As such, they provide direction and guidance for as long as they seem serviceable or until they conflict with other equally valid views.

When a customary medical practice, such as routinely prolonging the life of dying patients, even in the face of futility, no longer seems sensible to some, the question of goals arises. What is the *purpose* of the practice? To answer this question requires that we examine the rationale for doing what we had long considered the best way to treat dying patients, even though, admittedly, we were harming them in the process. Essential values – rescue the perishing, do no harm – are pitted against each other. At this point, we must step back and ask: What are we trying to accomplish? What is the end in view toward which end-of-life care practices should be directed?

Dialogue and debate of just this sort has been occurring in commissions, committees, congregations, courts, and at countless bedsides of the dying over the past four decades. As a result, practices that are reasonable and sensible in preventing premature death are increasingly considered inappropriate in caring for dying patients. Now that we are clear about the goal of such care, we are finding better ways to reach it.

This story contains an object lesson in how we might proceed to clarify other putative goals of medicine. Recalling Hans Jonas's (1903–1993) admonition to beware of "automatic utopianism" (see Chapter 16), there are likely to be no universal principles and few bright lines demarcating medicine's legitimate scope and limits. Instead, thinking through and getting clear about medicine's ends and purposes will happen policy by policy, practice by practice, and procedure by procedure in open dialogue and debate.

SUMMATION

This chapter explored some ways of thinking about the goals of medicine. Beginning with a discussion of the two principal ways of specifying medicine's *raison d'être* – the social constructionist approach and the essentialist approach – it examined how these two seemingly incompatible approaches might be kept in balance. In particular, it discussed how a mid-1990s study by the Hastings Center found common ground between these two camps by pointing toward four broad notions that can serve as guideposts along the path toward determining modern medicine's goals and limits. Then, with a focus on enhancing human traits and end-of-life issues in America, it considered how our understanding of the goals of medicine has evolved in recent years. Overall, though, this chapter attempted to emphasize that defining the goals of medicine is a task still very much in progress.

EXERCISES FOR CRITICAL THINKING AND CHARACTER FORMATION

QUESTIONS FOR DISCUSSION

1. What are your goals when you visit a doctor? How do you communicate these goals to your doctor?
2. What, in your opinion, are your doctor's goals? How does your doctor communicate these goals to you?
3. In the mid-1990s, the Hastings Center outlined four broad goals of medicine: (1) disease prevention and health maintenance and promotion; (2) relief of pain and mitigation of suffering caused by disease or injury; (3) care and cure of those with an ailment, and care for those who cannot be cured; and (4) avoidance of premature death and the pursuit of a peaceful death. What do you think of these goals? What, given the opportunity, would you change?
4. How has technology influenced our thinking about the goals of medicine? How do you think it will influence our thinking in the future?

SUGGESTED WRITING EXERCISES

Over the past few decades, economically developed societies have entered an unprecedented era of mass longevity and aging. As we have seen in this chapter and elsewhere, however, mass longevity comes with a price tag, since many older people now experience periods of disability, frailty, dementia, and pain, as well as technologically prolonged deaths. Think about how we care for the old and what goals – both spoken and unspoken – are at issue. Then spend fifteen to twenty minutes writing about some of the challenges that the issue of aging brings to the discussion about the goals of medicine.

SUGGESTED VIEWING

On Our Own Terms: Moyers on Dying (2000)

FURTHER READING

Daniel Callahan, *False Hopes: Why America's Quest for Perfect Health is a Recipe for Failure*

Robert Martensen, *A Life Worth Living: A Doctor's Reflections on Illness in a High-tech Era*

ADVANCED READING

David Barnard, Anna Towers, Patricia Boston, and Yanna Lambrinidou, *Crossing Over: Narratives of Palliative Care*

Robert A. Burt, *Death Is That Man Taking Names: Intersections in American Medicine, Law, and Culture*

Eric J. Cassell, *The Nature of Suffering and the Goals of Medicine*

Jonathan Glover, *Choosing Children: The Ethical Dilemmas of Genetic Intervention*

Philip Kitcher, *The Lives to Come: The Genetic Revolution and Human Possibilities*

John Passamore, *The Perfectibility of Man*

Michael J. Sandel, *The Case Against Perfection: Ethics in the Age of Genetic Engineering*

JOURNALS

American Journal of Hospice and Palliative Medicine
Journal of Medicine and Philosophy
Mortality

15 Health and Disease

The conservation of health ... is without doubt the primary good and the foundation of all other good of this life.[1]

– René Descartes

Health is the absence of disease.[2]

– Christopher Boorse

Health is a state of complete physical, mental, and social well-being, and not merely the absence of disease or infirmity.[3]

– World Health Organization

ABSTRACT

This chapter explores concepts of health and disease at the crossroads of philosophy, history, and social science. Beginning with a discussion of how these concepts have important consequences in our everyday lives, it examines various holistic conceptions of health and healing; the tension between biomedical and normative conceptions of health and disease; and the special challenge posed by mental illness. Then, with a focus on the rise of narrative medicine and the recent distinction between "disease" and "illness," it considers how we might think about health and disease in the twenty-first century.

INTRODUCTION

We all want to be healthy. Yet rarely, if ever, do we stop to ask *why* we want to be healthy or what we mean by health. As the French surgeon René Leriche (1879–1955) put it in 1936, "Health is life lived in the silence of the organs."[4] It is something we take for granted – until we lose it. Once the organs break their blissful silence, we want to know why we are feverish, exhausted, or in pain. That is, we are preoccupied with disease. Perhaps that is why medical thought and practice focus more on disease than on health. But, whatever the reasons, health is more desired than understood. And disease is discussed more than health.

Concepts of health and disease have important consequences in everyday life. They directly or indirectly affect the treatment and the goals of health care; the assignment of social roles; the availability of health insurance and distribution of health care resources; and social judgments about those who are labeled healthy or sick. For the last century or so, Western society has brought more and more of life under the purview of medicine. Many behaviors and experiences that were previously understood in religious and moral terms are now understood as medical problems. The implications of this process of "medicalization" (see Chapter 2) are complex. For example, if alcoholism, homosexuality, drug addiction, menopause, or even aging are considered diseases, then they are more likely to be seen as worthy of medical research and care. And those "afflicted" with these diseases are less likely to be judged as morally deficient. On the other hand, they are subject to the surveillance and control of medical management. They may also be stigmatized as pathological and rendered less likely to take responsibility for living own their lives without the assistance of medical experts.

This chapter discusses concepts of health and disease at the crossroads of philosophy, history, and social science. That is, we will locate philosophical debates about health and disease in the context of medicalization; the history of disease; and social criticism of ideology and biopower. First, we discuss holistic concepts of health along with their social and philosophical critics who raise a number of key questions. Should health be construed merely as the absence of disease? Or should it be defined in broader terms that include meaning, purpose, and well-being? What is health good for? Is it possible to be "against health"? Next, we analyze the primary philosophical debate – between the biomedical and the normative models – about the nature of disease, followed by a discussion of the crucial distinction between disease and illness. Finally, we examine why mental health and mental illness pose the greatest challenge to the view that there can be a single, universal concept of either health or disease.

HOLISTIC CONCEPTS OF HEALTH AND HEALING

Holistic concepts of health have an enduring linguistic history. In English, the word *health* originally meant wholeness and the verb *to heal* means to make whole. Ancient Greece had two words that meant "health" – *hygeia* and *euxia* – and both connoted a sense of living well and caring rightly for one's body. The work of healing, then, means restoring wholeness or function.

Holistic concepts of health are based on the intuitively appealing idea that health is more than the absence of pathology or disease; that it involves aspects of meaning and purpose that are essential to human flourishing. The World Health Organization, formed after World War II, famously proclaimed that health is "a state of complete, physical, mental, and social well-being, and not merely the absence of disease or infirmity."[5] More recently, a Task Force of the American Association of Medical Colleges (AAMC) claimed in 1999 that, "Health is not just the absence of disease but a state of well-being that includes a sense that life has purpose and meaning."[6]

The WHO's utopian definition reflects the optimism of an era that aspired to eradicate infectious disease. Most critics consider it inflated and unrealistic.[7] Not only does the WHO's definition of health create an impossible ideal, they argue, but it also creates disappointment among physicians and patients. There is simply no way to measure "a state of complete ... well-being" or to know when it has been achieved. In addition, the WHO definition also supports the modern Western view that health is the highest good – a troubling implication that the philosopher Daniel Callahan (1930–) has nicely captured with the phrase "the tyranny of survival."[8]

Holistic definitions have also been criticized for being too broad to guide the formation of health policy. Part of the problem is the attempt to define health positively (as a measure of well-being) rather than negatively (as the absence of disease). Furthermore, the WHO defines *all* elements of social well-being – wealth, legal capacity, political power, social prestige – as a part of health. Is it always the case that wealthy people are healthier than the poor? If health is a state of complete physical, mental, and social well-being, can anyone ever be healthy? In contrast, if no one is truly healthy, is everyone ill? Does health become a regulative ideal that we are compelled to pursue but will always fail to achieve?

Despite these difficulties, there remains the enduring view that the definition of health must include elements of meaning and purpose or wholeness. For most of the twentieth century, a biomedical model of health and disease prevailed. In this model, medicine consisted of scientific diagnosis and treatment of pathology. But the last quarter of the twentieth century witnessed a renewed emphasis on the art of medicine, on the physician as healer, and on the religious and spiritual dimensions of health. From this perspective, it is not sufficient simply to address disease. The effective clinician relates to the patient as a whole person, and the quality of that relationship affects the outcome of medical care. According to Edmund Pellegrino (1920–2013), scientific knowledge is applied to the care of specific individuals as "a right and good healing action."[9] Physician writers such as Howard Brody and Eric Cassell (1928–) have claimed that healing – the restoration or recreation of meaning, identity, or purpose – is the central work of medicine.[10] In his classic work *The Nature of Suffering and the Goals of Medicine*, for example, Cassell defines healing as the restoration of wholeness in a patient whose identity and social life have become fragmented.[11] In this view, the individual patient, not the doctor, stands in a position of empowerment to define his or her health needs. The doctor becomes a partner in finding ways to meet those needs.

Others have more recently called for a definition of health that, in addition to the physical, mental, and social dimensions of human life, also includes the animate and inanimate environment. The French philosopher and physician Georges Canguilhem (1904–1995), for instance, has insisted that human health cannot be separated from the health of our planet's biodiversity.[12] Human beings do not exist in a biological vacuum but just the opposite, in a mutually dependent environment that includes microorganisms, insects, animals, and our diverse ecosystem. Thanks to the science of climate change, we now understand only too well the contingency of human well-being on the "health" of the earth's systems of energy exchange.[13]

In addition to critics from within clinical medicine, others have warned of the social and cultural dangers of a preoccupation with health, however defined. "Health," declared Ivan Illich in the 1970s, "is the most cherished and destructive certitude of the modern world. It is a most destructive addiction."[14] This "addiction," fed by for-profit medicine, hospitals, pharmaceutical companies, self-help products, and a vast array of consumer products, overwhelms critical thinking about health and the goals of medicine. In the rush to stay youthful, healthy, and vigorous, consumers fail to ask what health is *for*.

In order to avoid these pitfalls, Leon Kass (1939–) counsels us to avoid the "false" goals of medicine. The first of these illusory goals, he argues, is the insatiable drive toward happiness or pleasure.[15] Kass attributes the false goal of happiness to the open-ended character of some contemporary notions of mental health, which consider frustration, anxiety, or unsatisfied desires to be marks of ill health rather than part of the human condition. Another false goal is "social adjustment" – creating a "healthy" society devoid of crime, poverty, or laziness – that in Kass's view lies outside the purview of doctors. Responsibility for creating a "healthy society" and healthy lifestyles, he argues, rests with policymakers, public health professionals, parents, clergy, teachers, and judges. And finally, Kass argues that we should avoid the goal of prolonging life indefinitely or escaping death altogether. To be alive and healthy are not the same. We are born with two inescapable "diseases" – aging and mortality – and, for Kass, medicine should be concerned with reconciling itself to these conditions rather than transcending them.

Another line of criticism comes from those who warn against "health" as a cultural enforcer of existing forms of domination. "Health," as Jonathan Metzl writes, "is a term replete with value judgments, hierarchies, and blind assumptions that speak as much about power and privilege as they do about well-being."[16] When we see someone smoking a cigarette and remark, "smoking is bad for your health," what do we really mean? Often, what we really mean is "you are a bad person because you smoke." Likewise, the comment "Obesity is bad for your health" may be less about a medical problem than about the implicit assumption that the person is lazy or weak of will. These values are easily wrapped into public health advertisements. One recent Michigan campaign, for instance, shows children left alone in homes or in cars, where they are helplessly left to breathe the second-hand smoke of their parents. "When you smoke around your kids," the narrator explains, "it's like they're smoking."[17] While the commercial rightly points out the dangers of smoking, it links the act with personal traits – negligence, irresponsibility – implying that the disease of smoking decays not only the body but also the soul.

Indeed, many forms of popular media – television, film, magazines – stealthily attach values to health that go unnoticed. Magazines such as *Health*, *Men's Health*, *Women's Health*, *Cosmopolitan*, and many others all share the assumption that health is intimately tied to a person's appearance and their sexual and athletic performance. They tout the importance of proper body image under the label of a "healthy" lifestyle: nice skin, toned abs, bulging biceps, even plastic surgery. In presenting these physical practices as part of a healthy lifestyle (rather than as the product of cultural narcissism) these and other "health" magazines actually construct certain bodies as desirable and others as unwanted or repulsive.

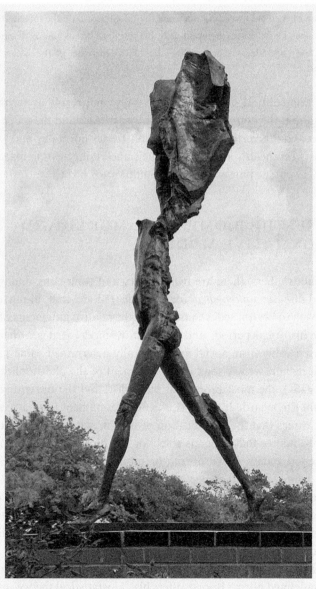

Figure 15. *Winged Victory* (Winged Woman Walking X), 1995, Stephen De Staebler 1933–2001, University of Houston, Moores Opera House, Courtesy Stephen De Staebler Estate.

Could she fly? Why would someone with wings be striding forward as this figure does? How could someone who appears to have suffered so much ruin appear so forceful? Does the absence of the figure's head suggest that it is mindless? Or could it refer to ancient sculptures, which, over the centuries, have lost heads, arms, feet, and other parts and yet still have the power to inspire us? Ancient sculptures often represented human perfection. What sort of ideal does this figure represent?

Speaking of his sculpture, artist Stephen De Staebler said, "We are all wounded survivors, alive but devastated selves, fragmented, isolated – the condition of modern man. Art tries to restructure reality so that we can live with the suffering." Is this the way a physician, an orthopedist, for example, would describe a patient's condition?

No physician or medical test could diagnose the diseases or cure the injuries this figure displays. How does De Staebler's figure fit into this chapter's discussion of disease, which happens to the body, and illness, which is the individual's experience of the disease?

Within this cultural climate, each new research result or technology raises questions about the boundaries of health and disease and the scope of medicine. We are less and less certain about what constitutes normalcy and where to draw the line between health and disease. Such uncertainty is one reason that some philosophers pursue purely scientific definitions of health.

DISEASE: THE BIOMEDICAL MODEL AND THE NORMATIVE MODEL

Among philosophers, there are two primary and competing understandings of health and disease: a *biomedical* (or *naturalist*) model that, in pursuing a value-free approach to health, seeks to transcend the relative judgments of a particular culture or historical period; and a *normative* model that sees health and disease as inseparable from social and culturally determined value judgments. To review this debate, we will look at the argument of the philosopher Christopher Boorse (1946–), the most prominent naturalist, and the dissenting response of H. Tristram Englehardt Jr. (1941–), the most prominent normativist.

Boorse argues that the classification of human states as healthy or diseased is an objective matter that depends solely on the biological facts of nature rather than value judgments, social norms, or subjective considerations.[18] As a result, disease is defined without respect to the implications for its bearer – whether the impact on an individual is good or bad, happiness generating or otherwise. A state of disease is taken simply to be one that interferes with proper or normal physiological functioning. Conversely, health is the absence of disease or the presence of proper physiological functioning.

But what constitutes "proper functioning?" How does one measure a deviation from an undefined norm? Boorse offers his "biostatistical theory" as a value-free way of differentiating between healthy body states and diseased body states.[19] The premises of this theory are that a healthy condition is normal, that disease is abnormal, and that the normal is derived from a statistical average. As he puts it, "the average person – or at least the average heart, lung, kidney, thyroid, etc. – must be normal, or we would have no way of telling what the normal person or organ should be like."[20] Any impairment of normal, natural functions – e.g., breathing, excretion, digestion – is considered a state of disease. Normality is thus defined statistically along a continuum of pathology and health.

In Boorse's model, a person, organ, or biological system is healthy only if it is functioning in a manner at or above the statistically normal level of functioning for entities of that type. Similarly, an entity is diseased if it is functioning at a level below the statistically normal level of functioning for entities of that type. The disease label is applied once it falls more than a certain distance below the population mean – a distance that, as Boorse himself admits, is to some extent arbitrary, since the precise line between disease and health cannot be determined.[21] Nevertheless, Boorse declares that his biostatistical model "looks in every way continuous with theory in biology and the other natural sciences, and I believe it to be value-free."[22]

Boorse acknowledges that his value-free theory of health is both controversial and radical. In fact, most writers on the subject have challenged the notion that disease can be understood in exclusively biological terms.[23] The *normativist model* sees health as a concept that both describes factual conditions and contains an assessment of whether these conditions are good or bad. As H. Tristram Englehardt (1941–) puts it, referring to Boorse's biostatistical method: "Statistical and functional analysis is ultimately a matter of values and, thus, invention – not only description."[24] In Englehardt's opinion, to see a phenomenon as a disease, deformity, or disability is to see something wrong with it. While this judgment is not a moral one – the question is not whether a person is good or bad, innocent or evil – it nevertheless involves an aesthetic consideration of human form and function. "That is a beautiful sunset" is a similar aesthetic judgment to "that is an ugly body," which has its roots in a sense of anatomical, physiological, and psychological achievement and realization.[25] Diseases, illnesses, and deformities can thus be seen as failures to achieve an expected state.

In other words, we see the world through our social expectations and through knowledge systems that are historically and culturally conditioned. These contexts – the Western medical tradition, for example – shape our understanding of conditions like heart disease, cancer, depression, homosexuality, or AIDS. The consensus on what "counts" as disease – what should be considered socially permissible or repugnant – changes radically over time and across culture. Indeed, by classifying various conditions or behaviors as disease, medicine has often disguised and reinforced existing power relations and/or prevailing moral values. In the American South before the Civil War, for example, Dr. Samuel A. Cartwright (1793–1863) described the disease "drapetomania" as a mental illness that caused black slaves to flee captivity.[26] Slightly more than a century later, psychiatrists at Ionia State Hospital in Michigan diagnosed blacks who espoused Civil Rights ideas with schizophrenia.[27] The political uses of disease concepts in psychiatry have also been closely connected with repressive goals and political agendas of certain governments. From the 1960s to the 1990s, for instance, the abuse of psychiatry for political purposes was reported to be systematic in the Soviet Union and other Eastern European countries.[28]

In addition, masturbation was once seen as a serious disease for which castration, excision of the clitoris, and other invasive therapies were employed. Individuals were even determined to have died of masturbation, with postmortem findings "substantiating" this claim. Similarly, homosexuality – which had long been considered morally repugnant – was labeled as a psychiatric disease in the 1950s, when the first edition of the American Psychiatric Association's *Diagnostic and Statistical Manual (DSM)* was published. Psychiatric classification was so closely aligned with the unquestioned cultural definition of normal as heterosexual that gays and lesbians were forced to hide their identities or face ostracism, discrimination, and forced medical treatment. At psychiatric meetings in the 1950s and the 1960s, gay and lesbian psychiatrists met in secret and even risked their jobs if they revealed their sexual orientation. Not until 1973 was homosexuality declassified in the second edition of the *DSM*. As the examples of drapetomania, masturbation, and homosexuality demonstrate, by framing social or moral transgressions of cultural norms as a matter of scientific objectivity or "fact," societies have used concepts of disease to impose social and political control.

Finally, the very act of naming something a disease or of calling a person "sick" has profound social implications. Consider the reaction of a person who has just been told that they have serious heart disease. Their experience of lived reality is transformed. A brief shortness of breath walking up the stairs, once dismissed as a normal moment of fatigue, now becomes a sign of disease. Previously innocent activities – eating, sleeping, exercising, recreation – now become serious matters of health, if not of life and death. One must now take medication, pills, and conform to a new diet in order to lower salt and cholesterol intake. The individual's view of life and her role in society has been fundamentally reshaped. Her life will never be the same.

To call a person "sick" then, is not only to inform her that she has a disease; it may also cast her into a "sick role" in which certain societal expectations are altered.[29] Some of these might include: (1) excusing ill individuals from some or all of their usual responsibilities (especially work); (2) considering them not responsible for their illness, although their behavior may have actually caused the disease; and/or (3) expecting them to seek out experts to treat their illness.

Essentially, the normativist position asks, What values shape concepts of health and disease, and to what extent are these concepts culturally determined? Contrary to Boorse, Englehardt insists that a value-free account of disease cannot exist because diseases are defined not only by their causes, but also by effects that gain significance within a cultural context. Nevertheless, the naturalist and the normativist positions need not always be seen as mutually exclusive. Many examples of disease – e.g., ischemic stroke, appendicitis, or cardiac arrest – suggest that value-laden meanings may be less important than urgent diagnosis and treatment using the best statistical evidence available.

THE SPECIAL CASE OF MENTAL ILLNESS

Mental health and mental illness pose the greatest challenge to the view that there can be a single, universal concept of either health or disease. Broadly speaking, the debate over mental illness concerns whether it is an objective phenomenon rooted in the body or a subjective phenomenon rooted in the mind, or various combinations of both. The idea that "insanity" is fundamentally different from other illnesses – that it is a disease of the mind rather than the body – is relatively new. Prior to the eighteenth century, "insanity" or "melancholia" were considered bodily illnesses similar to most other diseases.[30] Thanks to Descartes' (1596–1650) earlier famous dictum "I think, therefore I am," however, the mind was increasingly seen as distinct from the body. In addition, the development of private madhouses and large public asylums in the nineteenth century took the care of the mentally ill out of the hands of general physicians. By the mid-twentieth century, the terms "disease of the mind," "disorder of the mind," and "mental illness" were commonplace.

The linguistic distinction between mental and physical illnesses remains common today. Both laypersons and some medical professionals assume that, as a disorder of the mind rather than the body, mental illness is fundamentally different from other illness. There is a further, damaging assumption that the symptoms of mental disorders are in some sense less "real" than those of other disorders, which are rooted in physical, visible lesions of the body rather than merely "in the mind." From this perspective, it is tempting to regard "mental illness" as evidence of a certain lack of moral fiber or to assume that people with mere mental illnesses ought to be able to control themselves and, through an act of willpower, "snap out of it." For the psychiatrist Thomas Szasz (1920–2012), who represents an extreme version of this view, mental illness is merely a "myth."[31] What psychiatrists and society call mental illness, claims Szasz, is actually the challenges of one's life – struggles that are altogether normal.

Most psychologists and scientists today, however, assert that there is no separating mental from physical disease. As Nobel Laureate Eric Kandel (1929–), professor of Bain Science at Columbia puts it: "All mental process are brain processes. The brain is the organ of the mind. Where else could [mental illness] be if not in the brain.... Schizophrenia is a disease like pneumonia. Seeing it as a brain disorder destigmatizes it immediately."[32] Why, then, do we insist on distinguishing between mental and physical illness? A compelling answer appears in the fourth edition of *The Diagnostic and Statistical Manual of Mental Disorders (DSM)*, the authoritative publication of the American Psychiatric Association for more than sixty years. The goal of the *DSM* is to provide a common language and standard criteria for the classification of mental disorders. But finding precise language to solve this problem remains elusive. As the authors of the *DSM-IV-TR* put it:

> [T]he term mental disorder unfortunately implies a distinction between 'mental' disorders and 'physical' disorders that is a reductionistic anachronism of mind/body dualism. A compelling literature documents that there is much 'physical' in 'mental' disorders and much 'mental' in 'physical' disorders. The problem raised by the term 'mental disorders' has been much clearer than its solution, and, unfortunately, the term persists in the title of *DSM-IV* because we have no found an appropriate substitute.[33]

Debates about naming and classifying "mental illness" persist even within psychiatry and psychology – so much so that, when the fifth edition of the *DSM* was released in 2013, biologically based psychiatrists criticized the volume because it categorized diseases based on clusters of symptoms that were not tied to brain malfunction and drug therapies aimed at correcting them. Shortly afterward, the National Institute of Mental Health (NIMH) announced that it would no longer fund research based on *DSM* symptom clusters.

While neuropsychiatry improves our understanding of the biological basis of major mental disorders, the distinction between brain and mind remains essential. The brain may be the seat or cause of disease, but the human experience of mental disease is always filtered and shaped by environment and personal experience. Put another way, although there is an essential neural substrate to mental functioning, the brain does not explain all of the mind. In the next section, we will see that the distinction between "disease" and "illness" can shed light on this problem in psychiatry and in other aspects of medical care.

As contemporary psychiatrists and neuroscientists continue to shed light on the biological connections between the body and the mind, a rich assortment of personal writing about the experience of mental illness has emerged over the past quarter century. These autobiographical works or "pathographies," discussed in Chapter 7, describe the experience of depression, bipolar disease, and many other conditions. They break down cultural stereotypes by describing illness in descriptive, personal ways. Novelist William Styron (1925–2006), for instance, wrote his powerful memoir *Darkness Visible* in the wake of his experience with terrible depression. He suggests that depression, and mental illness in general, is wrongly dismissed by the public as less severe or important than physical illness (see Chapter 7 for more discussion of Styron). In *An Unquiet Mind*, Kay Jamison (1946–), a noted psychiatrist and expert in bipolar disease, wrote a moving memoir about her own experience of bipolar disease, also known as manic-depression. "Manic-depression," she writes, "distorts moods and thoughts, incites dreadful behaviors, destroys the basis of rational thought, and too often erodes the desire and will to live. It is an illness that is biological in its origins, yet one that feels psychological in the experience of it; an illness that it unique is conferring advantage and pleasure, yet one that brings in its wake almost unendurable suffering and, not infrequently, suicide."[34]

Elsewhere, Jamison has argued for an association between artistic creativity and manic-depressive temperaments.[35] Drawing from a rich tradition of artists including George Byron (1788–1824), Herman Melville (1819–1891), Ernest Hemingway (1899–1961), Virginia Woolf (1882–1941), and many others, Jamison challenges the normative association of health as positive and disease as negative. Mental illness can lead to great outpourings of creativity; it can lead, even in the midst of great pain, to moments of strange beauty. Russian novelist Fyodor Dostoevsky (1821–1881) captures some of this complexity in *The Idiot*, where the epileptic protagonist Prince Myshkin vacillates between interpreting his disease as a religious experience and as a disease. Before the "sadness, spiritual darkness and oppression" that accompanies an epileptic attack, Myshkin enjoys a few seconds of inexpressible ecstasy during which "his mind and his heart were flooded with extraordinary light; all his uneasiness, all his doubts, all his anxieties were relieved at once; they were all merged in a lofty calm full of serene, harmonious joy and hope."[36] Myshkin's efforts to understand his pre-epileptic sensations take the form of an unresolved contest between religious and medical explanations, thus questioning any clear-cut line between health and disease. As the great French writer Marcel Proust (1871–1922) put it – speaking, perhaps, with himself in mind – "Everything great comes from neurotics. They alone have founded religions and composed our masterpieces."[37]

CARING FOR THE PERSON

Given the strident disagreement between various conceptions of health and disease, and especially diseases of the brain, what common ground exists to aid in care of the patient as person? Here, efforts to bridge the gulf between biological science and human experience have been strengthened by the philosophical distinction between "disease" and "illness." According to Leon Eisenberg (1922–2009), the difference between disease and illness can be summed up in this way: "Patients suffer 'illnesses'; physicians diagnose and treat 'diseases' ... illnesses are *experiences* of disvalued changes in states of being and in social function; diseases, in the scientific paradigm of modern medicine, are *abnormalities* in the *structure* and *function* of body organs and systems.[38] Disease – what happens to the body – is understood through science. Illness – what the person experiences – involves an engagement with one's body that is not only physiological, but also social and experiential.

The distinction between disease and illness is especially important in the context of medical humanities. Without discounting the importance of the biological, much of the field centers on how individuals experience health, disease, suffering, and dying. As George Engel (1913–1999) insisted in 1980, clinical medicine is not only biomedical but also psychological and social: "The traditional biomedical view, that biological indices are the ultimate criteria in defining disease, leads to the present paradox that some people with positive laboratory findings are told that they are in need of treatment when in fact they are feeling quite well, while others feeling sick reassured that they are well, that is, they have no 'disease.'"[39] Health and illness, in other words, cannot be understood with lab results alone but only by attending to the patient's larger psychological and social environment. Engel's biopsychosocial model of medicine is an attempt to bridge the gulf between science and experience, which, as we noted in the introduction, is a central function of medical humanities.

In addition to Engel's path-breaking work, scholars and clinicians in the last twenty years have come to see religion and spirituality as key factors in understanding disease and facilitating health and healing. It may seem like too much to try, as some have suggested, to expand Engel into a "bio-psycho-social-spiritual" model, but there is no doubt, as we see in Section Four, that religion and spirituality are central both to understanding health and disease and to caring for patients.

From the perspective of caregiving, it is helpful for clinicians to remember the distinction between treating diseases and caring for persons who are ill. And it is here that patient narratives, which (as we saw in Chapter 4) had been dismissed as subjective and unreliable since the nineteenth century, are now understood as indispensable to good patient care. As Rita Charon (1949–) noted, narrative competence – the ability to evoke and interpret a patient's verbal account of his or her illness, taking into account a host of factors – is important both for diagnosing disease and for healing illness.[40] Serious disease or illness is a major disruption in the story a patient tells herself about her life. It is almost as if the patient says, "doc, my story's broke."[41] Helping her recover from illness involves helping her tell a new story in the context of medical treatment ("I can bear the burden of dialysis. As hard as it is, I will be able to live and enjoy my family while I wait for a kidney transplant"). The doctor might help the patient to ask, How have I been trained to think of my body, modern medicine, and doctors? How does my disease involve my family, my job, or other levels of society? Providing opportunities for conversations about such questions makes possible emotional and spiritual *healing*, whether or not physical *curing* (to use another important distinction) is possible.

Narrative medicine thus recognizes that a purely biomedical approach to medicine cannot help a patient find meaning or healing in the face of serious, disabling, or terminal disease. Along with their medical expertise, doctors can listen to their patients in order to better understand and help reconstruct their life stories. To return to the distinction previously mentioned, a narrow attention to what happens to the body (disease) cannot wholly account for the lived experiences of patients who struggle with illness. Ideally, treating disease and caring for persons who are ill go hand in hand.

Philosophy of medicine, like philosophy in general, flourishes not by giving correct answers but by engaging in fruitful debates. This is especially true when considering definitions of health and disease. As we have seen, health is more generally desired than understood and disease occupies more of our personal, biomedical, and philosophical attention. Health can be defined broadly, as in the WHO definition, or narrowly as in Boorse's view of health as the absence of disease. The central debate surrounding disease is whether it can be defined universally, using value-free, biomedical, and statistical terms, or whether concepts of disease cannot be separated from historical and cultural norms and values. In the main, philosophers and scholars have sided with the latter view. Mental illness confuses the whole debate because its experiential, cultural, and historical components coexist with an unquestionable neurological substrate, leading to the ongoing debate about the relative influence of the "mental" and the "physical" in mental illness. Finally, the distinction between "disease" (what happens to the body) and "illness" (the individual's experience of disease) offers a valuable bridge between objective science and personal experience. This distinction reminds physicians and health care professionals that attention to both the diseased body and the ill person is the goal of humanistic care of the patient.

SUMMATION

This chapter explored concepts of health and disease at the crossroads of philosophy, history, and social science. Beginning with a discussion of how these concepts have important consequences in our everyday lives, it examined various holistic conceptions of health and healing; the tension between biomedical and normative conceptions of health and disease; and the special challenge posed by mental illness. Then, with a focus on recent conceptual distinctions and the rise of narrative medicine, it considered how we might think about health and disease in the twenty-first century. Overall, this chapter emphasized that a narrow attention to what happens to the body cannot wholly account for the lived experiences of patients who struggle with illness, and that a greater awareness of various forms of health and disease this can enhance both treatment of disease and care for individuals who are ill.

EXERCISES FOR CRITICAL THINKING AND CHARACTER FORMATION

QUESTIONS FOR DISCUSSION

1. How do you know when you are sick? Is it when you feel sick or when a doctor gives you a diagnosis?
2. Do you agree with Thomas Szasz that mental illness is a "myth"? Why or why not?

3. Do you think that obesity is a disease? If so, who is responsible for its prevention and cure?

SUGGESTED WRITING EXERCISE

Write, for about twenty minutes, on what it means to be healthy. After you finish, reflect on your response. How does your own view compare to the different understandings of health in the chapter? Does your definition tend to be broad (like the WHO's) or narrow (like Christopher Boorse's)?

SUGGESTED VIEWING

The Biggest Loser (television series, 2004 –)

FURTHER READING

Fyodor Dostoevsky, *The Idiot*
Mark Haddon, *The Curious Incident of the Dog in the Nighttime*
Kay Jamison, *An Unquiet Mind*

Men's Health (periodical)
William Styron, *Darkness Visible*

ADVANCED READING

Christoper Boorse, "A Rebuttal on Health," in *What is Disease?*
Arthur Caplan, Tristram Englehardt, Jr., and James McCartney, *Concepts of Health and Disease: Interdisciplinary Perspectives*

Eric Cassell, *The Nature of Suffering and the Goals of Medicine*
Thomas Szasz, *The Myth of Mental Illness: Foundations of a Theory of Personal Conduct*

JOURNALS

Disability Studies Quarterly
Journal of Medicine and Philosophy

16 Moral Philosophy and Bioethics

The real work of bioethics, more often than not, is in listening, reading, and watching carefully in order to judge what is important and what is not.[1]

– Carl Elliott

ABSTRACT

This chapter explores the emergence of bioethics as a distinctive form of moral philosophy. Beginning with a discussion of the public's mounting unease with the applications and implications of "big" science and "rescue" medicine, it examines the birth of bioethics in the 1960s and the subsequent contributions of key thinkers such as K. Danner Clouser, Daniel Callahan, Tom L. Beauchamp and James F. Childress, Robert M. Veatch, and H. Tristram Engelhardt Jr. Then, with a focus on contemporary exchanges between recent ethical approaches, it considers how we might address some of the moral challenges facing medicine in the twenty-first century.

INTRODUCTION

As we have seen in previous chapters (4, 6, and 14) concerns about the ethics of clinical and research medicine began to surface in the 1960s. Revelations of abuse led to a call for public mechanisms to govern medical research involving human subjects. Surgical and pharmacological advances in the transplantation of vital organs generated new uncertainties about the definition and determination of death. And public unease mounted regarding the use of new technologies that often seemed to prolong life at the expense of dignity in dying. Medicine was becoming morally unsettled.

Before the 1960s, medical ethics was considered the province of physicians alone. Guided by professional norms, codes of ethics, and the moral authority of medicine, doctors typically made treatment decisions based on their own judgment. New advances in medicine and biotechnology, however, raised issues that could not be resolved by the traditional moral authority of physicians or with the outmoded intellectual tools of medical ethics. Increasingly, patients expressed a desire to be included in decision making regarding their medical care, and the public grew skeptical about the unchecked professional discretion of biomedical scientists. This chapter surveys some of the public involvement and intellectual ferment that accompanied the birth of a distinctive form of moral philosophy – bioethics – in the last three decades of the twentieth century.

THE BIRTH OF BIOETHICS: CONTROVERSY AND SCANDAL

To some extent, bioethics was born in response to controversy and scandal. In 1962, *LIFE* magazine published an article by journalist Shana Alexander (1925–2005) describing the proceedings of a lay committee appointed by the local county medical society in Seattle to decide who should get access to the newly effective life-saving technology of kidney dialysis. In "They Decide Who Lives, Who Dies,"[2] Alexander noted that among the criteria to which the committee appealed in making life-or-death decisions were age (under forty-five), state of residence (Washington), family considerations (preference for heads of households), church membership, and likely future contributions to society. By virtue of its large readership, the *LIFE* article provoked widespread public consternation and heralded the need for serious consideration of how to maximize fairness in the allocation of limited medical resources.

CASE STUDY: THE LIFE OR DEATH COMMITTEE

The meetings of the Life or Death Committee are held in the small, ground-floor library of a nurse's residence hall in downtown Seattle. The room is actually only a few hundred feet away from the three-bed Kidney Center where John Myers and his fellow patients come to be hooked up to their life-giving machines. But save for the comings and goings of the white coated doctors, there is absolutely no traffic between the two rooms. Neither the patients nor the committee wish any such confrontations. Their relationship is far too intimate for casual informality. To protect the integrity of their work, the members of the committee do not disclose exactly how many meetings they have held or how many patients they have considered. But neither do they wish to conceal the way they try to reach a decision, and all seven members have contributed to the preparation of the following facsimile. The dialogue has been pieced together from the memories of the people who spoke it. If the exchanges as recorded here seem stilted, the people are nonetheless real, as are the five patients under discussion, and the dynamics of the debate are wholly accurate. The lawyer, who is the committee's chairman, has just called the meeting to order.[3]

LAWYER: The doctors have told us they will soon have two more vacancies at the Kidney Center, and they have submitted a list of five candidates for us to choose from.

HOUSEWIFE: Are they all equally sick?

DR. MURRAY: (John A. Murray, M.D., Medical Director of the Kidney Center.) Patients Number One and Number Five can last only a couple more weeks. The others probably can go a bit longer. But for purposes of your selection, all five cases should be considered of equal urgency, because none of them can hold out until another treatment facility becomes available.

LAWYER: Are there any preliminary ideas?

BANKER: Just to get the ball rolling, why don't we start with Number One – the housewife from Walla Walla.

SURGEON: This patient could not commute for the treatment from Walla Walla, so she would have to find a way to move her family to Seattle.

BANKER: Exactly my point. It says here that her husband has no funds to make such a move.

LAWYER: Then you are proposing we eliminate this candidate on the grounds that she could not possibly accept treatment if it were offered?

MINISTER: How can we compare a family situation of two children, such as this woman in Walla Walla, with a family of six children such as patient Number Four – the aircraft worker?

STATE OFFICIAL: But are we sure the aircraft worker can be rehabilitated? I note he is already is too ill to work, whereas Number Two and Number Five, the chemist and the accountant, are both still able to keep going.

LABOR LEADER: I know from experience that the aircraft company where this man works will do everything possible to rehabilitate a handicapped employee ....

HOUSEWIFE: If we are still looking for the men with the highest potential of service to society, I think we must consider that the chemist and the accountant have the finest educational backgrounds of all five candidates.

SURGEON: How do the rest of you feel about Number Three – the small businessman with three children? I am impressed that his doctor took special pains to mention this man is active in church work. This is an indication to me of character and moral strength.

HOUSEWIFE: Which certainly would help him conform to the demands of the treatment ....

LAWYER: It would also help him to endure a lingering death ....

STATE OFFICIAL: But that would seem to be placing a penalty on the very people who perhaps have the most provident ....

MINISTER: And both these families have three children too.

LABOR LEADER: For the children's sake, we've got to reckon with the surviving parents opportunity to remarry, and a woman with three children has a better chance to find a new husband than a very young widow with six children.

SURGEON: How can we possibly be sure of that? [4]

1. Read the dialogue carefully and try to piece together the logic. What are the criteria for choosing one candidate over another?
2. Would you serve on the Life or Death Committee? Why or why not?
3. Why do you think Alexander's article provoked widespread consternation?

Shana Alexander's article was followed by signal events and widespread public interest: in abuses in clinical research; the ethics of transplantation; racism in government-sponsored research; and decision making in caring for impaired newborns. Four years after the publication of Alexander's *LIFE* magazine story, an article titled "Ethics and Clinical Research" appeared in the prestigious *New England Journal of Medicine*. Its author, prominent Harvard anesthesiologist Henry K. Beecher (1904–1976), presented the results of a literature review that revealed numerous ethical lapses in experiments with human subjects.[5]

The next year, South African surgeon Christiaan Barnard (1922–2001) performed the world's first heart transplant, raising a host of ethical questions (see Chapter 6), including who should have access to this new procedure. Once it became technically feasible to transplant vital organs, conflict-of-interest questions arose. Traditional medical ethics enjoined physicians to do what was best for and avoid harm to patients in their care. But how to do this when what is best for one patient depends on the death of another person? In these circumstances, was it morally sufficient for the transplant surgeon alone to determine the death of the organ donor, as had been the customary practice?

The scope of physician discretion in life-or-death decision making surfaced in yet another context in the early 1970s in what came to be known as the Johns Hopkins baby case in which parents requested that life-saving surgery be withheld from their newborn with Down's syndrome. The ensuing controversy over appropriate care of impaired newborns and about who should be involved in such decisions ranged widely through the medical journals and the popular press.[6]

In 1972, the *New York Times* broke the story of the Tuskegee Syphilis Study in which a group of illiterate African American men in Alabama were unwitting subjects in a U.S. Public Health Service study of syphilis. Because the researchers wanted to follow the full course of the "natural history" of syphilis, the men were not offered curative treatment when it became available.[7]

In the 1970s, the federal government established several commissions that put forth moral principles, federal guidelines and requirements and laws, which came to regulate both research and clinical care. In 1974, following the Tuskegee scandal, Congress created the first of these, known as the National Commission for the Protection of Human Subjects of Biomedical and Behavioral Research. The National Commission produced a series of reports, including *Research Involving Prisoners* (1976), *Research Involving Children* (1977), *Psychosurgery* (1977), *Disclosure of Research Information* (1977), *Research Involving Those*

Institutionalized as Mentally Infirm (1978), *Institutional Review Boards* (1978), and *Delivery of Health Services* (1978).

Near the end of its tenure, the Commission also published *The Belmont Report,* articulating the principles it deemed fundamental to the conduct of biomedical and behavioral research involving human subjects: respect for persons, beneficence, and justice.[8] These principles were accompanied by applications that eventually came to regulate the conduct of federally sponsored research: informed consent; assessment of benefits and burdens; and selection of subjects. These principles proliferated throughout the bioethics literature and, as noted by Commissioner Albert R. Jonsen (1931–), one of the drafters of The Belmont Report, "grew from the principles underlying the conduct of research into the basic principles of bioethics."[9]

BIOETHICS AND PHILOSOPHY

Given their long history of addressing moral questions, one would have expected philosophers to play a central role in addressing the controversial ethical quandaries arising in biomedicine. But in the United States at mid-century, moral philosophy as an existential and practical enterprise was more or less moribund. Anglo-American philosophers in the first half of the twentieth century had been principally preoccupied with analyzing the logic of moral discourse with mathematic-like precision, with the aim of clearing up the vagueness and ambiguity of ordinary language.[10] Conceived thus, the scope of philosophical deliberation about moral questions was necessarily limited. Philosophers were mostly in dialogue with other philosophers.[11]

This was not the case, however, with continental European philosophers who were accustomed to engaging in broad-ranging inquiry into questions of meaning and responsibility in the cultural context of modernity. In a seminal 1973 article, Hans Jonas (1903–1993) observed that pre-modern ethics set out from some basic beliefs: that the human condition was given; that the range of human action for good or ill was therefore narrowly circumscribed; and that, in that light, the human good was "known in its generality" and largely uncontroversial.[12] However, with the advent of modern science and our acquisition of novel technological powers, the nature of human action had changed. "The qualitatively novel nature of certain of our actions has opened up a whole new dimension of ethical relevance for which there is no precedent in the standards and canons of traditional ethics."[13] In a world in which the circumstances of the human condition were believed to be largely impervious to human intervention, "the question was only how to relate to the stubborn fact."[14] But as modern Western society acquired new knowledge and exercised the power to alter nature, the human condition turned out to be more malleable than we had thought. This was both a promising and a problematic prospect, since decisions now had to be made in the absence of comforting metaphysical and moral constraints. "The promised gift [of new knowledge and power] raises questions that had never to be asked before in terms of practical choice, and ... no principle of former ethics, which took the human constants for granted, is competent to deal with them."[15] In Jonas's view, the new task of ethics was to counter the drift toward "automatic utopianism"[16] – doing something because it is doable and seemingly desirable at the moment. What Jonas called "automatic utopianism" paid scant attention to the value of an action in the long term or in a larger scheme of things, and it paid little attention to possible unintended consequences.

Jonas's reflections on the existential questions raised by big science and rescue medicine were uncommon. In the 1970s, when philosophers began to turn their attention to the relationship of philosophical ethics to medical ethics, most adopted a more circumscribed approach. "Medical ethics," wrote K. Danner Clouser (1930–2000), the first philosopher appointed to an American medical school faculty, "is simply ethics applied to a particular area of our lives – roughly the area touched by medicine .... 'Structuring' the issues is an analytic dissection ... perhaps the central contribution of medical ethics." Moreover, "structuring in itself does not necessarily mean making a decision on what to do in the situation. It simply lays out the issues, bringing the hidden problems and principles to the surface." Notable about Clouser's description is that doing medical ethics philosophically was understood to be *analytic* work that stops short of making ethical judgments.[17]

But philosophers in this new field did not all hold the same view of their job description. In the 1973 inaugural issue of the *Hastings Center Report*, Daniel Callahan (1930–), an influential founder of the field, articulated a more expansive view in calling for the creation of an interdisciplinary field of *bioethics* that would bring philosophers and theologians into dialogue with physicians and biomedical scientists to address pressing ethical issues in both science and medicine. Unlike Clouser's understanding of a medical ethics that analyzes problems without making ethical judgments, Callahan advocated a search for "a philosophically viable *normative* ethic [emphasis added] which can presuppose some commonly shared principles" and help "scientists and physicians make the right decisions"[18] – "normative" meaning an ethic concerned with fundamental questions of traditional moral philosophy: What should we be? What should we do? What roles should medicine and science play in society? Callahan's vision of bioethics was that of an ongoing dialogue in pursuit of guidance in thinking through moral questions arising in anticipation of, and in the wake of, scientific, medical, and technological advances.

The year 1979 saw the publication of Tom L. Beauchamp (1939–) and James F. Childress's (1940–) *Principles of Biomedical Ethics,* which, along with its sister document *The Belmont Report,* would become immensely influential.[19] Beauchamp and Childress introduced their book thus: "Many books in the rapidly expanding field of biomedical ethics focus on a series of problems such as abortion, euthanasia, behavior control, research involving human subjects, and the distribution of health care. Rarely do these books concentrate on the principles that should apply to a wide range of biomedical problems .... Only by examining moral principles and determining how they should apply to cases and how they conflict can we bring some order and coherence to the discussion of these problems. Only then can we see that there are procedures and standards for deliberation and justification in biomedical ethics that parallel those in other areas of human activity."

This principles-and-applications approach, which came to be called "principlism," became henceforth a touchstone for a still nascent bioethics, which would be based on the *prima facie* principles of autonomy (respect for individuals' right to make choices and decisions based on their personal values and beliefs), nonmaleficence (an obligation to refrain from causing harm), beneficence (forms of action intended to benefit others), and justice (fair and equitable treatment in light of what is due) – with the principle of autonomy first among equals.[20] Most philosophers considered autonomy the most important principle because it provided a justification for the exercise of self-determination and choice for patients – that is, protecting them against the traditional unilateral power of physicians in decision making.

PROCEDURALISM AND ITS LIMITS

No sooner had applied bioethics provided principles and a procedure for identifying and adjudicating moral conflicts than critics began to note the limits of a procedural approach in health care contexts. Principlism is predicated on a view that moral responsibility is tantamount to rule responsibility. It is essential that there be rules to govern decision making and principles to serve as arbiters when rules conflict.[21]

This view comports well with the concept of a social contract, which assumes that self-interest is fundamental to social relations. The social contract framework underlies applied bioethics and construes the relationship between doctor and patient as one of mutual *self*-interest. Some critics point out that by associating freedom with negative liberty (the freedom not to be interfered with) and by grounding autonomy in this concept of freedom, the social contract framework fails to adequately equip doctors and patients for a relationship in which mutuality and trustworthiness play a significant part. In the conscientious practice of caring for the sick, it is not merely the freedom to be left alone but the engagement of patients and caregivers that shapes ethical problems and should guide their resolution.

As the principles-and-applications method of applied bioethics became increasingly prominent in journal articles and classrooms, other critics questioned the rationale for privileging the principles of autonomy, nonmaleficence, beneficence, and justice, and probed principlism's view of the moral self. Beauchamp and Childress engaged their critics in lively debate, often taking their critics' views into account in subsequent editions of their groundbreaking text.[22]

Other principlists believed that an overarching moral theory was needed in which to anchor appeals to principle. To this end, Robert M. Veatch (1939–) proposed as a theoretical construct a "triple contract" which would derive from: (1) the basic social contract between society and the medical profession; and (2) the contract between individual patients and physicians. These contracts, or covenants as Veatch calls them interchangeably, would put patients and physicians on morally equal footing, thus preventing or at least discouraging physician paternalism. Veatch stipulated that a covenant is "a particular kind of contract – one emphasizing moral bonds and the spirit of fidelity." In contract theory, he writes, "humans are viewed as autonomous agents, as ends in themselves .... It is their nature to possess the capacity for rational and free choice and to make covenantal relationships both as individuals and as moral communities."[23]

But covenants and contracts are, arguably, two distinct kinds of social exchange that set out from dissimilar starting points with divergent ends in view, and ought not to be conflated. Whereas covenants are historically rooted in communal and interpersonal practices of exchanging promises, contracts are artificial constructs, quid pro quo calculations of mutual advantage.[24] When applied to doctor-patient encounters, a covenantal perspective emphasizes the give and take of the relationship, while a contractual perspective emphasizes the freedom of exchange.

H. Tristam Engelhardt Jr. (1941–) offered a different kind of comprehensive theory for bioethics. In *The Foundations of Bioethics*, Engelhardt argues that because traditional sources of moral authority are ineffectual in a secular pluralist society, "it is hopeless to suppose that a general moral consensus will develop regarding any of the major issues in bioethics." Needed instead is a new foundation on which to build a structure for settling moral differences peaceably. The cornerstone of that foundation will be not a common morality but an uncoerced common agreement to a morality of mutual respect and tolerance uncommitted to any particular concrete moral view.[25]

According to this theory, physicians' primary moral responsibility is "that of explaining to patients the geography of possible outcomes of therapeutic interventions and their consequences and allowing patients to choose among those possibilities." And the task of ethical analysis is to "display the logical content of those possibilities."[26]

Engelhardt's theory legitimates a conception of patient-physician relations that privileges individual freedom and posits patients as autonomous maximizers of self-interest. It is a view shared by Veatch but one that is at odds with the experience of patients and health care professionals for whom fellow feeling and mutual regard are central to their relationship. As William F. May (1928–)

understood, "ethicists do not adequately respect or protect the moral being of patients if they simply clear out a zone of liberty free from medical interference but fail to lead the patient to discuss the moral uses to which the patient puts his liberty .... Respect must include a willingness to engage the patient and the patient's family in a moral give and take, a sometimes painful mutual deliberation, judgment, and criticism, and an occasional accounting for one another's view, on both sides, in the professional exchange."[27]

A formidable challenge to both methodological principlism and theorizing came from casuistry, or case-based inductive (bottom-up) reasoning, which was proposed as an alternative to deductive (top-down) applied ethics. Confronted with a morally problematic case, a casuist has recourse to provisionally settled opinions, or maxims, about similar controversial past cases. Maxims – for example, "a competent patient has the right to refuse treatment" – resemble principles but differ in being illuminative rather than prescriptive. Maxims aid moral reflection by drawing on received wisdom regarding analogous cases; they point toward what may be the most fitting resolution of a novel dilemma. This is not an application of the known to the unknown but an extension of received "rules of thumb" which provide general guidance to the work of practical moral reasoning in medicine.[28]

Over the course of the 1980s and 1990s, a lively exchange of ideas took place among feminist ethicists,[29] narrative ethicists,[30] religious ethicists,[31] sociologists and anthropologists,[32] and virtue ethicists[33] – all of whom, their differences notwithstanding, variously shared a sense of the central significance of contextual, experiential, relational and social elements in deliberations about moral matters.

CONCLUSION

Following the formative events of 1960s and 1970s, philosophy rediscovered its ethical voice and took its place as a discipline in scholarly and public debates about ethical issues in science and medicine. Medicine's pressing practical problems awakened moral philosophy from its metaethical preoccupations and, in so doing, "saved the life of ethics."[34] In his influential 1982 essay bearing that title, Stephen Toulmin (1922–2009) reiterated Aristotle's insight that ethics is a *practical* craft whose usefulness resides in thoughtful attention to the particularities of situations and relationships. Its work is done in conversations aimed not at a definitive or universally true solution but at a *reasonable,* humanly livable, resolution. To the extent that it has reappropriated this insight, bioethics generally has become less rationalistic, less procedural, and more interdisciplinary. But as Daniel Callahan points out, to fulfill its promise bioethics will need to return to questions about the *ends* of science, medicine and technology; it will need to set bioethics in the larger debates about what is good for both human beings and humanity [35]

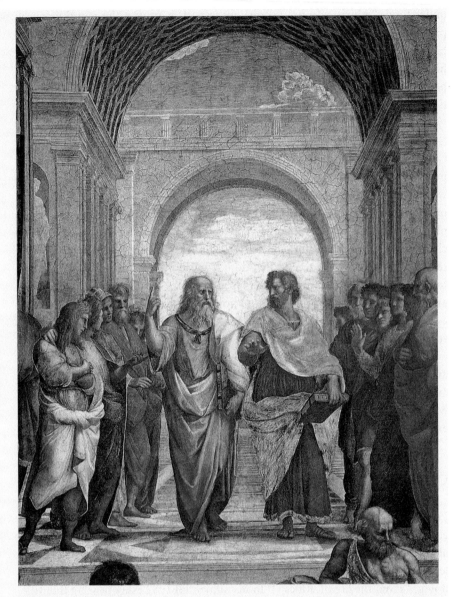

Figure 16. *Aristotle and Plato: detail from the* School of Athens *in the Stanza della Segnatura, 1510–11 (fresco) (detail) Raphael (Raffaello Sanzio of Urbino) (1483–1520)/Vatican Museums and Galleries, Vatican City/The Bridgeman Art Library.*

Are the central figures in this painting in concord with one another or in dispute? Is either figure depicted in a way that suggests he is the dominant person, or subordinate? What brings them together compositionally, what do they have in common? How are the figures to either side responding to the central figures – with admiration, with contempt?

The title tells you that the setting is Greece, and the dress of the figures that it is ancient Greece. Both figures are philosophers. Which is Plato and which is Aristotle? Plato argued for the existence of ideal or universal forms that are not part of particular things. In contrast, Aristotle argued that knowledge was derived from observation of the concrete and particular.

Which of these philosophers would agree with Stephen Toulmin's argument, summarized in this chapter, that "ethics is fundamentally a practical endeavor whose usefulness resides not in a search for general principles and their theoretical foundations but in attention to the particularities of situations and the human relationships constituting them?" How would the other philosopher respond?

The *School of Athens* is one of the most important masterpieces of Renaissance art. It is large, sixteen by twenty-five feet, colorful, and filled with portraits of philosophers and artists. You will find reproductions, descriptions, and interpretations of it in many articles and books, and on the Internet.

SUMMATION

This chapter explored the emergence of bioethics as a distinctive form of moral philosophy. Beginning with a discussion of the public's mounting unease with the applications and implications of "big" science and "rescue" medicine, it examined the birth of bioethics in the 1960s and the subsequent contributions of key thinkers such as K. Danner Clouser, Daniel Callahan, Tom L. Beauchamp and James F. Childress, Robert M. Veatch, and H. Tristram Engelhardt, Jr. Then, with a focus on contemporary exchanges between recent ethical approaches, it considered how we might address some of the moral challenges facing medicine in the twenty-first century. Overall, this chapter has emphasized the central significance of contextual, experiential, relational, and social elements in deliberations about moral matters.

EXERCISES FOR CRITICAL THINKING AND CHARACTER FORMATION

QUESTIONS FOR DISCUSSION

1. What are your fundamental values? Where did they come from? How did you learn them? Have you ever had to reassess your values?
2. What values are most important to you in your encounters with doctors? What values would you like your doctor to have?
3. As discussed in this chapter, Tom L. Beauchamp and James F. Childress argue for a principles-and-applications approach to bioethics with the *prima facie* principles of autonomy, nonmaleficence, beneficence, and justice its watchwords. What do you think of their approach? What do these principles mean to you?
4. How did technology stimulate the development of bioethics? What are the dangers of what Hans Jonas called "automatic utopianism"?

SUGGESTED WRITING EXERCISES

Imagine that you are speaking with someone who is from a culture different from your own and who has values that you do not fully understand or agree with. How would you begin a dialogue with this person? How would you articulate your values to them and how would you attempt to understand their values in a way that does more than just dismiss them? Would your answers to these questions change at all if, in this situation, you were either a doctor or a patient? Think about these questions, and then spend fifteen to twenty minutes writing about how you would approach the situation.

SUGGESTED VIEWING

The Cider House Rules (1999)
A Clockwork Orange (1971)
Gattaca (1997)

How to Die in Oregon (2011)
Million Dollar Baby (2004)

FURTHER READING

Judith Andre, *Bioethics as Practice*
Robert Baker, *Before Bioethics: A History of American Medical Ethics from the Colonial Period to the Bioethics Revolution*
H. Tristram Engelhardt, Jr., *Bioethics and Secular Humanism*

Albert R. Jonsen, *The Birth of Bioethics*
Gilbert C. Meilaender, *Body, Soul, and Bioethics*
David J. Rothman, *Strangers at the Bedside: A History of How Law and Bioethics Transformed Medical Decision Making*

ADVANCED READING

Carl Elliott, *A Philosophical Disease: Bioethics, Culture, and Identity*
Renee C. Fox and Judith P. Swazey, *Observing Bioethics*
Albert R. Jonsen and Stephen Toulmin, *The Abuse of Casuistry: A History of Moral Reasoning*

William F. May, *The Physicians Covenant: Images of the Healer in Medical Ethics*
Stephen Toulmin, *The Place of Reason in Ethics*

JOURNALS

Cambridge Quarterly of Health Care Ethics
The Journal of Medicine and Philosophy
Kennedy Institute of Ethics Journal

Narrative Inquiry in Bioethics: A Journal of Qualitative Research

ORGANIZATIONS AND GROUPS

American Society for Bioethics and Humanities http://www.asbh.org/ American Society of Law, Medicine, and Ethics

http://www.aslme.org/ Public Responsibility in Medicine and Research
http://www.primr.org/

17 Medicine and Power

Power is not something that is acquired, seized, or shared, something that one holds on to or allows to slip away; power is exercised from innumerable points, in the interplay of nonegalitarian and mobile relations.

– Michel Foucault[1]

ABSTRACT

This chapter explores the topic of medicine and power in the context of race, gender, and class. Beginning with a discussion of quantitative methods of addressing medicine and power, it then examines Michel Foucault's description of how knowledge/power objectifies human beings by means of dividing practices, scientific classification, and subjectification; John Money's description of how gender identity is "completely malleable"; Mary Daly's description of how American gynecology is part of a larger tradition of the social control of women's bodies and minds; and various issues raised by the Tuskegee Syphilis Study. Then, with a focus on contemporary research in emergency rooms, it considers some of the challenges facing us in the twenty-first century.

INTRODUCTION

There are a number of ways one could address the topic of medicine and power along the lines of race, gender, and class. One way would be to look at pay differences between male and female physicians. A 2011 study on newly trained physicians in New York State focusing on the years 1999–2008 found a $16,819 pay differential between male and female physicians.[2] What is striking about this study is that it examined the starting salaries of physicians leaving residency programs, meaning that confounding variables such as experience and rank were thus accounted for, at a time when one would expect all things to be equal. Previous commentators have attributed pay differences in medicine, when they are observed, to the fact that women tend to pursue lower paying specialties. But this study controlled for specialty choice, hours worked, and other such variables and found that the difference still holds. For example, newly trained male physicians in pediatrics made, on average, $125,343 when they began their career, while newly trained female physicians in pediatrics only made $116,950; and newly trained male physicians in emergency medicine made $218,767, while newly trained female physicians in emergency medicine only made $206,114. The authors speculate that female physicians may be seeking business practices that are "family friendly" (i.e., business practices that are less demanding), but, if this is the case, one might ask why women, to a greater extent than men, seek these practices.

Another way to address the topic of medicine and power would be to examine health care disparities across the globe. In his widely cited 1990 essay, "More Than 100 Million Women Are Missing," economist Amartya Sen (1933–) points out that the ratio of women to men is 1.05 or 1.06 in Europe and North America but the ratio is 0.94 in certain parts of Asia and Africa.[3] This is curious because women, Sen observes, tend to outlive men when given the same level of medical care (for example, the 2011 preliminary data from the Center for Disease Control in the United States indicates that the life expectancy for women is 81.1 years and for men is 76.3 years[4]). So one would expect that there would be more women than men in the world. This, however, is not the case. In 2012, the world population was 7,003,554,291 (3,526,050,280 male, 3,477,504,011 female).[5] Sen calculates that some 100 million women are "missing" on account of gender bias, and he suggests that one expression of this bias is that men have better access to goods such as medicine and thus outnumber women in the world. Sen's calculations have been subject to debate,[6] but his point with regard to women's health still stands.

These ways of addressing the topic of medicine and power (i.e., by comparing physician salaries and health disparities) are quantitative or social scientific; this chapter, in contrast, addresses the topic of medicine and power from a humanities perspective by exploring the links between knowledge and power in medicine. In a sense, this chapter is a continuation of Chapter 15, which demonstrates that concepts of health and disease are shaped by cultural values. Here we explore the subtle workings of power along such lines as race, gender, and class and introduce the thought of Michel Foucault (1926–1984) as one way of thinking about power in medical humanities. We begin by introducing some of Foucault's key ideas and then apply these ideas to topics in medical humanities. Our point here is not to explore Foucault's writings on medicine and psychiatry – as found, for example, in *The Birth of the Clinic*[7] or in *Madness and Civilization*[8] – but rather to introduce a way of asking questions in medical humanities.

Michel Foucault

Foucault was a French philosopher associated with the Collège de France who focused on the history of thought. Specifically, he was interested in studying how language functions in various contexts to demonstrate the ways in which knowledge production serves particular political interests. For Foucault, knowledge cannot be separated from power. Indeed, as the epigram of this chapter suggests, Foucault thought that power is ubiquitous and everywhere. He argued that, while we cannot escape power relations, we should try to keep altering them.

Foucault's thought is difficult to introduce. For this reason, we turn to Paul Rabinow (1944–), an expert on Foucault, who wrote an introductory essay on Foucault's thought.[9] Rabinow notes that Foucault explored the link between knowledge and power by studying three ways in which human beings are objectified: (1) dividing practices; (2) scientific classification; and (3) subjectification. Dividing practices involve separating individuals or groups from other individuals or groups, such as the poor from the rich, the insane from the sane, and the criminals from the law-abiding citizens.

Scientific classification resembles dividing practices (indeed, Rabinow points out that Foucault held that one can only distinguish between dividing practices and scientific classification at the analytical level). The key idea with regard to scientific classification is that modes of inquiry, such as biology and anthropology, also divide human beings. For example, various disciplines are employed in classifying some as sick and others as well, some as Hispanic and others as Asian, and some from the Occident and others from the Orient. Foucault's point is that both literal dividing practices as well as abstract scientific classification are related to power. While it is easier to see how domination is related to the confinement of prisoners, domination is also a part of scientific classification (though, Rabinow notes, this relation is "more oblique"[10]). An exemplary text in this tradition of inquiry is Edward Said's (1935–2003) *Orientalism*,[11] a modern classic in post-colonial studies, where Said traces the ways in which Western conceptions of the Middle East (e.g., historical and anthropological scientific classifications of "the Orient") have been used to justify Western imperialism.

But Foucault's most creative interest, Rabinow points out, involved exploring the ways in which human beings are made into "subjects," what Foucault refers to as processes of subjectification. Foucault is interested in how various social and intellectual forces cultivate self-formation in individuals. In other words, what does it mean to think of oneself as "heterosexual" or "homosexual"? The claim here is that these categories have not always existed, meaning that (1) the idea that a person would identify as a "homosexual person" is a relatively recent phenomenon; and (2) the personal, subjective experience of identifying as straight or gay *did not exist before these categories* were posited (this does not mean that straight or gay people did not exist once upon a time, say, before the nineteenth century; it just means that people did not think of themselves in these categories because the categories did not exist). In other words, the idea of sexual orientation has created new possibilities for subjectivity. Similarly, new possibilities for gendered experience changes over time because cultural constructions of masculinity and femininity change over time. In *The Body Project*, for example, Joan Brumberg (1944–) traces the history of American girls' self-formation with regard to femininity by examining their diaries; she found, by extensively reading diaries, that some 100 years ago American girls from all over the country where concerned with cultivating inner beauty whereas today they are preoccupied with cultivating outer beauty.[12]

Foucauldian Category	Examples
Dividing Practices	Isolation of lepers; confinement of poor; institutionalization of persons with mental illness; imprisonment of socially deviant
Scientific Classification	Creation of "objective" categories in various disciplines (e.g., biology – alive or dead; economics – productive or unproductive; Middle Eastern studies – Occident or Orient; medicine – normal or abnormal)
Subjectification	Creation of possibility for active cultivation of subjective experiences and identities (e.g., gay/straight; masculine/feminine; modern psychological self-awareness)

What is most original about subjectification, Rabinow points out, is that, in cases of dividing practices and scientific classification, the subject is passive, but in cases of subjectification, the subject is active. In other words, in subjectification, persons actively create their own identifies by playing out and playing into the cultural scripts that they are given.

FOUCAULDIAN INTERROGATIONS IN MEDICAL HUMANITIES

We now want to apply Foucault's thought in medical humanities. We do so by analyzing various topics in medical humanities through the lens of Foucault's three modes of objectification (i.e., dividing practices, scientific classification, and subjectification). The topics that we focus on involve issues of race, class, and gender. This chapter is an example of medical humanities as moral critique and political aspiration.

The John Money Controversy

In "The Five Sexes, Revisited," Anne Fausto-Sterling (1944–) notes that in the 1950s clinical researchers at Johns Hopkins University revolutionized thinking about sex and gender.[13] John Money (1921–2006), a psychologist, led the way. They argued that gender identity is "completely malleable" for the first eighteen months after birth. This provided psychological justification for the medical management of and surgical intervention on infants who presented with so-called ambiguous genitalia (or intersex conditions, also known as disorders of sex development) for any number of biomedical reasons, such as gonadal dysgenesis, congential adrenal hyperplasia, partial or complete androgen insensitivity syndrome, or hypospadias.[14] The Intersex Society of North America defines "intersex" as "a general term used for a variety of conditions in which a person is born with a reproductive or sexual anatomy that doesn't seem to fit the typical definitions of female or male."[15]

An ideal test case presented itself to Money and his colleague to test the theory of gender malleability.[16] Twin boys were born in Canada in 1965. Neither was born with an intersex condition. But one of them, Bruce, was severely injured on account of a circumcision accident during which his penis was severely burned. In 1967 Bruce's parents heard about Money's thesis by means of a television program, and they contacted him to see if Bruce could be reassigned as a girl. Money agreed. He arranged for Bruce's penis and testes to be removed, and Bruce was renamed Brenda. If successful, Money's claim that gender identity is a matter of nurture, and not nature, would seem to be very strong if one boy of a pair of male twins could be reassigned successfully as a girl.

So Bruce became Brenda. The family traveled to Johns Hopkins each year for follow ups. Money gave presentation after presentation and he wrote paper after paper about the case, claiming confirmation of his theory. He became somewhat of a celebrity in sexology. As Brenda approached puberty, Money encouraged her to take female hormones so that she would grow breasts; she reluctantly agreed. But being a girl never felt quite right to Brenda (she would, for example, attempt to urinate while standing). She did not know the truth about her body until she was fourteen, when a psychiatrist determined that it was time for her to know the truth. When she found out, she stopped taking female hormones and instead began taking testosterone. She began wearing male clothing and renamed herself David.

So Brenda became David. David subsequently arranged to have surgery to reattach his penis and testes in prosthetic form. In 1990 David married Jane Fontane. He suffered from depression throughout his adulthood and committed suicide in 2004. In the meantime, Money continued writing papers on the success of the case. The complications of the case were not brought to light until 1997 when two psychiatrists who had been consultants on the case published a paper that revealed that the case was an utter failure.

DISCUSSION: THE CASE OF DAVID REIMER

Even though David Reimer was not born with an intersex condition (his medical condition, as noted, was due to a circumcision accident), his case is often invoked when thinking about intersex conditions (also known as disorders of sex development), conditions where infants are born with so-called ambiguous genitalia. Sometimes corrective surgeries are performed to "fix" these infants. What power relationships are being assumed and perpetuated by means of this practice? Is not the idea that human beings are *either* male or female a created vocabulary that enables a particular kind of understanding of the human body? If the vocabulary does not fit the bodies that we see, why is it that bodies, rather than vocabulary, should change?

Foucault, as noted, is interested in how ideas function. So, one might ask, how has the scientific theory of gender malleability functioned both in the case of David and in wider society? The idea of gender malleability, at first glance, seems to be a liberating one. This point of view suggests that one's gender identity and one's gender performance are not given by God or by nature but are learned. And if gender identity (e.g., how one defines one's own gender, such as thinking of oneself as a man, a woman, or as transgendered) and gender performance (e.g., how intimates one's gender to others through bodily practices, such as wearing gender-specific clothing) are things that we learn, it seems to follow that society ought to be accepting of a wide range of gender expressions. This seems to be a progressive idea, not a form of domination. Yet the effect of the idea of gender malleability did not create a more accepting society with regard to persons of so-called disorders of sex development but, rather, a society in which the medical intervention for disorders of sex development was performed more regularly (which, of course, has financial implications). In this sense, society became less, not more, accepting of difference on account of the idea of gender malleability. The idea of gender malleability gave Bruce's parents and his doctors the power, in the form of scientific knowledge and medical authority, to form, quite literally, his body.

Body Projects for and of Women

Mary Daly (1928–2010) was a highly creative radical lesbian feminist philosopher who taught at Boston College for more than thirty years.[17] She began her career as a Christian theologian but eventually de-converted from Christianity and subsequently referred to herself as "post-christian" because she viewed Christianity as hopelessly sexist and androcentric. She was well known for not allowing men to talk in her classes in feminist theory.

In *Gyn/Ecology*, Daly has a chapter on American gynecology.[18] This chapter follows a chapter on Chinese foot-binding (a practice where the feet of women are wrapped in a tightly bound state such that the feet become deformed) as well as a chapter on what she calls African genital mutilation[19] (practices where various parts of a girl's genitals are removed), practices, Daly argues, that are performed for the sake of "beauty." In the chapter on American gynecology, she argues that the history of American gynecology is a part of a larger tradition of the social control of women's bodies and minds – a tradition that can be observed both cross-culturally and historically – and that this tradition of patriarchy and misogyny continues into the present. "It is essential," she writes, "to see that the specialized treatment for women known as gynecology arose in the nineteenth century as a direct response to ... feminism" in America.[20]

Daly begins her argument by qualifying what she means by "gynecology." She writes:

> I use the term *gynecology* broadly to all those professions – including psychiatry and the other psychotherapeutic fields – which specialize in the "disease and hygiene" of women's bodies and minds. I use the term *gynecologist* to refer to all members of those professions whose beliefs and behaviors are motivated by loyalties to their patriarchally identified fields rather than by concern for women.[21]

Daly concedes that some specialists are sometimes helpful but adds that "such genuine helpfulness occurs *in spite of* the pervasive intent, ethos, and method of their professions."[22] Her point is that "gynecologists," as defined above, control women by preoccupying them in unnecessary ways that, in effect, privilege men because such medicine takes up the time and energy of women. Consider this advice from one physician:

> Self-examination, regular examination by a qualified breast surgeon, mammograms, xerograms, and thermograms still remain the best defense against breast cancer.[23]

Daly comments: "This is, of course, an effective formula for keeping women in a state of ... preoccupation."[24] In recent years, there has been lively debate concerning overtreatment (especially the overuse of mammograms[25]), but most of this literature has focused on evidence-based outcomes and on healthcare costs. Daly's concerns are focused more directly on the ongoing political liberation of women.

Daly offers a number of historical observations to support her argument that American gynecology emerged as a direct response to nineteenth-century feminism. Some of the most compelling include:

1. The "father of gynecology," J. Marion Sims (1813–1883), experimented on vulnerable women, such as slaves, so that he could perfect his techniques for white women;
2. The first Women's Rights Convention in America was held in 1848, and, around this time, Charles Meigs (1792–1869) instructed his (male) students that by studying the female organs they would be able to understand and to control the hearts, minds, and souls of women;
3. A decade after the first Women's Rights Convention, the "clitoridectomy" was invented by Isaac Baken Brown (1811–1873) and was advocated as a cure for female masturbation in the United States; and
4. In 1873, female castration – that is, the removal of the ovaries – was invented by Robert Battey (1828–1895) to cure female insanity.

These historical facts do cast the practice of gynecology in a macabre light. Daly's argument can be summarized as follows: When American women in the nineteenth century were beginning to demand equal treatment, their "acting up" was diagnosed as hysterical, and surgery was offered as a medical solution. Medicine, then, functioned as a tool of patriarchy.

Some might dismiss this history as a part of an unfortunate past, something that no longer applies to us today. But Daly goes on to show that a more subtle

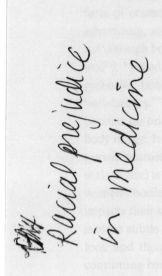

form of power exerts itself in the lives of contemporary American women in the form of cosmetic medicine. How? Women, by a variety of means but especially advertising, are formed into consumers in ways that men, by comparison, are not. Although body image has become an issue for boys and men in recent years as well, "inspired with inspired fixations," Daly writes, women check "to see if hair, eyebrows, lashes, lips, skin, breasts, buttocks, stomach, hips, legs, and feet are acceptable." Foucault's notion of subjectification is especially relevant here because one is "forcing" women to obsess about all of these issues related to body image. It is also important to note that, while women themselves value and crave cosmetic medicine, desire for women's bodies (especially heterosexual male desire) is also shaped by advertising, and this desire for particular kinds of women's bodies, in turn, asserts another kind of pressure on women that directly impacts their sexual and romantic relationships. Oppression or domination here is quite subtle because women internalize certain images about how they should look and then work to conform by dieting, obsessive exercising, surgery, and consuming beauty products. When viewed alongside African genital mutilation, one might be able to see that issues of gender have not been "solved" in America. External practices that are limiting in Africa, Daly points out, correspond to internal formations that are also limiting in America.

Medical Apartheid and the Distinction between Prejudice and Racism

African Americans have been exploited in a variety of ways for centuries in the United States. This was most obviously the case during slavery. Racism, however, persists today – well after slavery, well after the civil rights movement, well after affirmative action, and even after the election of Barack Obama, the first African American President of the United States. Racism is not simply a matter of the past.

It is helpful to make a distinction between racial prejudice and structural racism.[28] Racial prejudice is *personal* and concerns whether an individual dislikes or hates a particular group of people based on race or ethnicity, or believes that a particular group of people is inferior or superior based on race or ethnicity. The Ku Klux Klan, for example, is a group that is racially prejudiced, as its members believe that African Americans are inferior to Caucasian Americans. Structural racism is different. Structural racism is *social* and concerns the extent to which a society privileges some and disenfranchises others. If differences exist between races or ethnicities along the lines of, say, access to care, health outcomes, incarceration rates, education, and social and economic class, then the society is racist structurally speaking even if no one in the society is at the individual level racially prejudiced. For example, the U.S. Census Bureau reports that the median income for all families in the United States was $61,521 in 2008. The median family income for whites was $65,000, while the median income for blacks was $39,879. The percentage of children in the United States living below the poverty line was 18.5 percent for all races in 2008, though the percentage of whites living below the poverty line was 15.3 percent while it was 34.4 percent for blacks.[29] These data suggest structural disadvantages for blacks – disadvantages that will likely affect their education, their income, their health, and the course of their lives.

Sometimes racial prejudice and structural racism overlap: "[I]t was cheaper to use niggers than cats," Henry Bailey noted in 1977, "because they were everywhere and cheap experimental animals."[30] Bailey was referring to his neuroresearch at Tulane University in New Orleans, research that was funded by the Central Intelligence Agency (CIA). Today, it is less common to hear officials talk in blatantly prejudiced ways, but the structural disadvantages that were present in 1977 still persist to some degree, as indicated by the data above.

A formidable group, these twelve Boston doctors were photographed in 1850. The stiffness of their poses was partly due to the required exposure time – more than 10 seconds required by the daguerreotype process, invented in 1839. Following the direction of this chapter, how would you interrogate the points from which this group exercised power among themselves as well as in relation to their patients and to society in general? Do you think they are as uniform in their opinions and perspectives as their dark suits suggest?

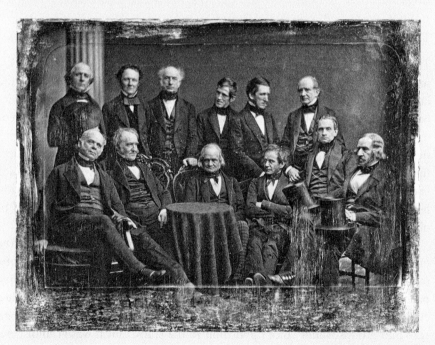

Figure 17. *Boston Doctors,* ca. 1850. Albert Sands Southworth 1811–1894. Daguerreotype, 16.5 x 21.6 cm (6 1/2 x 8 1/2 in.). Gift of I. N. Phelps Stokes, Edward S. Hawes, Alice Mary Hawes, and Marion Augusta Hawes, 1937 (37.14.39). The Metropolitan Museum of Art, New York, U.S.A. Image copyright © The Metropolitan Museum of Art. Image source: Art Resource, NY.

As we have seen in Chapter 2, new knowledge about disease has historically been retracted from the bodies of persons of color. In *Medical Apartheid*,
Harriet Washington chronicles the history of human subjects research in light
of racism. She writes about exploitation on plantations, the display of black
bodies during surgical procedures in the antebellum clinic, the Tuskegee Syphilis
Study, radiation experiments on African Americans, research on black prisoners, and current research in emergency rooms and in Africa. This history is vast.
And there are many excellent books that engage it: for example, James Jones's
(1943–) *Bad Blood*,[31] Eileen Welsome's *The Plutonium Files*,[32] Todd Savitt's
(1943–) *Medicine and Slavery*,[33] Allen Hornblum's (1947–) *Acres of Skin*,[34] Susan
Reverby's *Examining Tuskegee*,[35] and John Hoberman's (1944–) *Black and Blue*.[36]
We commend Washington's book to those who want an introduction to this history, but we also want to point out that Washington is writing as a journalist,
not as a scholar, and one reviewer of the book has sharply criticized the book
for a number of incorrect facts.[37] We believe, however, that the strength of the
book – putting much of this history into a single, readable volume – outweighs
the weaknesses of getting this or that fact wrong. Here we present two case studies discussed in Washington's book (the Tuskegee Syphilis Study and contemporary research in emergency rooms), and we supplement her presentation with
relevant scholarly sources.

The Tuskegee Syphilis Study

The Tuskegee Syphilis Study (discussed in several other places in this book –
see the index) is universally mentioned when addressing the topic of race and
medicine. As previously noted, in 1932 the United States Public Health Service
began a study in Macon County, Alabama, to observe the natural progression of
untreated syphilis in African Americans, and the study lasted until 1972. During
these forty years of experimentation, subjects were enrolled and led to believe
that they were being treated for "bad blood." But in fact they were being studied
and *not* treated. Penicillin became widely available in the 1950s but was withheld from the men in the study so that the natural course of syphilis could be
observed – until death.[38]

The study was not kept a secret. Indeed, health care professionals involved
presented papers and articles about their research. Physicians, for example, presented at the American Medical Association. Allan Brandt notes that the first
paper published about the study appeared in 1936, and a paper was published
every four to six years until the study was disrupted.[39] From time to time, persons and groups would voice opposition to the study. But it wasn't until Peter
Buxtun, an employee of the Public Health Service, took action that the study
was stopped.[40]

There were numerous ethical violations in this study: (1) the subjects enrolled
in the study were a vulnerable population; (2) the subjects were induced to enroll
in the study by means of free hot meals and small amounts of money; (3) health

care professionals lied to the subjects about the nature of the study; (4) the study did not offer the subjects any direct benefit, and, indeed, once penicillin became available, the study prevented the subjects from receiving any potential benefit from taking the drug because they were considered ineligible to receive penicillin; and (5) prior to penicillin, the standard of care for the treatment of syphilis (arsenotherapy) was withheld from them.

Some have defended the Tuskegee Syphilis Study, arguing that, by 1950 (when, as noted, penicillin became widely available), penicillin would not have helped the subjects in the study because they would have reached the advanced stages of syphilis (tertiary syphilis) by this point. Others have argued that the standard of care of the day (arsenotherapy) did more harm than good, and so the study was *good* for these men because they were spared from harm. Still others have argued that these men, because they were poor, would never have been treated anyway – that is, with or without the study, their fates would have been the same. And still others deny any racial component to the study, that, in effect, the study "just happened to be in a black community."[41]

These defenses of the Tuskegee Syphilis Study enable us to ask Foucauldian questions in a clear and straightforward manner. What medical and scientific assumptions enabled African Americans to be singled out and enrolled? At the time, some believed syphilis affected the neurological systems of whites but the cardiovascular systems of blacks, and the study was therefore designed to test this hypothesis. The research was also framed as "a study in nature" and not as an experiment. Framing the study in this way enabled the researchers to assume a passive role. In other words, this logic suggests that the researchers were not actively doing any harm by means of an experiment but were merely observing nature. A Foucauldian perspective would query the function of the vocabulary of knowledge here: Whose interests are being served by this vocabulary? One might also ask, How do assumptions about race and sexuality – blacks (both men and women) were assumed to be more sexual and less moral than whites[42] – intersect with this "study in nature"? Or one might question assumptions relating to economic class. It wasn't, after all, rich African Americans who were enrolled in the study but poor ones. What "science" enabled these practices?

A Foucauldian perspective here would emphasize that it was not a lack of committees or a lack of oversight that led to this scandal, but that it was the link of knowledge and power, the very discourse of science. A key lesson from Tuskegee Syphilis Study, we suggest, is not that we need stringent institutional review boards and other such bureaucratic checks (though, to be sure, these review boards are important) but that we need to examine, on an ongoing basis, *how* our current research interests are related to power.

Contemporary Research in Emergency Rooms

In recent years, researchers in emergency rooms have been testing the effects of artificial blood substitutes such as PolyHeme and Hemopure. Washington points out that the development of such a substitute would constitute a signif-icant achievement with many health benefits. Blood transfusions, for example, would be easier and safer, as there would be no need to match blood types, and the risk of transmitting viruses would be avoided as well. There would no longer be a shortage of blood in large cities or in rural areas, as artificial blood substi-tutes can last for two years, much longer than blood can be stored. But the ethics of this research is questionable, Washington argues, because patients who are in need of blood transfusions in the emergency room are often unconscious and therefore do not have the opportunity to consent to this research.[43]

Instead of obtaining individual consent in emergency room research, one practice has been obtaining "community consent." For example, if a given indi-vidual does not want to be enrolled in such a study in one's own community and should happen to need a blood transfusion, one would need to wear some kind of marker such as a bracelet that indicates that one does not want to be a part of the study to prevent oneself from being enrolled while unconscious.[44] Advocates for this research justify it without initial consent on the grounds that the risk to individuals is minimal while the potential gains for society are great – that is, we need more effective ways of treating trauma victims. While this may be true, Washington invites us to ask, Who is it that will be bearing this "minimal risk"? Will those who bear this "minimal risk" turn out to be poor or vulnerable in some other way?

CONCLUSION

In this chapter, there are a number of theorists that we could have used to think about power. We could have used, for example, S. Kay Toombs (1943–),[45] Havi Carel,[46] or Fredrik Svenaeus.[47] But because Foucault is such a towering figure in the humanities, we felt it best to introduce his thought rather than other think-ers; graduate students in medical humanities should explore these other thinkers in detail. Also, there are many other topics that we could have focused on, such as contemporary debates over AIDS research in Africa; the underfunding of the study of women's health; the Guatemala Syphilis Study; and rhetoric surround-ing the health care reform debate in the United States – this list could be greatly expanded. We invite readers to consider more thinkers as well as more topics for interrogating medicine and power. We also invite readers to consider the links between knowledge and power within medical humanities.

SUMMATION

This chapter explored the topic of medicine and power in the context of race, gen-der, and class. Beginning with a discussion of quantitative methods of address-ing medicine and power, it examined Michel Foucault's description of how knowledge/power objectifies human beings by means of dividing practices, scientific classification, and subjectification; John Money's description of how gender identity is "completely malleable"; Mary Daly's description of how American gynecology is part of a larger tradition of the social control of women's bodies and minds; and various issues raised by the Tuskegee Syphilis Study. Then, with a focus on contemporary research in emergency rooms, it considered some of the challenges facing us in the twenty-first century. Overall, though, this chapter has attempted to emphasize how many of the seemingly objective practices of medicine are, in fact, embedded in complex networks of knowledge/power.

EXERCISES FOR CRITICAL THINKING AND CHARACTER FORMATION

QUESTIONS FOR DISCUSSION

1. What cultural scripts do play a role in your life? Are they helpful or unhelpful?
2. In what ways does medical education cultivate the selves of medical students and/or premed students?
3. In what ways are medical scripts liberating, and in what ways are they constricting?
4. How do medical scripts play into other operations of power in a given society?

WRITING EXERCISE

Sometimes the negative effects of actively playing into a cultural script can be seen as destructive, such as when young women internalize the ideal of the supermodel and then denigrate themselves for not achieving this ideal. Boys, too, in recent years have been struggling with masculine ideals about male body image. Write a personal journal entry (three paragraphs) about your feelings toward your body. You do not need to share this with anyone.

SUGGESTED VIEWING

Cider House Rules (1999)
Hermaphrodites Speak! (2008)

Miss Evers' Boys (1997)

SUGGESTED LISTENING

"911 is a Joke," Public Enemy
"A Boy Named Sue," Johnny Cash

"Lola," The Kinks

ADVANCED READING

Judith Butler, *Gender Trouble*
Michael Foucault, *The Birth of the Clinic*
John Hoberman, *Black and Blue: The Origins and Consequences of Medical Racism*
Deborah Lupton, *Medicine as Culture: Illness, Disease and the Body*

Ellen Moore, Elizabeth Fee, and Manon Parry, eds., *Women Physicians and the Culture of Medicine*
S. Kay Toombs, *The Meaning of Illness*
Cornell West, *Race Matters*

JOURNALS

International Journal of Feminist Approaches to
　Bioethics

Medical Anthropology Quarterly
Signs

ONLINE RESOURCES

AMA Website on Eliminating Health Disparities
http://www.ama-assn.org/ama/pub/physician-resources/
public-health/eliminating-health-disparities.page
Judith Butler on Gender
http://www.youtube.com/watch?v=Bo7o2LYATDc
Cornell West on the Role of Philosophy

http://ed.ted.com/on/0iY9k6uU
International Network on Feminist Approaches to
Bioethics (FAB)
http://www.fabnet.org/
Race and Culture/Ethnicity Affinity Group of ASBH
http://www.asbh.org/

18 Just Health Care

A decent medical-care system that helps all the people cannot be built without the language of equity and care.[1]

– Rashi Fein

ABSTRACT

This chapter explores the issue of equity in the organization and distribution of health care. Beginning with a discussion of various presidential attempts to establish greater equity, it examines what Paul Starr calls "the American health care trap" as well as the reasons why America, alone among postindustrial democracies, has failed to enact a universal health insurance program. Then, with a focus on recent work in the field, it considers how we might find our moral and political compass amidst the complex network of actors and institutions that determine how we organize and distribute health care.

INTRODUCTION

In Chapters 11 and 12, we discussed the virtue of *care* in doctor-patient relationships. But what of *equity*, or fairness, in the organization and provision of health care? This chapter critically examines the requirements of justice in the allocation and distribution of health care services.

Justice is considered one of the primary virtues of a good society. Beliefs about justice help *constitute* social relationships in a society and, in turn, *reflect* those beliefs in the relationships thus constituted. Two conceptions of justice tend to predominate in modern thought: to each according to one's *need;* and to each according to one's *merit* or contribution. Debates about justice generally occur at points of tension between those who believe that justice is principally a *formal* matter of rules and procedures (treating people justly means consistently and fairly applying relevant rules to them); and others who are committed to the idea that the *substantive content* of justice should be empirically determined (do people have what they need to live a decent life?).

Modern democracies typically combine aspects of these two conceptions by privileging either the provision of social resources responsive to *need*, or market mechanisms to determine *merit*. Even in societies where hunger and homelessness are tolerated, few would deny that some needs (e.g., for food and shelter) are "basic," meaning one can't live without their being met. Is health care a basic need? If so, how should a decent society go about meeting it?

EARLY STRUGGLES

America has struggled for decades with the question of how to distribute and pay for quality health care services for its citizens. Here is an excerpt from a presidential State of the Union Address. "Action thus far taken falls far short of our goal of adequate medical care for all our citizens. If we are to deal with the problem realistically and in its true dimensions, action is required on a broader scale. Technical resources have been greatly increased, but as a nation we have not yet succeeded in making the benefits of these scientific advances available to all those who need them. The best hospitals, the finest research laboratories, and the most skillful physicians are of no value to those who cannot obtain their services. Our objective must be two-fold: To make available enough medical services to go around, and to see that everybody has a chance to obtain those services. We cannot attain one part of that objective unless we attain the other as well." One would not be faulted for thinking that this statement is of recent origin but it is, in fact, from President Harry Truman's 1949 State of the Union Address.[2]

For complicated political reasons, the Social Security Act, which had become law in 1935 during Franklin D. Roosevelt's presidency, made no mention of *health* security. When FDR took office in 1933, "the Great Depression had altered political priorities. With millions out of work and a grass-roots movement among the elderly demanding help from government, unemployment relief and old-age pensions became more urgent than health insurance." Nonetheless, despite strenuous efforts made by the Roosevelt administration to include health insurance in deliberations about the Social Security Act of 1935, "the AMA went into high gear to oppose any action, and key congressional leaders made it clear that health insurance would get no consideration."[3]

Roosevelt subsequently made two attempts at a national insurance program. In 1937 he tested the political waters for a proposal to provide federal support for maternal and child health, the disabled, the poor and the general public, and for hospital construction. But again, the American Medical Association mobilized against any such idea, and congressional leaders followed suit. In his 1944 State of the Union address, Roosevelt called for "an 'economic bill of rights' to fulfill hopes for the security that Americans were fighting for in

World War II. Among those were a 'right to adequate medical care' and 'a right to adequate protection from the economic fears of sickness.'"[4]

Three months later the president was dead, as was any prospect for comprehensive national health reform for the following two decades.

1940s–1970s

Shortly after becoming president in 1945, Truman urged Congress to establish a national health insurance system to ensure adequate medical coverage for all citizens. Public reaction was initially sympathetic, but reception in Congress was less so. Faced with strong organized opposition from the proposal's opponents, who successfully labeled Truman's efforts "socialized medicine," the idea of a national health insurance program was scuttled.[5]

During John F. Kennedy's short-lived presidency in the early 1960s, momentum for health care coverage for the elderly gathered steam in response to the ever-rising cost of hospital care. After Kennedy's assassination, Medicare became a centerpiece of President Lyndon B. Johnson's Great Society initiatives, and in 1965 Johnson signed into law a compulsory hospital insurance program under Social Security (Medicare Part A), an insurance program covering physicians' fees (Medicare Part B), and a joint federal-state insurance program for low-income individuals (Medicaid).

In 1970, Massachusetts Senator Edward Kennedy and Representative Martha W. Griffiths of Michigan introduced the Health Security Act, calling for all extant public and private health plans to be consolidated in a single, federally operated comprehensive health insurance system. Key components of the plan were a cost-controlled national budget, from which funds would be allocated regionally, and incentives for prepaid group practice.[6]

In response, the Nixon administration countered with a proposal of its own to expand the small number of nonprofit health maintenance organizations (HMOs) already in operation, such as the successful Kaiser-Permanente prepaid group practice, and to encourage profit-making corporations to join in the expansion effort. President Nixon signed the Health Maintenance Organization Act into law in late December 1973, explaining that its purpose was to "provide initial Federal development assistance for a limited number of demonstration projects, with the intention that they become self-sufficient within fixed periods."[7]

The HMO Act was far less than the comprehensive insurance program that reformers had hoped for, but it did advance the cause. Moreover, Nixon announced his intention to submit a bill to the next session of Congress creating a national health insurance system. In a message to Congress on February 6, 1974, he described national health insurance as "an idea whose time has come in America." But the Watergate scandal quickly consumed the administration's attention, and six months later Nixon resigned the presidency.

1980s

Ronald Reagan ran for president to "get government off our backs," and included in his first budget after taking office provisions for cutting federal health programs, including Medicaid. By this time, as Paul Starr puts it, "the health-care industry was already becoming more of a field for corporate enterprise primarily because of the profitable opportunities created by the absence of effective cost controls in either private insurance or government programs."[8]

Although circumstances varied, and many different factors were at play in the defeat of these reform efforts, there were two notable constants: (1) Americans' traditional wariness about government overreach, and (2) organized medicine's relentless opposition to any reform that might threaten the profession's sovereignty over all things medical. In 1982, Starr opined that, "In its rejection of 'big government' the public seems to be expressing a desire to return to older and simpler ways. Similarly, the medical profession, in protesting against government regulation, wants a return to the traditional liberties and privileges of private practice. But ... in medical care, the reliance on the private sector is not likely to return America to the status quo, but rather to accelerate the movement toward an entirely new system of corporate medical enterprise."[9] Ironically, in steadfastly opposing government involvement in organizing a national health insurance system, organized medicine opened the door to corporate dominance.

1990s

Soon after assuming the presidency in 1993, Bill Clinton made health care reform a central goal of his administration. Despite a modest increase in Medicaid eligibility, the uninsured population had risen to 38.6 million in 1992, an increase of 5.2 million from 1989. Health care costs seemed out of control. Employers were trimming benefits. Insurance premiums were on the rise, limiting increasing numbers of Americans' access to care. Public opinion strongly favored fundamental reform.

Clinton's plan was ambitious, some said audacious. "The federal government would establish a right to affordable health care, provide much of the financing, and set a limit to the rate of growth of expenditures ...."[10] In light of rising costs and deteriorating coverage, Clinton advocated a system of universal, comprehensive coverage featuring consumer choice based on price competition among private health plans. Each private health plan would deliver a package of uniform benefits (managed competition) under a ceiling on health spending. The president's personal commitment to the reform effort was evident when he appointed Hillary Rodham Clinton to chair the President's Task Force on National Health Care Reform and named his close advisor Ira Magaziner as its director.

Clinton unveiled the framework for his plan in a rousing speech to a joint session of Congress on September 22, 1993. He began by outlining the problems prompting the need for reform. Then, turning to the proposed remedy, the president invoked the notion of security and, in a particularly effective symbolic gesture, held up a laminated card resembling a driver's license, saying, "Under our plan, every American would receive a health security card that will guarantee a comprehensive package of benefits over the course of an entire lifetime, roughly comparable to the benefit package offered by most Fortune 500 companies. This health security card will offer this package of benefits in a way that can never be taken away .... With this card, if you lose your job or you switch jobs, you're covered. If someone in your family has unfortunately had an illness that qualifies as a preexisting condition, you're still covered. If you get sick or a member of your family gets sick, even if it's a life-threatening illness, you're covered. And if an insurance company tries to drop you for any reason, you will still be covered, because that will be illegal. This card will give comprehensive coverage. It will cover people for hospital care, doctor visits, diagnostic services like Pap smears and mammograms and cholesterol tests, substance abuse, and mental health treatment."[11] The speech was generally well received, and public reaction was positive. Momentum for reform seemed to be building. Early endorsement of significant reform by key interest groups and a cautious bipartisan spirit in Congress pointed toward the possibility of progress.

But soon fissures appeared. Congressional Democrats needed the support not only of moderate Senate Republicans and conservative House Democrats but also of influential business leaders. To complicate matters, the Democrats themselves were not of one mind about the shape reforms should take. Some favored universal health care without managed competition; others wanted managed competition without universal coverage. As the wrangling dragged on and the bill became more complicated, momentum flagged.

Meanwhile, the health care industry launched a nationally televised advertising campaign featuring a concerned couple, "Harry and Louise," sitting at their kitchen table and worrying that the Clinton health plan would cramp consumer choice. "They choose, we lose" was the ad's punch line. Business leaders began to back away from their earlier commitment to reforms, Senate Republicans' support evaporated, and reform legislation soon slipped out of reach.[12]

Another factor in the defeat of the Clinton plan is what Paul Starr calls "the American health policy trap." In spite of the fact that a growing minority of citizens are financially unprotected in sickness, the health care system nonetheless satisfies enough people to make it difficult to change. The key elements of the trap are employer-provided insurance whose beneficiaries are unaware of its high cost; government programs that cover groups such as the elderly and veterans who vote; and a vast financing system that enriches the health care industry, creating powerful interests averse to change.[13]

2000s

Passage of the Patient Protection and Affordable Care Act in early 2010 marked a milestone on the road to universal health care. The law provides for an increase in the number of Americans eligible for Medicaid, estimated by the nonpartisan Congressional Budget Office to be about 16 million, and better benefits for Medicare beneficiaries, especially for preventive care. Primary care physicians treating Medicaid and Medicare patients are to be paid at a higher rate than previously. Children are to remain covered under their parents' health insurance policies until they reach the age of twenty-six. Private insurers must cover people with preexisting conditions and are barred from canceling the policies of sick people and from placing caps on payments to policyholders. Private insurers are required to spend 80 to 85 percent of premium revenues on medical claims.[14] The law also includes provisions for rewarding quality of care.[15] Most observers agree that reducing the growth rate of federal health care expenditures is essential for any sustainable health reform. The new law contains a number of provisions for moving in that direction over the long term.

In the fall of 2013, when people first began signing up for the insurance under the Affordable Care Act, serious glitches appeared in the website and programs designed to facilitate enrollment. Other problems of cost and access developed as well. If these problems are resolved and the ACA is fully implemented, expansion of coverage will have been achieved and health security strengthened for millions of Americans, moving the country closer to the goal of universal health care. Nonetheless, much unfinished work lies ahead. Upwards of 30 million citizens will remain uninsured and millions more underinsured. And the challenge of reining in health care costs will continue to loom large.

Who's in darkness, Who's in light in this dramatic scene? Are there any elements in the picture that you associate with a particular time and place? Is a rescue taking place, or are the figures in the water being abandoned? Who appears to be in charge of the lifeboat, and where is his gaze directed? What appears to engage the interest of most of the other figures in the boat? What could account for the position of the viewer? As the viewer, what might account for your perspective, where might you be standing? Do you feel that you are in a position to take part in the action?

How would the scene be different if there were more detail, if there were a full range of middle tones rather than stark black and white? How would the scene affect you if it were in full color and you could see the faces of the figures? By reducing the detail – and thus the information in the picture, has the artist given it more or less of a grip on our imaginations?

Turning to the topic of this chapter, "Just Health Care," imagine that the painting represents the parties to the efforts to reform health care and that the lifeboat represents health insurance. Would the figures in the boat be healthy or ill? Would the figures in the water be

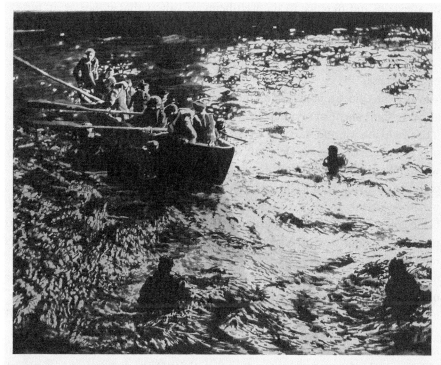

Figure 18. *Between Darkness and Light,* 2005, Mary McCleary 1951–, Courtesy Moody Gallery, Houston TX © Mary McCleary 2005.

uninsured? Are they healthy or ill? As the viewer, how might you determine which of the figures in the water deserve to be in the boat? How might you determine if some figures in the boat should be in the water? What concerns might the figures in the lifeboat and the figures in the water have in common?

A MORAL FAILURE?

Analyzing nearly a century of health care reform efforts in America, David Rothman explores the question of why the United States, alone among postindustrial democracies, has failed to enact a universal health insurance program. Many factors have come into play including, as previously noted, the American commitment to limiting governmental authority, as well as the political power of health insurance companies, hospital corporations, labor unions, pharmaceutical conglomerates, and organized medicine all defending their financial stake in the existing system. Such political exigencies aside, however, there is, Rothman observes, a confounding social context for this failure: "what is under discussion is essentially a *moral* failure [italics added], a demonstration

of a level of indifference to the well-being of others that stands as an indict-
ment of the intrinsic character of American society .... How could Americans
ignore the health needs of so many fellow countrymen and still live with themselves? How could a society that prides itself on decency tolerate this degree
of unfairness?"[16]

Americans place a premium on individualism and independence. They generally give short shrift to interdependence and abhor dependence. However, when
it comes to disease and sickness, all citizens (and noncitizens) are vulnerable and
may be in need of help. As Deborah Stone perceptively observes, "help is the way
we live. We are born needing help, we die needing help, and we live out our days
getting and giving help. Help and gratitude connect people. Without them, life
would be terribly lonely. *Not* belonging is misery. Getting help and, better yet,
being able to *count on* help make us part of the human family."[17] The organized
provision of, and equitable access to, quality health care is a decent society's
response to the needs of the sick.

Thinking in terms of social needs and values has largely fallen out of favor
over the last three decades, which Michael J. Sandel (1953–) calls "the era of
market triumphalism."[18] During this era, "without quite realizing it, without
ever deciding to do so, we drifted from *having* a market economy to *being* a market society. The difference is this: a market economy is a tool – a valuable and
effective tool – for organizing productive activity. A market society is a way of
life in which market values seep into every aspect of human endeavor. It's a place
where social relations are made over in the image of the market."[19]

American society and culture are thoroughly commercialized, awash in consumer goods. But a society is more than an economy, and health care is not like
consumer goods which are subject to supply and demand. It is, rather, a public,
social good, which cannot be adequately provided in an economy solely based
on private markets. As Benjamin Barber (1939–) puts it, "The market is finally
an instrument of private goods, which necessarily overshadow public goods.
Consumer judgment is private judgment (what do *I* want?), while public good
demands a degree of public judgment (what do *we* need?). If the demands of
both can be accommodated, a blend is possible, but where the two are in opposition, as is often the case, the private must trump the public .... Consumers
simply are not the same thing as citizens."[20]

Health care is an irreducible social good. It is intrinsically good, indivisible,
and held in common.[21] Unlike commodities, social goods like health care and
education, public safety and equal treatment under the law, are things that we as
citizens value not only for our survival but for our flourishing and our integrity
as well. Health care is a good that is constitutive of who *we* are as citizens of a
democracy grounded in social equality and respect for individuals in communities. When Americans look away from tens of thousands who have no health
insurance, and thousands more who are underinsured, they are leaving many
fellow citizens unnecessarily exposed to the ravages of sickness. Leaving the

provision of health care to the marketplace condones the separation of "haves" who are deemed deserving from "have nots" who are considered unworthy of respect and care. It defies what Michael Walzer (1935–) calls "the social and moral logic of provision," according to which "Once the community undertakes to provide some needed good, it must provide it to all the members who need it in proportion to their needs."[22]

In 1975, Howard Hiatt (1925–) asked provocatively who is responsible for making the decision to apportion society's medical resources that will benefit not some, but all members of the society.[23] Drawing on the metaphor of "the commons" – a patch of grazing land set aside in medieval villages to be shared by all the local farmers – Hiatt observed that today we lack a well-conceived methodology for governing access to the *medical* commons. Instead, we have appeals for resources for routine support of ongoing research, education and patient care, and haphazard raids on the commons by various disease-entity and organ-system lobbies. Needed, Hiatt argued, is a framework for setting reasonable and responsible access to a system of communal provision.

A JUST FRAMEWORK

In 1983, the President's Commission for the Study of Ethical Problems in Medicine and Behavioral Research, offered such an ethical framework in its report, *Securing Access to Health Care: The Ethical Implications of Differences in the Availability of Health Services.* The six core propositions of the framework are as serviceable today as when they were drafted:

1. Because differences in the need for health care are, for the most part, undeserved and beyond an individual's control, society has an ethical obligation to ensure equitable access to health care for everyone.
2. This societal obligation is not exclusive but is balanced by individual obligations, that is, individuals ought to pay a fair share of the cost of their own health care.
3. All citizens should have access to an adequate level of care that should be thought of as a floor below which no one ought to fall rather than as a ceiling above which no one may rise.
4. When private forces are sufficient to enable equitable access, there is no need for government involvement, although the federal government has the final responsibility for ensuring that health care is available to everyone.
5. The cost of achieving equitable access ought to be shared fairly at a national level and should not fall disproportionately on particular practitioners, institutions, or residents of particular communities.
6. Efforts aimed at containing costs should not focus on limiting access to the least well-off members of the society.

The commission argued for an adequate level of care below which no one should fall. The commission understood health care as a public good because of its special role in "relieving suffering, preventing premature death, restoring functioning, increasing opportunity, providing information about an individual's condition, and giving evidence of mutual empathy and compassion."[24] This special importance distinguished health care from commodities that could be bought at individual discretion within the constraints of the purchaser's budget. As a common good, it should be equitably shared at an adequate level by everyone.

SECURITY AND SOLIDARITY

Arguments for achieving a just distribution of health care services have been advanced from a variety of theoretical vantage points – contractarian, egalitarian, libertarian, and utilitarian.[25] Here we will focus briefly on mutuality and sociality as starting points for thinking about equity, as articulated by Larry Churchill. In two books, *Self-Interest and Universal Health Care* (1994) and *Rationing Health Care in America* (1987), Churchill argues that the primary goals of an ethically sound health care system are security and solidarity. In his view, these two goals are linked and complementary. Security refers to personal well-being, whereas solidarity is a sense of community. In matters of illness and health, solidarity emerges from awareness of a common vulnerability; it encourages support for a shared system of benefits and responsibility that creates personal security.

Churchill's argument draws on the eighteenth century Scottish moral philosopher David Hume (1711–1776)[26] for whom prudent self-regard is not selfishness but a studied sense of what is likely to be good for me and mine in the long term. Such enlightened self-regard, Churchill argues, curbs the exercise of immediate self-interest and leads to the recognition that only if I back benefits that others need, are others in turn likely to support programs that I too may need. Everyone must be assured access to health care if I am to remain secure in the conviction that I will continue to enjoy freedom of access. "The needs of others are ... part of my own security."[27]

From this perspective, justice is impeded by a short-term view of self-interest unconstrained by social reciprocity. But how does one come to understand enlightened self-interest and the need for social reciprocity? Churchill addresses this question in the language of sympathy and rights. Drawing again on Hume, and also Adam Smith (1723–1790),[28] he adduces the notion of sympathy, construed as the natural human affinities characteristic of social life. Although we have a strong sense of what sets people apart, there are countless ways in which we are drawn to each other, rely on each other, and help each other. Churchill advocates the deliberate cultivation of what we have in common in support of a social ethic grounded in solidarity and enlightened self-interest.

Churchill makes a case for a universal right to equitable access, based on need alone, and regardless of ability to pay, to all the effective health care a society can reasonably afford.[29] His view challenges us to specify the *scope* of the right, to articulate the meaning of "equitable" and "reasonable," including setting reasonable limits to a right to access. Churchill uses the term "limit" as a moral concept to encourage us to reconsider the way we think about fairness in the provision of health care. The emphasis is not on amounts of money or units of service ("my share") but on sharing a finite resource that we all hold in common. What is required is clarity of mind and heart about what health care is and what it should be for. Without a sense of the purposes the American health care system is supposed to serve, we will not be able to know whether we are achieving our aims. Churchill concludes: "The chief issue in health care reform is not finding the right mix of economic adjustments, it is finding our moral and political compass."[30]

SUMMATION

This chapter explored the issue of equity in the organization and distribution of health care. Beginning with a discussion of various presidential attempts to establish greater equity, it examined what Paul Starr calls "the American health care trap" as well as the reasons why America, alone among postindustrial democracies, has failed to enact a universal health insurance program. Then, with a focus on recent work in the field, it considered how we might find our moral and political compass amidst the complex network of actors and institutions that determine how we organize and distribute health care. Overall, this chapter emphasized that health care is an irreducible social good that is constitutive of who we are as citizens of a democracy grounded in social equality and respect for individuals in communities.

EXERCISES FOR CRITICAL THINKING AND CHARACTER FORMATION

QUESTIONS FOR DISCUSSION

1. Throughout this chapter, you have read about several different definitions of justice. What do you find useful or problematic in these definitions? What does justice mean to you?
2. During the health care debates of the 1990s, the health care industry launched a nationally televised advertising campaign urging against reform efforts. What are some of the various interests that influence health policy today?

3. This chapter begins with an epigraph from Rashi Fein: "A decent medical care system that helps all the people cannot be built without the language of equity and care." Do you agree with this? Why or why not?
4. What, in your opinion, are some of the challenges we face today when thinking about the just distribution of health care?

SUGGESTED WRITING EXERCISE

What, in your opinion, would a just health care system look like? How does your system depart from the current system in the United States? What are some of the obstacles that might prevent your ideal system from becoming a reality? Think about these questions, and then spend fifteen–twenty minutes writing about your idea of a just health care system.

SUGGESTED VIEWING

Escape Fire: The Fight to Rescue American Healthcare (2012)
Money and Medicine (2012)

Sicko (2007)
The Waiting Room (2012)

FURTHER READING

Jonathan Cohn, *Sick: The Untold Story of America's Health Care Crisis – and the People Who Pay the Price*

Paul Farmer, *Partner to the Poor: A Paul Farmer Reader*, ed. Haun Saussy

ADVANCED READING

Seyla Benhabib, *The Rights of Others: Aliens, Residents, and Citizens*
Norman Daniels, *Just Health: Meeting Health Needs Fairly*

Leonard M. Fleck, *Just Caring: Health Care Rationing and Democratic Deliberation*
Michael Ignatieff, *The Needs of Strangers: An Essay on Privacy, Solidarity, and the Politics of Being Human*

JOURNALS

Health Affairs
Journal of Health Politics, Policy, and Law

ORGANIZATIONS AND GROUPS

America's Health Insurance Plans
http://www.ahip.org

PART IV
Religion and Medicine

PART OVERVIEW
Religion and Medicine

Part 4 of this book deals with religion. The subject of religion as well as insights from religious studies and theology are underrepresented in medical humanities. In contrast, history of medicine, literature and medicine, and philosophy and medicine – Parts 1, 2, and 3 of this book – have long been established in medical humanities. This is not the case with religion and medicine. Indeed, some medical humanists have noted this absence and have invited religious studies scholars and theologians to contribute to the field. Writing in an editorial for *Medical Humanities*, Stephen Pattison observes, "My own discipline, religious studies and theology, has not been particularly fully represented in these pages. This, I believe, is unfortunate."[1] Pastoral theologians have made similar calls.[2]

Yet it would be inaccurate to say that religion has been ignored in medical humanities and in bioethics. In Chapter 22, we note that nearly all of the "founders" of bioethics had some ties to religion and that many of them were theologically trained but that in time, as bioethics became "secularized," as Daniel Callahan (1930–) puts it,[3] it became more problem- and policy-oriented as well as institutionalized and formalized. But medical humanities (in contrast to bioethics), with its pedagogical emphasis on educating humane doctors, did not secularize. If anything, spirituality is more important and recognized today in medical education than, say, forty years ago.[4] Moreover, founding as well as contemporary medical humanists and bioethicists such as Larry Churchill (1945–),[5] Leigh Turner,[6] Courtney Campbell,[7] Gilbert Meilaender (1946–),[8] Laurie Zoloth (1950–),[9] Andrew Lustig,[10] Daniel Sulmasy,[11] Paul Ramsey (1913–1988),[12] Richard McCormick (1922–2000),[13] William May (1928–),[14] David Smith (1939–),[15] Albert Jonsen (1931–)[16] wrote from, or were informed by, theological perspectives about the relevance of such concepts as suffering, meaning, healing, mutual regard, other-directedness, dialogue, empathy, caring, identity, and justice to patient care.

We explore this history in more detail in Chapter 22, but it is worth pointing out that the Society for Health and Human Values, which would later become the American Society for Bioethics and Humanities, was launched by Ronald

McNeur (1920–2005). McNeur was a New Zealander with a graduate degree in mathematics who, after returning from service in World War II, procured a doctoral degree in religious studies, became pastor of a Presbyterian church in the Bay Area of San Francisco, developed a series of lectures in which he attempted to "re-interpret the Christian faith for the scientific age," and then in 1959 took up the post of university pastor at the University of California, San Francisco Medical School. Over the next ten years, McNeur was the driver of the movement (then called "health and human values") during the period when it was conceived as a nonsectarian ministry. Verlyn Barker (1931–) also played a key role.[17] McNeur became executive director of the Society for Health and Human Values at its birth in 1969 and remained a thoughtful, low-key, influential presence in the Society's work until Edmund Pellegrino succeeded him and established an Institute on Human Values in Medicine.[18]

It is also worth noting that two of the coauthors of this book, Nathan Carlin (a junior scholar) and Ronald Carson (a senior scholar who served as president of the Society for Health and Human Values), were trained as theologians. Reflecting on his vocation, Carson writes:

> With hindsight, I realized that taking up my calling as a theologian in … medical humanities marked a move into a secular setting in which the life story that had formed me, and that I was critically appropriating, was one story among others and had no place of privilege. But it was (and is) my way of making sense of things. It indelibly informs my work.[19]

Carlin feels his own vocation unfolding in a similar manner. And we suspect that many of the persons listed above could identify with Carson's reflections. Also, it should be noted that this list is not meant to be exhaustive; rather, our point here is that, while there is more room for religious studies scholars and theologians to contribute to medical humanities as Pattison suggests, there is nevertheless a rich foundation on which to build. And there seems to be more freedom in medical humanities than in bioethics in this regard precisely because medical humanities is less formalized than bioethics.[20]

Today there also are a number of places where the subject of religion is regarded as important in medical contexts, such as (1) epidemiology of religion and health (a subject we address in Chapter 20); (2) existential and spiritual issues related to suffering, especially at the end of life (a subject we address in Chapter 23); and (3) and clinical matters of "cultural competency" in patient care (a subject we address in Chapter 19). The epidemiological, the existential, and the clinical are all places where matters of religion and spirituality have been explored in medical humanities writing. Some of the major questions of the field or area of religion and medicine can be put this way:

- In what ways do various religious beliefs, experiences, and practices intersect with particular health outcomes?
- In what ways do persons and communities draw on religion and spirituality to cope with, and to make sense of, disease and illness?

- How can physicians and other health care professionals best attend to matters of religion and spirituality in the context of patient care?
- What is the relevance of the religious faith and/or spirituality of caregivers for the practice of medicine?

These questions are all practical in some way. They address the ways in which religion is (or is not) good for health, the ways in which religion helps (or does not help) persons and communities cope and find meaning, the ways in which physicians and other health care professionals can provide better patient care, and the ways in which physicians and other health care professionals maintain meaning in the face of suffering. Other questions, such as learning about topics in religion and medicine simply for the sake of learning (such as studying the anthropology of religion and medicine in medieval Spain or in nineteenth-century Africa), also are important topics in religion and medicine, but, for reasons of space, we do not include such material in this section of the book.

A major purpose of this section of the book is to pull together material from other fields to establish this subfield or area – i.e., religion and medicine – within medical humanities. This approach is precisely how other fields and disciplines have come into being. Religious studies, for example, emerged out of many other fields, such as philosophy of religion, psychology of religion, theology, history of religions, sociology of religion, and so forth. Also, it is worth noting that one chapter in this section is different from the rest. Chapter 21, which focuses on religious experience and mental health, is intended not to pull together material from other fields but is intended to offer methods from religious studies. Specifically, in this chapter idiographic methods in psychology of religion are employed as a model to demonstrate how medical humanists might pursue new topics in religion and medicine.

19 World Religions for Medical Humanities

The fact that religion can be and often remains divisive is not a good reason for excluding it from the conversation.[1]

– David Smith

Medicine needs a scientific basis – but it also needs a soul.[2]

– Daniel Sulmasy

ABSTRACT

This chapter explores the world's five great religious traditions: Hinduism, Buddhism, Judaism, Islam, and Christianity. Beginning with a discussion of some of the challenges involved in cultural competency education, it examines why it is important to address religion and spirituality in patient care in general; the central tenets of each religious tradition; and the ways in which these tenets often inform peoples' understanding of health and illness. Then, with a focus on clinical practice, it considers three ways of addressing religion and spirituality in patient care.

INTRODUCTION

What should one do when a patient who is a Jehovah's Witness refuses a life-saving blood transfusion? How can one make sense of the heated debates among Roman Catholics and secular bioethicists on the ethics of end-of-life care? What should health care professionals know about the world's religious traditions? These types of questions often fall under the rubric of cultural competency education, which has become increasingly common in health professional schools. There are a number of guides or textbooks on the topic.[3] Many of these define "culture" and "cultural competency" in some way, provide a model of cultural competency (e.g., the Purnell Model for Cultural Competence), and then apply that model to various groups such as "People of German Heritage," "People of South Asian Heritage," and "People of African Heritage" to derive clinically relevant material for health care professionals. Such models often report whether, for example, a disease is more prevalent in a given group or whether certain cultural assumptions or behaviors are likely to be in conflict with Western biomedicine.

There are important critiques of cultural competency education. One critique is that, because the time spent on it is so brief, this kind of education in health professional schools spreads misinformation rather than promoting "critical awareness."[4] In other words, sometimes a little knowledge can do more harm than good. Knowing, for example, that many Jehovah's Witnesses often refuse life-saving blood transfusions does not mean than *all* Jehovah's Witnesses do, because some such patients might only voice their disagreements with their tradition in private (i.e., not in front of other family members).[5] Another critique is that this kind of education can lead to an increase of stereotyping,[6] the opposite effect of the intention of this education.[7] Even if the information taught is correct, there is still the problem of unintentionally inculcating an undesirable change in attitudes. For example, knowing that a given group suffers disproportionally from, say, diabetes could lead some health professionals to become "jaded" toward this group because they experience these patients as "non-compliant."[8] A third critique, which follows from the previous two, is that learning "facts" about groups of patients could lead to less patient-centered care. As Patricia Marshall writes,

> [I]n the fields of bioethics and biomedicine, applications of the "culture" concept are often simplified and do not provide a nuanced account of the full implications of cultural systems for healthcare or medical morality .... The consequence is a view of "culture" that is reified, too often reducing culture to a list of behavioral traits or customs that might be easily applied to individuals from diverse ethnic groups.[9]

These critiques hold a lot of weight when the advice being given in the name of cultural competency is not rooted in sophisticated anthropological work.

What is culture? Clifford Geertz (1926–2006), a highly regarded anthropologist, offered this definition: culture is "a system of inherited conceptions expressed in symbolic forms by means of which [people] communicate, perpetuate, and develop their knowledge about and attitudes toward life."[10] Culture, in other words, is the world in which one grows up. It is everything around us; it is the way we see things. Ideas about reality influence how we perceive our surroundings, and these ideas in turn inform our behavior. The study of these influences and perceptions is the work of anthropologists. To do anthropology well, Geertz emphasized the importance of "thick description," what he defined as the process of "sorting out the structures of signification."[11] This might be more plainly stated as paying serious and rigorous attention to context.

An oft-cited illustration used to explain what thick description is involves interpreting the experience of being winked at. Geertz notes that a person being winked at cannot understand the meaning of a wink without context, because winks can connote flirtation, irony, irritation, or something else entirely (winks can be involuntary). Because behaviors have meanings in contexts, it is not possible to interpret behavior outside of context. It follows that because medicine – along with everything else – is practiced in a context, the various behaviors that can be described in medicine cannot be understood without attention to context. Whereas many professional models of cultural competence fail to appreciate the significance of context, a model for excellent anthropological work in medicine can be observed in the writings of Arthur Kleinman (1941–), a medical anthropologist who was greatly influenced by Geertz.[12]

This chapter is not a chapter in medical anthropology. It does not do thick description of religious experience and medicine. But we do offer more than lists. This chapter attempts to provide a foundation for students to begin to think about religion and medicine by doing two things: (1) offering background information, both historical and clinical, on the five great religious traditions; and (2) offering practical advice on how to address religious and spiritual issues in patient care. We begin by addressing the rationale for teaching and learning about religion and spirituality in medical humanities.

SEVEN REASONS TO ADDRESS RELIGION AND SPIRITUALITY IN PATIENT CARE

In *Spirituality and Patient Care*, Harold Koenig offers six reasons for addressing religion and spirituality in patient care: (1) many patients report that they want their health care professionals to know something about their religious or spiritual background; (2) patients often use religious or spiritual beliefs and practices in order to cope; (3) patients who are hospitalized are sometimes separated from their religious communities and, therefore, could benefit from chaplaincy services; (4) religious beliefs can affect medical decision-making as well as compliance; (5) there is a substantial amount of evidence to suggest an association between religion and health; and (6) religious involvement may be related to support-systems in patients' communities.[13] Christina Puchalski offers an additional reason: taking spiritual histories can help clinicians understand their patients better by helping them attend to spiritual suffering.[14]

WORLD RELIGIONS FOR HEALTH CARE PROFESSIONALS

What is "religion"? What is "spirituality"? Many religious studies scholars have pointed out that defining religion is very difficult.[15] Koenig defines religion as "an organized system of beliefs, practices, and rituals of a community ... designed to increase a sense of closeness to the sacred ... and to promote an understanding of one's relationship to and responsibility for others living together in a community." He defines spiritualty as "a more generic personal quest for understanding answers to ultimate questions about life and its meaning ... and may or may not lead to religious beliefs, rituals, or the formation of a community."[16] This is only one way to define these terms; there are many others. Indeed, there are no authoritative definitions.[17]

The world's five great religious traditions are Hinduism, Buddhism, Judaism, Christianity, and Islam. This chapter focuses on each of these traditions. The following discussion will be split roughly equally between describing some of the basic features of these traditions and conveying information relevant to patient care.

Hinduism

Hinduism is the world's third largest religion with about 850 million adherents. It seems to have arisen in the Indus Valley around 1500 BCE. One distinctive feature of Hinduism is that it has no single religious founder (such as the Buddha), no single sacred text (such as the Qur'an), and no single central authority (such as the Pope). While there is great diversity among Hindus with regard to beliefs as well as practices, the *Vedas* (a collection of various sacred writings) tend to inform much of what Hindus practice and believe.[18]

Hindus often believe in a single, impersonal God (Nirguna Brahman). But because it is difficult to conceive of an impersonal God, the idea of a personal God (Saguna Brahman) arose, and this personal God is often imagined in three ways: as Creator (Brahma), as Preserver (Vishnu), and as Destroyer (Shiva). Manoj Shah and Siroj Sorajjakool note that Brahma, Vishnu, and Shiva are not three separate gods but are three manifestations of Saguna Brahman: "Ultimately, Hinduism asserts one Supreme God and the goal of believers is to merge with this God."[19]

Two key ideas in Hinduism are *samsara* and *karma*. *Samsara* refers to the cycle of birth, death, and rebirth (reincarnation), and *karma* refers to a law of causation that is linked to moral actions. Just as physics asserts that for every action there is an equal and opposite reaction, karma asserts that all moral actions have consequences but that sometimes the consequences of actions are realized in the next life. Hindus believe that the *atman* (often translated as soul) is immortal, while the body is mortal. The ultimate goal of Hinduism is *moksha* or liberation from samsara, and ways to achieve moksha include ridding oneself of karma by practicing various forms of yoga and by living a moral life. The idea that the soul is immortal combined with the idea that souls can be reincarnated as other forms of life such as plants or animals leads to a basic attitude of nonviolence and respect for all life. In some religious traditions of India that grow out of Hinduism, such as Jainism, some persons will only eat fruit that has fallen from trees because they believe that actively picking fruit from a tree is a form of violence.[20]

Hindu beliefs can affect how Hindus think about debates in bioethics. Regarding death and dying, for example, on the one hand euthanasia and physician-assisted suicide are often discouraged because suffering is sometimes understood to be the result of karma. On the other hand, prolonging life with artificial life support is also often discouraged because this is seen as disrupting the pattern of samsara. A similar logic influences how many Hindus think about abortion. Relatedly, some Hindus also oppose organ donation on the grounds that the karma from a donor's organ could affect the karma of the recipient.[21]

Ayurveda, a medical tradition in India concerned with health and longevity, arose in India in the sixth or fifth century BCE. Shah and Sorajjakool note that Ayurvedic medicine has eight basic categories: (1) general principles, (2) pathology, (3) diagnosis, (4) anatomy and physiology, (5) prognosis, (6) therapeutics, (7) pharmaceutics, and (8) treatment protocol. Ayurvedic medicine attempts to cultivate a balance among the body, the mind, and the soul, and it attempts to do this by means of such techniques as regulating diet, implementing exercise, and altering perception.[22]

Prakash Desai notes that "Hindu medicine never became divorced from the rest of life's pursuits, especially not from religious practice, as did medicine in the West."[23] Because Hinduism is more of a tradition (a way of life) than a faith (a system of beliefs), persons live out their traditions in ways that are not always conscious. This includes practices related to Ayurvedic medicine. For example, in *Shamans, Mystics, and Doctors* Sudhir Kakar (1938–) relates a personal experience in this regard. Kakar notes that he has used a tongue scrapper all of his life, a practice that he believes to be uniquely Indian, one to which he had attached no religious significance. It was only later in life while reading the first book of *Caraka Samhita* as a scholar of religion that he discovered that his daily practice of tongue scrapping has its roots in Ayurvedic medicine.[24]

Various scholars note that Ayurvedic medicine asserts that, on the one hand, there are external toxins that can create imbalance among the basic constitution of individuals. This tradition asserts that because people are made up of *vata* (wind and ether), *pitta* (fire and water), and *kapha* (water and earth), eating bad foods or breathing polluted air can create an imbalance within an individual. On the other hand, there are also internal factors, such as feelings of depression and anxiety, that can create imbalance.[25] One writer on Ayurvedic medicine notes that "an excess of *fire* will produce fever, redness, burning, smells, and discoloration; an excess of *wind* will produce paralysis, cramps, fainting, deafness, and joint pains; and the symptoms of aggravated moisture are drowsiness, lethargy, swelling, and stiffness."[26] Individuals are made of different constitutions, and so treatment varies based on one's constitution. For example, a person whose constitution leans toward vata responds well to hot beverages, whereas a person whose constitution leans toward pitta responds well to cold beverages. As a way of restoring balance, there is a practice called *panchakarma*, which consists of various procedures such as purging.[27]

Shah and Sorajjakool point out some key facts about Hinduism that health care professionals should know: (1) patients sometimes interpret disease as the result of *karma* (this belief can affect various aspects of clinical care, such as self-reports of pain); (2) the treatment of disease might include various practices from Ayurvedic medicine; (3) many Hindus are lacto-vegetarians, which affects both diet and medications; and (4) there are holy days in which Hindus commonly fast. Other practical advice that they offer for health care professionals includes removing one's shoes when entering an Indian household, not using one's left hand when interacting with persons from South Asia (the left hand is socially unclean), not placing Hindu scriptures on the floor, and noting the exact time of birth for Hindu children.[28] Koenig notes that many Hindus prefer obstetric services to be performed by female clinicians; bodies of the deceased are usually cremated (and that, after death, bodies are often not left alone until they have been cremated); and prayer for health is often not emphasized as in other traditions such as Christianity.[29] Purnell notes that a common complication for Western health professionals when caring for Hindu patients involves a difference in emphasis in the goals of medicine. While Ayurvedic medicine tends to focus on prevention, Western biomedicine tends to focus on restoration; the clinical upshot is that Hindu patients often engage in various forms of self-medication/self-care about which Western health professionals should inquire.[30]

Buddhism

Buddhism is a religion of India that grew up in the context of Hinduism. Unlike Hinduism, Buddhism does have a founder: Siddhartha Gautama (the Buddha). Gautama was born around 565 BCE to wealthy parents in modern day Nepal. Legend has it that nine months before he was born his mother had a dream in which she saw a white elephant (a symbol of holiness) entering her. The legend also holds that Gautama could walk immediately when he was born and that flowers grew in the place of his first footsteps. These stories, obviously, are meant to attest to his remarkable conception and birth. His mother died shortly after he was born.

As the story goes, a sage told Gautama's father that Gautama would become either a great king or a great holy man. Because his father wanted him to become a great king (and not a great holy man) he shielded his son from all things religious. He also sheltered him from the world. And so young Gautama grew and took a family and bore a son of his own. But as fate would have it, it seems as though Gautama was destined to become a holy man. One day he took a journey outside of his palace and he saw, for the first time, sickness, old age, and death. He was greatly disturbed by the suffering that he saw and so took upon himself the religious life to find out why there is suffering and how it might be overcome. He tried the path of meditating, but this did not yield the answers. He then tried the path of asceticism, but this, too, did not yield the answers.

And so he embraced components from both approaches, which he called "the middle way." He decided to sit under a tree until the mysteries of suffering were revealed to him. Under this tree, he became the enlightened – that is, he became the Buddha.[31]

What did the Buddha teach? He is best known for his Four Noble Truths. The first noble truth is that all of life is suffering. Some might regard this truth as a pessimistic philosophy of life. But Kathleen Gregory (1946–) writes, "To live within these conditions from which none of us can escape, Buddhism suggests, is not to be pessimistic, but to have a 'healthy attitude' of mind."[32] The second noble truth is that the cause of suffering is desire; the third noble truth is that the suffering can be relieved by giving up desire. The fourth noble truth is that desire can be given up by following the Eightfold Path, which means practicing correct views, intent, speech, conduct, means of working, endeavors, mindfulness, and meditation.[33]

Another key insight of the Buddha is the idea that nothing is permanent. The things people generally want in life – youth, health, pleasure, money, safety, friends, family, power – never stay the same. People age, friends get sick, pleasure fades, stock markets crash, family members die, and power and safety come and go. The Buddha taught that we need to cultivate detachment from all things in order to avoid suffering. Another key idea is the notion that there is no self. This teaching holds that the self, just like all things, is not permanent or real in any ultimate sense.[34]

What is the upshot of these basic beliefs for clinical practice? Siroj Sorajjakool and Supaporn Naewbood suggest that three key ideas affect how many Buddhists think about health and disease. First, since Buddhists see a strong connection between mind and body, as health is understood to be "the harmonious balance of the body, mind, emotion, and the spiritual dimension and therefore is not merely the absence of disease."[35] Health, then, is ultimately a spiritual matter. Second, as in Hinduism, disease is sometimes understood to be the result of karma from immoral actions in one's current or previous lives. Hindus and Buddhists also hold collective understandings of karma (e.g., industry polluting the environment can cause both collective and individual suffering). Third, because Buddhism teaches a respect for all life and advocates nonviolent ways of being, many Buddhists oppose abortion. But some Buddhists, Peter Harvey notes, believe that abortion is acceptable if it is done out of compassion (e.g., to save the mother's life).[36] As the Dalai Lama has said, "If the unborn child will be retarded [sic] or if the birth will create serious problems for the parent, these are cases where there can be an exception. I think abortion should be approved or disapproved according to each circumstance."[37]

Sorajjakool and Naewbood also offer some practical clinical advice. They note that there is great diversity among beliefs and practices of Buddhists (the main divisions are Mahayana Buddhism and Theravada Buddhism), and that even within a given school of thought there will be considerable diversity. They also note that many Buddhists practice various dietary restrictions. Some practice vegetarianism, while others will not eat onions or garlic. Paying attention to religious items such as sacred threads is important, and such items ought not to be removed without the patient's permission. Regarding death practices, Buddhists often let the body lie for a period of time, sometimes until a Buddhist monk leads the body to the temple for funeral rites.[38] Clinically speaking, this would mean not moving the body immediately after death in the intensive care unit. Koenig writes that, "It is extremely important to provide as much peace and quiet as possible for the dying person, since state of mind at the moment of death is believed to affect the quality of the next life."[39]

Judaism

The father of the Jewish faith is said to be Abraham, who lived around 1750 BCE. God, or YHWH (pronounced *Adonai*), called Abraham into a covenantal relationship, meaning that if Abraham would obey God's commands then God would multiply Abraham's progeny. Abraham's descendants became known as Hebrews. After some time, they fell into slavery in Egypt. While enslaved, Moses, another major figure in Judaism, led them out from their enslavement. Jews believe that the Law (or Torah) was subsequently given to Moses from God around 1125 BCE on Mount Sinai. Other key events in Jewish history, as recounted in the Hebrew Bible, include the militaristic conquest of Canaan sometime after the death of Moses; King David's rule (circa 1000 BCE); and the Babylonian Exile in the sixth century BCE. The Rabbinic Period of Judaism (63 CE to 500 CE), distinguished by the fact that it was inaugurated by the destruction of the Second Temple by the Romans, was characterized by transforming Judaism from a religion oriented around temple rituals to a religion focused on the interpretation of texts. Another key feature of the Rabbinic Period is that Jews were expelled to move all over the world (this is sometimes referred to as the Diaspora). For hundreds of years Jews lived as minorities among Christian and Muslim populations, often facing discrimination and persecution. A notable exception to this was the Golden Age of Spain (900 CE–1200 CE) where Jews held prominent positions in the royal courts. The most infamous persecution in modern times was the Holocaust (1938–1945), where 6 million Jews were killed by the Nazis during World War II. In 1948, the state of Israel was established to provide Jews a home. The creation of this state and its borders was and still is rife with dispute and conflict because creating this home for Jews meant moving Muslims, sometimes with force, out of the land, and some Muslims have responded with force. What is striking – and unfortunate – is that both groups believe that this land is sacred, that God gave the land to them, and that God has authorized them to use force in order to defend it.[40]

What are the central beliefs and practices of Judaism? The first thing to note about Judaism is that it is a practice-oriented religion and not a belief-oriented religion. Judaism, it is sometimes said, is a religion of deed, not creed. Yet there are essential precepts in Judaism, such as (1) God is one, (2) God is transcendent, and (3) God has entered into a covenantal relationship with Jews. Judaism also upholds the sanctity of life and respect for the body, so much so that some sacred texts in Judaism (e.g., the Talmud) command Jews not to live in a town in which there is no physician.[41]

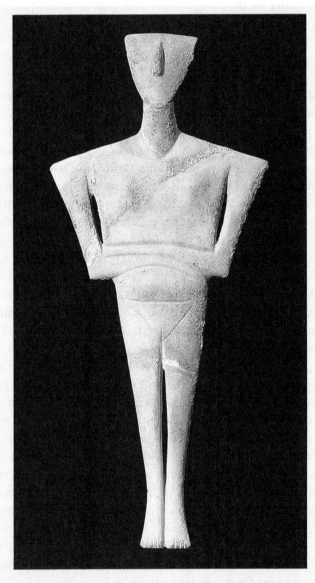

Figure 19. *Cycladic Idol from Syros,* ca. 2000 BCE. National Archaeological Museum, Athens, Greece. Photo Credit: Scala/Art Resource, NY.

How does this figure express the reserve you might experience when addressing a person from a different culture with beliefs different from your own? With its shield-like head and flat, angular anatomy, its arms crossed at the waist, this figure appears self-contained, even enigmatic. These characteristics are seen in European and American abstract sculpture of the early to mid-twentieth century. For comparison, search for sculptures by Henry Moore and Jacques Lipchitz. However, this figure was created more than four thousand years ago, in the Cyclades, a group of Greek islands in the Aegean sea. The figure, and others like it, has been enigmatic to archaeologists, who have found no evidence to determine if they are either idols or dolls.

Have you encountered any patients like this? Is she suffering or simply uncommunicative? How would you expect her to respond to diagnostic questions? What would you need to know to formulate questions this figure would respond to? For practice, review the questions recommended in this chapter and ask a few of them, out loud, to this figure. How does the figure's reticence make you feel? How would a patient who exhibits similar reticence make you feel?

Douglas Kohn points out that there are different sects or branches of Judaism, such as Orthodox, Conservative, and Reform. These different brands of Judaism attest to a wide range of beliefs, which is apparent on issues such as abortion. Kohn suggests, for example, that in the Hebrew Bible life is believed to have begun when an infant takes his or her first breath (cf. Genesis 2:7; Job 33:4; Ezekiel 37:10), and so, he reasons, abortion should not be regarded as the killing of a person but rather the destruction of a fetus (since fetuses do not breathe). And death, Kohn also points out, is believed to have occurred when a person stops breathing (in Hebrew, the word for "breath" and the word for "soul" is the same). Yet many Orthodox Jews oppose abortion, citing passages in the Torah that equate life not with breath but with blood (see Leviticus 17:11). Kohn points out that, even if the fetus can be regarded as human life by the logic of the Torah, it is certainly not on par with the life of children and adults, as the Torah is clear that the death of a fetus is not as great of a loss as the death of a person (Exodus 21:22; cf. *Oholt* 7:6).[42]

A key theological belief in Judaism is that the body is a gift from God and ought to be treated as such. Treating the body in a healthy manner is, therefore, a moral mandate. This leads some Jews to discourage things such as tattoos and body piercing. Historically, this also led some Jews to object to autopsies and embalming as well as organ donation.[43] Also, many Jews observe a dietary system called *kashrut*. The foods that are acceptable to eat are *kosher* and foods disallowed are *treif*. Animals with cloven hoofs, such as pigs and dogs, are treif, as well as fish that lack scales or fins such as catfish and shellfish. The Talmud also forbids mixing meat and milk from the same animal during a single meal. Many people believe that the rationale for these beliefs are related to health, but Kohn suggests that these restrictions arose out a "discipline for Jewish living" rather than a concern for health (the health outcomes of these various practices were unknown when they were prescribed). But some practices, such as the command to wash one's hands seven times a day, *did* lead to better health outcomes during, for example, the Black Death.[44] Today, circumcision is sometimes defended on the grounds of health outcomes (it is unclear if circumcision is beneficial, in terms of health outcomes, in developed countries, but it has been shown to be beneficial in reducing the spread of HIV/AIDS in Africa[45]). Yet Kohn also suggests that circumcision and other such practices may be "construed" as health practices today.

Kohn notes that there are a number of genetic diseases that are more prevalent among Jews than other groups. These include Tay-Sachs disease, Gaucher disease type 1, Bloom's disease, familial dysautonomia, and cystic fibrosis. Jewish couples, therefore, are often encouraged to undergo genetic testing prior to conceiving a child to consider various strategies for pregnancy. He also points out that some recent research suggests that breast cancer and ovarian cancer are more prevalent among Jews.[46] Koenig notes that Orthodox (and some Conservative) Jews believe that women are impure for a period of time after childbirth and menstruation, meaning that men will not touch their wives during these periods; that keeping kosher is very important; that a body should not be touched for some time after death (usually eight to thirty minutes); that Jews may not touch dead bodies on the Sabbath; and that the Sabbath begins on Friday evening and ends on sunset the following day. He notes that Reform Jews are more relaxed about many of these customs (some even eat pork), so it is, therefore, harder to make generalizations about Reform Jews and to offer clinical advice to health professionals.[47] As Dan Cohn-Sherbok (1945–) writes, "In the modern world, the Jewish community has fragmented into a wide range of different groupings, each with their own interpretation of the tradition ... [but] all Jews ... embrace the Jewish emphasis on caring for the sick and those who suffer."[48]

Christianity

Christianity is the world's largest religion. "Christian" means follower of Jesus Christ. Jesus of Nazareth was born about 2,000 years ago (circa 2 BCE). His father Joseph was a carpenter or some kind of tradesman. When Jesus was about thirty years old, he left his father's trade (assuming he worked with his father), was baptized by John the Baptist in the wilderness, and gathered his disciples. According to Christian sources, for a short period – either a year or three years (the Gospels disagree on the length of his ministry) – it is said that he traveled around what Christians call the Holy Land, preaching, teaching, healing, and performing miracles. The Gospels suggest that he was perceived to be a threat by religious (Jewish) and political (Roman) leaders, and so he was put to death under the supervision of a Roman official named Pontius Pilate. Most Christians believe that Jesus was resurrected from the dead three days later and that after a few brief appearances to his friends and followers he ascended into heaven. Before he ascended into heaven, Christian sources indicate that he commanded his followers to go into the whole world proclaiming the "good news" of salvation, baptizing them in the name of the Father, Son, and Holy Spirit (Matthew 28:16–20).[49]

There are three major branches of Christianity: Roman Catholic, Eastern Orthodox, and Protestant. Within Protestant Christianity, there are thousands of different denominations. This means that there is a great deal of variety regarding the specifics of what various Christians believe. Core beliefs that many Christians hold in common include the following: (1) God is one; (2) God is triune; (3) God is both immanent and transcendent; (4) Jesus Christ is the incarnation of God, who is both fully human and fully divine; (5) Jesus Christ became human to die (atone) for the sins of humanity; and (6) Jesus Christ was raised from the dead, thus conquering death and giving hope to all of humanity.[50] Alister McGrath points out that the idea that salvation is offered by Christ through the church is a core belief in Christianity, and that salvation has many meanings, such as healing, restoration, and rescue. He also points out that St. Augustine of Hippo, arguably the greatest theologian of the Western church, used medical images to argue that "the Christian church was to be conceived as a hospital – a place in which wounded and broken people might receive care and healing."[51]

Another core belief in Christianity, which is derived from Judaism, is that human beings are created in the image of God (Genesis 1:27); also, in the New Testament St. Paul asserts that the body is a Temple of the Holy Spirit (1 Corinthians 6:19–20) – these scripture verses in the Hebrew Bible and the Christian New Testament have led Christian theologians and ethicists to argue that human life is sacred. This conviction has sparked debate in areas such as contraception and abortion as well as end-of-life care.[52] Indeed, some of the most well-known cases in the history of bioethics have involved the tensions between secular bioethicists and Roman Catholic theological ethicists.[53]

In the Roman Catholic tradition, deriving from the writings of St. Thomas Aquinas, the notion of "intention" is especially important, as it informs what is called the doctrine or rule of "double-effect."[54] The doctrine of double-effect makes a distinction between foreseeable consequences and intended consequences. If, for example, the intent of an abortion is to end life, it is wrong. On the other hand, if the intent of a surgery is to save a mother's life – from, say, uterine cancer – and the consequence is the death of the fetus, the surgery can be viewed as morally justifiable. Is it wrong for health care professionals to hasten death by giving a large dose of pain medication? It is not necessarily wrong if the intent is to relieve suffering (so long as one does not intend to cause death). It should be noted, however, that there is internal debate within the Roman Catholic Church concerning the application of the doctrine of double-effect (some, for example, hold that abortion is only justified in cases of uterine cancer and ectopic pregnancy).

In recent decades, issues relating to sexuality have received a great deal of popular and scholarly attention with regard to Christianity. David Larson (1947–) notes that while Christians affirm that human sexuality has two functions – a unitive purpose (making love) and a procreative purpose (making babies) – Christians are divided as to whether it is morally permissible to separate these functions. Since, for example, gay men cannot procreate with each other, some Christians oppose so-called "homosexual practice."[55] Abortion also sometimes separates these purposes. As Larson observes, conservative Christians tend to oppose abortion (unless it is performed to save the mother's life) while liberal Christians affirm women's right to choose (though often with regret at the loss of the life of the fetus).[56]

In terms of clinical practice, a few words about diet are instructive. Many Christians, perhaps the majority, do not observe dietary restrictions on the grounds that St. Paul argued that all foods and drinks are acceptable (1 Corinthians 10:31). Yet some Christians abstain from alcohol, practice vegetarianism, and/or observe certain fasts.

Beliefs about the sacraments and other such beliefs also can impact clinical care. For centuries, the Roman Catholic Church unofficially taught that unbaptized babies that die would not go to heaven but would instead go to limbo, a place between heaven and hell. The upshot of this belief was that if there were any chance that a baby would die at birth a priest would be called to baptize the baby as quickly as possible.[57] Another sacrament in the Roman Catholic tradition is Holy Unction/Last Rites (also called the Anointing of the Sick), where a priest will perform certain rituals with the dying patient in order to help him or her cope. Koenig notes that Protestant pastors and ministers, while they do not practice the sacrament of the Holy Unction, often offer prayers at the bedside of sick patients and perform communion services. And he notes that some Christians, such as Roman Catholics, revere certain objects such as rosary beads and statues of the Virgin Mary, and that practices relating to baptism vary across denominations.[58]

Islam

Islam is a monotheistic religion founded by the Prophet Muhammad (570–632 CE) in the seventh century CE. He is believed to be the final Prophet in a long line of prophets, a line that includes Abraham, Moses, David, Jesus, and others. It is believed that the Prophet received a revelation from the angel Gabriel at the age of forty. This revelation is known as the Qur'an, the central sacred text of Islam. It also is believed that the Qur'an is the literal word of God (Allah), spoken by Gabriel to Muhammad in Arabic over a period of twenty-three years. The word "Muslim" means "one who submits to Allah." Because Gabriel spoke the language of Arabic to the Prophet, Arabic holds a special place among Muslims in a way that, for example, Greek (the language of the New Testament) or Aramaic (the language of Jesus) does not for Christians. Next to the Qur'an, the Sunnah is the second foundational doctrinal source. The Sunnah consists of written accounts of alleged words and deeds of the Prophet.[59]

There are two main groups of Muslims: Sunni and Shi'a. Sunni Muslims constitute the vast majority of Muslims (roughly 80 percent of all Muslims). The Shi'a split from the Sunni after the death of the Prophet because of disagreement as to who should succeed the Prophet. A third group of Muslims constitute the Sufis. Sufism represents the major mystical branch of Islam. Sufis also often identify as either Sunni or Shi'a. Within these basic groups, there are many subgroups.[60]

There are a diversity of beliefs and practices among Muslims. However, what is common to most is an affirmation of the Five Pillars of Islam. The first pillar is the *shahada*, or a verbal affirmation that there is one God and the Prophet is His messenger. The second pillar is *salat*, the practice of daily prayers (five prayers are to be said every day, facing Mecca). The third pillar is the giving of alms or charity (*zakat*). The fourth pillar is *sawm*, the practice of fasting during the holy month of Ramadan (a month to celebrate the revelation of the Qur'an to the Prophet). And the fifth pillar involves the obligation for Muslims to complete the *Hajj*, a religious pilgrimage to Mecca, at least once in their lives.[61]

Hamid Mavani notes that much of what Muslims believe about ethical issues relating to health and disease is similar to what Jews and Christians believe because all of these traditions are rooted in the faith of Abraham and thus have similar sentiments. However, as Aasim Padela points out, modern Islamic medical ethics writers ground their arguments in non-Judeo-Christian sources, such *Adab* literature and the *Shari'ah*.[62] Just as there is great diversity within Judaism and Christianity, there is great diversity within Islam. For example, just as Jews and Christians are divided on the ethics of abortion, so, too, are Muslims. But what is unique about Muslims is when they define ensoulment. While there is not an "official" definition, Mavani notes that many Muslims hold that ensoulment occurs around forty-five days after fertilization, meaning that many Muslims would especially oppose abortion after this period. Mavani also notes that Muslims tend to have a more positive view toward sexuality within marriage than many Christians because Muslims do not insist that the procreative and unitive functions of sex need to be combined.[63] Historically, many Christians, such as St. Augustine, have lamented the fact that sex is pleasurable at all, even in marriage.[64]

Basic attitudes toward ethical issues in end-of-life care are similar to those of Christians (allowing a patient to die is often viewed as acceptable whereas the active hastening of death is not). It also is believed that, since God is the author of life and death, both murder and suicide are wrong because they interfere with God's prerogative (Qur'an 3:145).[65]

Muslims have distinctive rituals of death and dying. Certain rituals are believed to help the soul leave the body, such as (1) the recitation of the shahada; (2)

seeking forgiveness from God; (3) reciting certain passages from the Qur'an such as Yasin and the Confederates; and (4) placing the soles of one's feet such that they face the Ka'bah in Mecca. Once the patient dies, he or she must be buried (not cremated) quickly, according to certain rituals. Specifically, the body must be washed, shrouded, and prayed over, and dead bodies are treated as though they were alive in that gender prohibitions relating to modesty still ought to be recognized. These rituals usually are not performed for babies less than four months old.[66]

Related clinical issues involve matters of modesty, prayer, and diet. Many Muslims do not eat pork or take medication derived from pigs. Many will only eat or use *halal* (i.e., permitted) products.[67] The injunction not to consume pork leads some, but not all, Muslims to reject certain medical devices such as certain biological heart valves that utilize material derived from pigs. Koenig notes that fathers of infants often whisper prayers into the ears of babies when they are born; that special fasting and prayers occur during the month of Ramadan; and that religious services are typically held on Friday.[68]

Concluding this section on world religions for health professionals, we would do well to remind ourselves that simply learning a list of do's and don't's with regard to religious traditions is inadequate. As Abdulaziz Sachedina (1942–) notes with regard to Islam, "Spiritual care begins in providing settings that permit, and preferably encourage, religious observance .... [and] also involves supporting appropriate decision-making. Healthcare practitioners need the capacity to provide patients and families with information that is appropriate to religious, communitarian ethical decision-making, and to respect the process such decision-making must take."[69]

HOW TO ADDRESS RELIGION AND SPIRITUALITY IN PATIENT CARE: THREE APPROACHES

We conclude by offering three models of how to attend to religion and spirituality in patient care. We present (1) a general list of advice derived from the previous discussion; (2) a list of questions suggested by medical anthropology; and (3) the "FICA" model of taking a spiritual history.

Some Clinical Advice

The clinical implications of our discussion of world religious traditions can be summed up as follows:

1. Ask about dietary needs.
2. Ask about fasting.
3. Ask about daily religious practices (such as prayer and meditation practices). Try to accommodate these needs as much as possible.

4. Ask about holy days and how they might be relevant to their care.
5. Be aware of modesty concerns, and accommodate them as much as possible.
6. Do not touch or remove objects that may appear to be sacred.
7. Ask patients if they are aware of any of their religious beliefs that may affect their care or clinical decision-making, such as prohibitions against blood transfusions or other medical procedures.
8. Ask patients and families how they prepare for birth, and what rituals are important to them.
9. Ask patients and families how they prepare for death, and what rituals are important to them.

Giving specific advice is a valuable tool, but it is no substitute for addressing existential and emotional issues and it can also fall prey to the critiques of cultural competency offered in the introduction of this chapter.

Arthur Kleinman's Model

Another approach, offered by medical anthropologist Arthur Kleinman, involves asking certain culturally sensitive, open-ended questions:

- What do you call your problem? What name do you give it?
- What do you think has caused your problem?
- Why do you think it started when it did?
- What does your sickness do to your body? How does it work inside you?
- How severe is it? Will it get better soon or take longer?
- What do you fear most about your sickness?
- What are the chief problems your sickness has caused for you (personally, in your family, and at work)?
- What kind of treatment do you think you should receive? What are the most important results you hope you will receive from the treatment?[70]

Joan Anderson et al. note that these questions do not have to be (and perhaps should not be) used as direct questions to be asked but could/should instead be used as "listening cues." When, for example, a patient mentions something about one of these questions, the physician can follow up with a question that probes a little deeper by asking for an elaboration or clarification.[71] The strength of this approach is that it does not require health care professionals to learn all of the intricate details about, say, Christian Science beliefs regarding illness and disease because these questions are open ended. A weakness is that it is not specific enough about spirituality and religion.

The FICA Model

Christina Puchalski has put forth a well-known method of taking a spiritual history, called "FICA."[72] It has received considerable attention in recent years, perhaps because of its applicability and recall-ability. "F" concerns asking patients about their *faith* (e.g., Are you religious? Do you attend religious services?). "I" concerns asking patients about the *importance* of their faith or belief (e.g., Are religious beliefs a significant part of your life?). "C" concerns asking patients about their faith *community* (e.g., Are there people from your religious community who can support you in your time of illness?). "A" concerns how patients would like their faith *addressed* in their care (e.g., Do you want your physician to attend to your faith concerns – if so, how?). Pulchalski has learned that simply being present goes a long way with patients and that it is important to refer to chaplains. She has also found that it is important to make time and space for activities such as ritual, prayer, guided imagery, and mediation. This model has a number of strengths: It is brief, specific to spirituality and religion, and is open-ended.

ROLE PLAYING

This is a role-playing exercise. Students should get into groups of three. One student should pretend to be an internal medicine physician, attending to Ms. Smith. The second student should play the role of Ms. Smith. The third student should simply observe. The role of the third student is to observe what seem to be helpful (and unhelpful) word choices. In other words, which word choices feel awkward, and which word choices seem to lead to more connection and sharing?

Ms. Smith is:

"[A] forty-seven-year-old single woman, in whom the sudden appearance of widespread metastatic breast cancer caused her to be hospitalized and near death .... But it is not primarily the weakness, profound anorexia, and generalized swelling, as distressing as these things are, that are the source of her suffering, but the loss of control an inability to prevent the evaporation of her career, whole brilliant promise had finally been realized a few months earlier."[73]

You, as her internal medicine physician, have seen Ms. Smith many times before, and you have a good relationship with her. You are prompted to take a spiritual history after hearing Grand Rounds on the topic.

Students should switch roles and do the exercise again. All three students should have a chance to play all three roles.

Debriefing Questions

1. How did Ms. Smith interpret her illness?
2. How did Ms. Smith talk about her work life?
3. What role did religion or spiritually play in Ms. Smith's life?
4. What did it feel like to be listening to Ms. Smith's story?
5. Did you, as the internal medicine physician, use any awkward phrases or words choices? If so, how would you reword what you said?

CONCLUSION

This chapter offered historical and clinical information on the five great religious traditions of the world, as well as practical advice on addressing religion and spirituality in patient care. While realizing the limits of cultural competency education, the purpose of this chapter was to help students to learn about religion and medicine. This chapter also mentioned, in passing, reasons why addressing religion and spirituality in patient care is important (e.g., there appears to be an association between religion and health). Subsequent chapters will explore such reasons further.

SUMMATION

This chapter explored the world's five great religious traditions: Hinduism, Buddhism, Judaism, Islam, and Christianity. Beginning with a discussion of some of the challenges involved in cultural competency education, it examined why it is important to address religion and spirituality in patient care in general; the central tenets of each religious tradition; and the ways in which these tenets come to inform people's understanding of health and illness. Then, with a focus on clinical practice, it considered three ways of addressing religion and spirituality in patient care. Overall, though, this chapter attempted to emphasize that religion and spirituality play an important part in many people's lives, and that a greater attention to this fact can help us to better understand and care for patients.

EXERCISES FOR CRITICAL THINKING AND CHARACTER FORMATION

QUESTIONS FOR DISCUSSION

1. What role does religion play in your life?
2. How might your own religious or spiritual commitments affect your worldview as a health care professional?
3. Some people think that there is not enough time to take spiritual histories, and that there are more important matters to which to attend. What do you think about this objection?

4. To what extent should requests made by patients based on religious commitments be accommodated? For example, if a female Muslim patient requests female caregivers, to what extent and under what circumstances, if any, should this request be accommodated?

SUGGESTED WRITING EXERCISE

In *Cross-Cultural Caring*, Nancy Waxler-Morrison and Joan Anderson describe a situation where a physician called a social worker about a case of potential child abuse.[74] A two-year-old Vietnamese boy presented with trouble breathing. When examined, a physician discovered bruises all over his back. When a social worker inquired about the case, she found that the family was practicing "spooning," a common treatment for colds in Vietnam that entails pressing a silver spoon up and down a child's back. The mother of the child said that they wanted to try this approach first because they did not have a lot of money to spend. From the perspective of the mother, write a letter to the social worker, explaining your side of the story.

SUGGESTED VIEWING

Stanford University's *World's Apart* Documentary Film Series

http://medethicsfilms.stanford.edu/worldsapart/

FURTHER READING

Karen Armstrong, *The Case for God*

Huston Smith, *The Illustrated World's Religions*

ADVANCED READING

Mark Cobb, Christina Puchalski, and Bruce Rumbold, eds., *The Oxford Textbook in Spirituality and Health*
Kathleen Culhane-Pera, Dorothy Vawter, Phua Xiong, Barbara Babbitt, and Mary Solberg, eds., *Healing by Heart: Clinical and Ethical Case Studies of Hmong Families and Western Providers*
Clifford Geertz, *The Interpretation of Cultures*

Arthur Kleinman, *The Illness Narratives*
Harold Koenig, *Spirituality in Patient Care*
Jing-Bao Nie, *Medical Ethics in China: A Transcultural Interpretation*
Siroj Sorajjakool, Mark Carr, and Julius Nam, eds., *World Religions for Healthcare Professionals*
Bryan Turner, ed., *Routledge Handbook of Body Studies*

JOURNALS

Anthropology and Medicine
Journal of the American Academy of Religion
Journal of Medicine and Philosophy

Journal of Religion and Health
Social Science and Medicine
Studies in Medical Anthropology

PROGRAMS

The University of Chicago Program in Medicine and Religion

https://pmr.uchicago.edu/

ONLINE RESOURCES

Karen Armstrong TED Talk
http://www.ted.com/talks/karen_armstrong_makes_her_
ted_prize_wish_the_charter_for_compassion.html
Onora O'Neill on Trust – Philosophy Bites
http://ec.libsyn.com/p/1/4/7/147bef66fc0b192f/Onora_
ONeill_on_Trust_originally_on_Bioethics_Bites.mp3?d1
3a76d516d9dec20c3d276ce028ed5089ab1ce3dae902ea1d
01c08233d0ce547046&c_id=4568869
The Center on Religions and the Professions
http://www.religionandprofessions.org/other-resources/
professional-associations-faith-groups/
Healthcare Chaplaincy

http://www.healthcarechaplaincy.org/
Health Ministries Association
http://www.hmassoc.org/
Interfaith Health and Wellness Association
http://www.ihwassoc.org/
Georgetown University's National Center for Cultural
Competence
http://nccc.georgetown.edu/body_mind_spirit/resources.
html
The George Washington Institute for Spirituality and
Health
http://www.gwumc.edu/gwish/index.cfm

20 Religion and Health

Our spiritual judgment ... must be decided on empirical grounds exclusively. If the fruits of life of the state of conversion are good, we ought to idealize and venerate it, even though it be a piece of natural psychology; if not, we ought to make short work with it, no matter what supernatural being may have infused it.[1]

– William James

ABSTRACT

This chapter explores the field of religion and health. Beginning with a discussion of the historical roots of the field, it examines the contributions of key authors Jeffrey Levin and Harold Koenig; the major approaches and instruments that have been used to study the relationship between religion and health; and the critics of these studies. Then, with a focus on clinical practice, it suggests that paying attention to the way that religion functions in patients' lives can help us to better care for patients.

INTRODUCTION

A woman traveled into town one morning to go shopping and began to feel ill. She felt pain in her bones, felt nauseated, and had a headache. She also felt as though she were going to faint. It occurred to her that these were symptoms of the flu. The woman then thought about the mind-cure techniques she had been learning, and decided to try them. After she returned home, she asked her husband to call a doctor to come the next morning, as she wanted to continue trying her mind-cure techniques during the night. She next describes one of the most beautiful experiences of her life:

> I cannot express it in any other way than to say that I did "lie down in the stream of life and let it flow over me." I gave up all fear of any impending disease; I was perfectly willing and obedient. There was no intellectual effort, or train of thought. My dominant idea was: "Behold the handmaid of the Lord: be it unto me even as thou wilt," and a perfect

confidence that all would be well, that all *was* well. The creative life was flowing into me every instant, and I felt myself allied with the Infinite, in harmony, and full of the peace that passeth understanding. There was no place in my mind for a jarring body. I had no consciousness of time or space or persons; but only of love and happiness and faith. "I do not know how long this state lasted, nor when I fell asleep; but when I woke up in the morning, *I was well.*"[2]

One might consider this account, found in William James's (1842–1910) *The Varieties of Religious Experience*, to be somewhat trivial, as James himself concedes, and one might also note, as James did, that the woman may have been deluded. However, how do we know that the universe and reality is not more complex than what science allows for – how do we know that techniques such as mind-cure do not work? Could it be that science gives us access to some domains of reality whereas religion gives us access to other domains of reality, and that no single system can fully account for the complexity of reality? James suggests that this might be the case.

Writing shortly before James, Francis Galton (1822–1911) was an early psychologist of religion who studied religion quantitatively (i.e., with statistics, questionnaires, and rating scales). He, like James, was interested in the fruits of religion but, in contrast to James, had a negative bias toward religion. He therefore sought to show, empirically, that religion does not provide benefits – health or otherwise. If prayer were associated with longevity, Galton suggested that male members of royal households should have longer lives than the average male because the public prays for these persons on a daily basis, but he observed the life span of male members of royal households from 1758 to 1843 and found that their lives were among the shortest of male members of affluent classes. He also studied the biographies of many eminent religious leaders (e.g., Martin Luther, John Calvin, and John Donne) and found that such persons tend to live shorter lives than other eminent men. And he found that religious buildings such as churches have no special protection, statistically speaking, against hazards such as earthquakes and fires.[3]

Galton's quantitative methods were not sophisticated, and his agenda certainly biased his observations. While today's empirical methods are much more sophisticated, bias still remains. Indeed, one of the largest financial supporters of the field of religion and health is the John Templeton Foundation. The back cover of the second edition of Harold Koenig's *Spirituality in Patient Care* reads:

> Templeton Foundation Press helps intellectual leaders and others learn about science research on aspects of realities, invisible and intangible. Spiritual realities include unlimited love, accelerating creativity, worship, and *the benefits of purpose in persons and in the cosmos.*[4]

This press, in other words, solicits research that will provide empirical support to the benefits of spirituality. Just as one can be skeptical of Galton's bias, one can be skeptical of the Templeton Foundation's bias and the research projects it funds. But, in fairness, it is important to note that the Templeton Foundation funded Herbert Benson's multimillion dollar study of prayer that found that *intercessory prayer had no effect* among 1,800 coronary-bypass surgery patients, a modern result consistent with Galton's previous findings.[5] The publication of this paper speaks to the integrity of the Templeton Foundation.

Foundations and individual researchers will always have a bias when it comes to religion – religion is simply too emotional a topic to be studied in an unbiased way. This suggests that the goal for researchers should not be to eliminate bias but rather to manage bias appropriately. This chapter tries to manage any potential bias by attempting to provide an even-handed introduction to the field of religion and health.

AN OVERVIEW OF RELIGION AND HEALTH

The field of religion and health, just like any other field, can be defined in various ways. We understand the field as a combination of empirical psychology of religion and epidemiology. If one were to choose a single text to represent the field, it would be *The Handbook of Religion and Health*, edited by Harold G. Koenig, Dana King, and Verna Carson.[6]

Common Topics and Sample Findings in the Field

There are a number of questions that are routinely asked in the field of religion and health. Does going to church have an effect on heart disease, hypertension, or cancer? Can healthy behaviors, such as not smoking, be correlated with religious affiliation? To what extent is religious involvement associated with disability? What are the health benefits of intercessory prayer? Do older adults who identify as religious or spiritual age better than those who do not identify as such? To what extent and in what ways does religion help individuals cope with various life stressors? Can meditation help individuals mitigate pain? These are but a few questions that intimate the nature of the field. The field attempts to find statistical associations – positive or negative – between various dimensions of religion and/or spirituality and specific measures of health.

In a 2012 literature review of the field, Hisham Abu-Raiya and Kenneth Pargament (1950–) offer a summary of some of its methodological issues as well as some of the key findings in recent years. The table below relays some of these findings.[7]

SAMPLE FINDINGS FROM RELIGION AND HEALTH STUDIES

Variable Measured	Positive Health Outcomes
Religious involvement (e.g., self-rated religiousness, endorsement of religious beliefs, participation in religious rituals)	Religious involvement is associated with lower hypertension, lower rates of substance abuse, lower rates of overall mortality
Religious motivation (i.e., intrinsic versus extrinsic)	Intrinsic religious motivation positively correlates with sociability, sense of well-being, and tolerance
Religious coping (e.g., negative or positive coping strategies)	Religious coping strategies are more important than available social support in helping patients adjust to a diagnosis of cancer

There are hundreds of studies attempting to investigate the links between religion and health; this table is only intended to intimate the kinds of associations that have been found.

Historical Roots of the Field

As noted, the field of religion and health can be seen as growing out of the discipline of psychology of religion. William Parsons dates the founding of psychology of religion to the 1880s and cites in this regard the pioneering work of William James, Sigmund Freud, G. Stanley Hall, C. G. Jung, Wilhelm Wundt, and others. Wundt, widely regarded as the founder of experimental psychology, developed with his students (especially Hall) a statistical approach to psychology of religion. Such empirical methods would eventually come to dominate the discipline of psychology.[8] Indeed, as Ralph Hood, Bernard Spilka, Bruce Hunsberger, and Richard Gorsuch point out, empirical (or quantitative) psychology – in contrast to conceptual (or interpretive) psychologies like those of Freud and Jung – emerged in the 1950s and set the discipline of psychology on firm scientific grounds. The empirical psychology of religion emerged as a part of this larger trend, out of which the field of religion and health also emerged.[9]

Institutionalizing the Field: Two Key Events

Another major event in establishing the field of religion and health involved the founding of the *Journal of Religion and Health* by the Blanton-Peale Institute in 1961. In the inaugural edition of the journal, George Anderson wrote an editorial laying out the journal's rationale to provide a space for the correlation of medicine, the behavioral sciences, theology, and philosophy around the subject of improving health:

> Man is more than a mere biological entity. He is matter harnessed to a spirit. Anthropology, sociology, theology, and medicine shed light on the nature of man and help to make him comprehensible; the behavioral sciences especially contribute valuable knowledge to a scientific understanding of human beings and to the total health of man. While it may be desirable to have a division of labor, it is obviously essential that there be a synthesis of goals. We must search for ultimate rationales and goals for those who work for the advancement of science and health.[10]

This journal continues to provide a venue for the latest research in the field.

Another major event was the publication of the *Handbook of Religion and Health*, first published in 2001. This volume is 700-plus pages in print and analyzes more than 1,200 studies and 400 review articles on religion and health. It marks the first attempt to gather the current literature on religion and health into a single volume. In the "Foreword" of the volume, Jeffrey Levin notes that there was a once a time when those studying the linkages between religion and health could have sat around a single conference table, but now (i.e., in 2001) this is no longer the case, thanks in large part to the editors of the handbook (especially Harold Koenig). Levin also notes that the field receives national and international attention in the media and many different fields hold conference panels on the topic. Because of this success, Levin writes, perhaps too optimistically, that "[a]s those of us who have labored in this field for many years have long suspected, the relationship between religion and health, on average and at the population level, is overwhelmingly positive. Now we can say, finally, that we know this to be true."[11]

Institutionalizing the Field: Two Key Authors

While there are many persons working in the field of religion and health, two names in particular stand out, names that we have already mentioned: Jeffrey Levin and Harold Koenig.

Larry Dossey credits Levin with establishing epidemiology of religion, noting that, while many persons see such a connection as obvious, many physicians have denied and sometimes even ridiculed such a relationship. "Levin's findings," Dossey writes, "have created immense interest in the medical profession because they rest on a powerful word: data."[12] Levin became interested in the epidemiology of religion as a graduate student at the School of Public Health at the University of North Carolina in Chapel Hill in the early 1980s. In a course titled "Culture and Health," he read two articles on the association of religion and health that suggested a positive association. Shocked and intrigued, he found the direction for his life's work.[13]

Levin employs the term "epidemiology of religion" and, in explaining what he means by this term, notes that epidemiologists make generalizations that "are generally expressed (1) on average, (2) across a population, and (3) all things being equal."[14]

SAMPLE SUBSTANTIVE FINDINGS FROM LEVIN'S *GOD, FAITH, AND HEALTH*[15]

Association	Finding
Religion and Heart Disease	In Missouri, death rate due to ischemic heart disease among Reorganized Church of Latter-Day Saints was 80 percent lower than other Missourians.
Religion and Blood Pressure	A study in California of non-religiously affiliated adults with Chinese, Filipino, and Japanese ancestry found that hypertension was double than those with religious affiliation. Similarly, a study of Buddhist priests in Japan found that these priests were half as likely to die from hypertension as other Japanese men.
Religion and Lung Cancer	A study at the University of Texas Medical Branch found that Jewish men are 60 percent less likely to die of lung cancer than non-Jewish men (i.e., Gentile men).
Religion and Longevity	Meta-analysis demonstrates that actively religious persons live longer than non-religious persons, even when controlling for behaviors that religions tend to proscribe (e.g., drinking and smoking).

Levin also notes that epidemiology cannot tell us if smoking caused Patient X's emphysema or if Patient X will get better if he stops smoking now. This is because epidemiology gives us information about populations, not about specific cases. While epidemiology cannot tell us anything about Patient X, it *can* tell us that emphysema is found in significantly greater rates among those who smoke as compared with those who do not. Similarly, epidemiological research has demonstrated that factors such as diet and exercise are associated with good health. Levin was one of the first persons to suggest, from a specifically epidemiological point of view, that religion could have a positive effect on health like diet and exercise.

Is this figure is praying? Isn't it too late? How might you interpret this drawing as more than simply ironic? Can you recall any recent disasters whose victims might have identified with this figure? Regardless of one's personal attitude toward religion, this chapter urges us to take the religious beliefs of patients seriously and to observe how religion functions in their lives. How can we determine if religion might be helping or hurting in a given situation?

How is this figure similar to or different from the skeleton contemplating a skull that accompanies Chapter 12? One difference is that Vesalius's skeleton is in direct contact with the skull it contemplated, while the object of this skeleton's prayer is outside the frame. Another difference is how each image was created. The artists Vesalius employed drew directly from cadavers and skeletons he prepared. This image appeared almost 200 years later in *Osteographia: Or, The Anatomy of Bones*, published in 1733 by William Cheselden, an English surgeon and teacher. For greater accuracy, Cheselden prepared skeletons, and then employed artists to copy them using a camera obscura, which is a large camera-like device that projects an image on a sheet of paper. Since Cheselden took such pains to be scientifically accurate, why do you think he would have included this figure that is appealing to something outside the scientific realm?

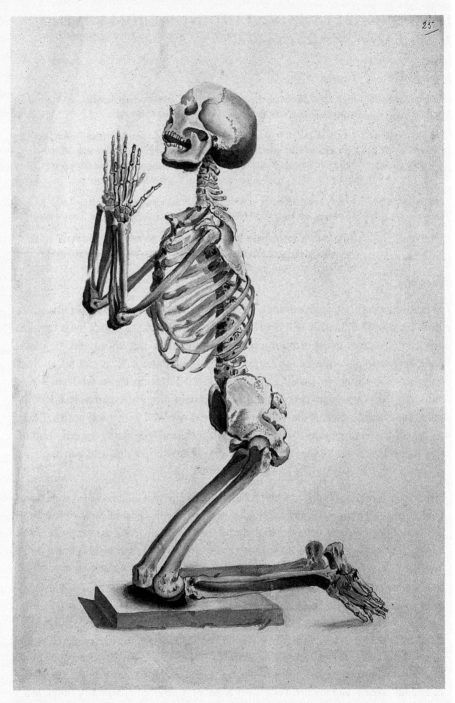

Figure 20. *Praying Skeleton*, 1733, William Cheselden 1688–1752, Wellcome Library, London.

Koenig, a psychiatrist, built on the foundation that Levin laid. In researching the literature on spirituality and health, he found hundreds of studies with a positive association. But he also discovered that many of these studies were weak in terms of methodology (most were cross-sectional studies) and that a major flaw in spirituality and mental health research in particular is that much of it is tautological (spirituality is often circularly defined as good mental health). Studies in recent years are much stronger methodologically, and they, too, are establishing a positive association. But Koenig also points out that religion can negatively impact health and has noted a common misconception about the implications of this research: "there is no evidence," he writes, "from clinical trials that if patients become more religious *only in order to be healthier* that better health will result. The research shows that persons who are religious may have better health outcomes. These persons are usually religious for religious reasons (not health reasons)."[16]

If Levin (as a doctor of philosophy) was instrumental in bringing the field of religion and health into the vision of mainstream medicine by identifying and theorizing the core issues, it was Koenig (as a doctor of medicine) who raised the status of the field in the eyes of physicians by launching a rigorously designed research program.

MEASURING RELIGION AND HEALTH: APPROACHES AND INSTRUMENTS

In a major review article, Daniel Hall, Keith Meador, and Harold Koenig analyze the major approaches and instruments that have been used to study the relationship between religion and health.[17] We present some of these to intimate how knowledge in the field of religion and health is produced.

Hall, Meador, and Koenig note that there are currently more than 100 psychometric instruments that attempt to measure "religion" and/or "spirituality." Often religion is measured in behavioral terms: How often does a subject go to church, pray, fast, sing in the choir, read sacred texts, and go on mission trips? How much money does a subject give to religious organizations? Questions such as these are often included as a single-item question or as multi-items on surveys or questionnaires. They also note that because these items are convenient to use, these types of questions have produced some of the strongest evidence for an association between religiousness and various positive health outcomes, such as longer life, lower disability, faster recovery from depression, and improved sense of satisfaction.

Despite the consistency of these findings, it is unclear what to make of them. Are these associations merely the result of the social connections provided by religious organizations?[18] Could there be a selection bias involved?[19] In doing such empirical research on religion and health, there is a tradeoff between reliability (i.e., the consistency of a measure, or the degree to which a measure will be reproducible) and validity (i.e., the accuracy of a measure, or the degree to which a measure corresponds with the world as it is). Measuring religious activity can achieve high levels of consistency and reliability, but is weekly church attendance a valid way of measuring religiousness?[20] What about people who are "spiritual but not religious," that is, persons who consider themselves deeply spiritual but are not affiliated with any religious institution?[21] Measuring religiosity according to institutional affiliation or involvement would not capture their spiritual commitment. Thus, a significant problem with this type of research (i.e., research that measures religious behavior such as attending church) is that, as the ways of measuring become more sophisticated (e.g., designing studies to account for unchurched spirituality), weaker associations can result.

Another way to measure religiousness is qualitative and focuses on an individual's personal religiosity. For example, such research might include questions such as "To what extent do you consider yourself a religious person?"[22] Hall, Meador, and Koenig note that these questions seem to be more valid in comparison with questions about weekly attendance at religious organizations, but the findings are not as reliable and consistent because there is an inherent subjectivity in such assessments.

Other approaches include measurements of religious motivation and orientation. Such approaches often draw on Gordon Allport's distinction between intrinsic and extrinsic religion (I/E) where a person who is extrinsically religious "uses" religion for instrumental reasons (such as when a person attends church to find a partner) while a person who is intrinsically religious is religious for the sake of being religious.[23] Allport and Ross developed a scale to measure religiousness in terms of intrinsic and extrinsic factors. Subjects mark levels of agreement with statements such as "I try hard to carry my religion over into all my other dealings in life" (intrinsic measure) and "One reason for my being a church member is that such membership helps to establish a person in the community" (extrinsic measure).[24] This approach has been heavily criticized by Kirkpatrick and Hood on the grounds that Allport's model lacks conceptual clarity.[25] In any case, it is worth pointing out that a number of tools have been developed in this tradition, such as the Santa Clara Strength of Religious Faith Questionnaire.[26]

DISCUSSION QUESTIONS

1. How do you define religion and/or spirituality?
2. If you are religious and/or spiritual, to what extent does your religiousness or spirituality affect your psychological well-being? Do you find that religion and spirituality helps you to cope? Or do you find that religion and/or spirituality makes you more anxious?

Other instruments have been developed to measure religiousness multi-dimensionally. These scales attempt to incorporate various types of measurement into a single instrument. Examples include Koenig's Duke Religion Index,[27] the Fetzer/NIA Multi-dimensional Measurement of Religiousness/Spirituality,[28] and the Spiritual Beliefs Inventory.[29] While these approaches are a significant advancement, there is still no consensus as to an appropriate definition of religion or to the number of dimensions that ought to be measured.

Hall, Meador, and Koenig point out that the previous types of measurements attempt to discriminate between religiousness versus non-religiousness. Another approach, however, includes studying the functional value of religiousness, such as studying the effects of religiousness on coping. Kenneth Pargament is widely regarded as the leading scholar in the area of religious coping. He has refined his work over the years by developing two influential scales: the RCOPE and brief RCOPE.[30] These scales attempt to measure the various ways in which subjects use religion to cope with illness. Other instruments, such as the Spiritual Well-Being Scale, measure religious well-being. Such instruments contain items such as, "I have a personally meaningful relationship to God."[31] Koenig has criticized these instruments on the grounds that they do not seem to measure anything distinctly religious but rather existential well-being in general.

Hall, Meador, and Koenig also review various instruments and approaches that are less widely used. Some involve "quest" scales, first developed by Gregory Bateson,[32] which focus on the extent to which an individual faces existential questions such as doubt. Others have focused on beliefs and values, such as beliefs about life after death. A significant amount of empirical work has focused on religious affiliation, but a problem with this approach is that no religious tradition is a monolith. Yet another approach involves measuring religious maturity. The most influential researcher in this area is James Fowler.[33] Yet another approach is that of taking longitudinal religious histories. Hall, Meador, and Koenig note that the best instrument available in this regard is the SHS-4. The value of these approaches is that they examine religiousness over time rather than at a single point in time. And, finally, there are instruments that attempt to measure religious experience, such as mystical or spiritual experiences.[34] The Daily Spiritual Experience Scale, for example, asks questions about feelings of inner peace and harmony.[35]

Hall, Meador, and Koenig conclude their review by noting the importance of context, emphasizing that it is important for empirical researchers to realize that there is no such thing as "religiousness-in-general" and that it is a misguided assumption to suggest that it does not matter *what* a person believes so long as they *do* believe. This sort of assumption rests on decontextualized religiousness, and such approaches lead to over-generalization. Empirical researchers, like good clinicians, need to be able navigate the tension between generalizablity and specificity.

CRITIQUE AND SKEPTICISM

The field of religion and health remains controversial. Despite the evidence that Levin, Koenig, and others have compiled by means of literature reviews (as well as by means of their own studies), some still maintain that a link between religion and health does not exist. They think that the methodological difficulties in measuring religion are too great to overcome. Others reject the field in principle on the grounds that they do not want to mix religion and science. Still others raise practical questions: Will patients feel guilty if they become ill or do not recover, interpreting their condition as due to a lack of faith? Some also maintain that religion is a matter that is too delicate for physicians to study.[36] And others, objecting on theological grounds, point out that God or the transcendent cannot be reduced to human constructs and numbers and that so-called "bad" outcomes may be a part of God's plan, that, in other words, the field of religion and health tends to reduce religion, inappropriately, to its functionality.[37]

Perhaps the most outspoken critic of the field is Richard Sloan. He has coauthored articles in medical journals – notably, *The Lancet* – and has also published a monograph expressing his skepticism.[38] Sloan's basic point is that the methodology that is attempting to establish a link between religion and health is weak, and in making his case, he examines a number of specific studies with weak methodology. Not surprisingly, Koenig has taken on Sloan's critiques in a number of papers, conceding that some studies have been weak methodologically but that (1) Sloan is selectively and unfairly presenting his evidence and (2) the field has been getting stronger methodologically in recent decades.[39]

Each of the objections raised here has merit. But it seems to us that the sheer number of studies suggesting an association between religion and health cannot be ignored and that it does not seem fair to reject all of them outright out of a negative bias toward religion; each study must be answered on its own terms. Perhaps, in the end, it will be discovered that the associations between religion and health – if these associations prove to stand the test of time – are the product of several factors: (1) religious traditions often discourage unhealthy behavior, such as drinking, smoking, and promiscuity; (2) involvement in religious communities provides individuals with social connections; and (3) religious practices and beliefs provide individuals with coping mechanisms and an overarching belief structure that helps them make sense of their lives, especially in times of health-related crisis.

CONCLUDING ADVICE FOR CLINICAL PRACTICE

Following William James, we believe that religion should be judged by its fruits. We suggest to students, therefore, that, no matter what their own attitudes toward religion may be, they ought to pay attention to how religion functions in the lives of their patients: Does religion seem to be helping or hurting in a given situation? If a patient seems to be employing negative religious coping methods, a chaplain should be consulted. If a patient seems to be employing positive coping methods, these methods should be strengthened by, for example, involving a local pastor, rabbi, or imam in patient care.[40]

SUMMATION

This chapter explored the field of religion and health. Beginning with a discussion of the historical roots of the field, it examined the contributions of key authors Jeffrey Levin and Harold Koenig; the major approaches and instruments that have been used to study the relationship between religion and health; and the critics of these studies. Then, with a focus on clinical practice, it suggested that paying attention to the way that religion functions in patients' lives could help us to better care for patients. Overall, though, this chapter attempted to emphasize that, despite the methodological difficulties involved in measuring the effect of religion on health, the sheer number of studies suggesting a link between them is too great to be ignored.

EXERCISES FOR CRITICAL THINKING AND CHARACTER FORMATION

QUESTIONS FOR DISCUSSION

1. To what extent can religion/spiritualty be measured?
2. What do you think about the associations that are consistently found between religion and health?
3. If the associations between religion and health are valid, what does this mean for clinical practice?
4. What are some possible ethical issues for health care professionals should they choose to discuss religion and/or spirituality with their patients?

SUGGESTED WRITING EXERCISE

Write, in as much concrete details as you can, about your worst experience or impression of religion. Write for fifteen minutes. Share your reflections. Now, imagine that you are a physician, and write for ten minutes about how your experience or impression might affect the way you respond to patients in the future should the topic of religion and/or spirituality arise in the clinical setting.

FURTHER READING

Jeff Levin, *God, Faith, and Health*

Richard Sloan, *Blind Faith: The Unholy Alliance of Religion and Medicine*

ADVANCED READING

Allan Brandt and Paul Rozin, eds., *Morality and Health*

Mark Cobb, Christiania Puchalski, and Bruce Rumbold, eds., *Oxford Textbook of Spirituality in Healthcare*

William James, *The Varieties of Religious Experience*

Harold Koenig, *The Handbook of Religion and Health*

Jeff Levin and Michele F. Prince, eds., *Judaism and Health: A Handbook of Practical, Professional and Scholarly Resources*

Kenneth Pargament, ed., *APA Handbook of Psychology, Religion, and Spirituality*

Kenneth Pargament, *The Psychology of Religion and Coping*

Joel Shuman and Keith Meador, *Heal Thyself: Spirituality, Medicine, and the Distortion of Christianity*

Thomas Plante and Allen Sherman, eds., *Faith and Health*

JOURNALS

Journal of Religion, Disability and Health

Journal of Religion and Health

ONLINE RESOURCES

Duke Center for Spirituality, Theology, and Health
http://www.spiritualityandhealth.duke.edu/
Harold Koenig on Faith and Health
http://www.youtube.com/watch?v=xspdcEY9WpE

Jeffrey Levin's website
http://religionandhealth.com
The John Templeton Foundation
http://www.templeton.org/

21 Religion and Reality

If the doors of perception were cleansed, everything would appear to man as it is, infinite.

– William Blake[1]

ABSTRACT

This chapter explores the relationship between religious experience and mental health. Beginning with a discussion of the general distrust of religious experience among health care professionals, it examines Sigmund Freud's reductionistic interpretation of a physician's religious experience; Andrew Sullivan's sympathetic interpretation of his own religious experience in the wake of learning that he was HIV+; Fred Frohock's agnostic interpretation of Helen Thornton's near-death experience; and William Styron's metaphorical interpretation of his depression. Then, with a focus on recent scholarship, it suggests some other ways of studying the intersections of religious experience and mental health.

INTRODUCTION

Donald, a divinity school student, was having problems. He was having difficulty concentrating in his classes and was having trouble sleeping. He went to see Sara, a therapist, for help. Things were going well between Donald and Sara until he found out that she was Jewish. Donald, a Lutheran Christian, insisted that if the therapy were to continue Sara would have to convert to Christianity. The director of the day treatment program called Nancy Kehoe, a Roman Catholic nun and a clinical psychologist, to help deal with the impasse between Donald and Sara. Donald explained:

> I like Sara, but then I found out that she is Jewish. I can't work with her because she is not a Christian. I have read a lot of Freud. I know what therapists think of people who have religious beliefs; they think that they are sick or that they should grow up and let go of their childish beliefs. My religion means everything to me.[2]

Kehoe notes that there was much truth in what Donald had said. Indeed, when this episode occurred in 1981, "[t]he entrenched belief in the mental health community then was that therapists could not and should not talk about religion with 'crazy people.'"[3] Kehoe mediated the discussion between Donald and Sara and helped him to articulate his fear that Sara would try to take his religious faith away from him. When Sara promised that she would not try to take away his faith, Donald was reassured enough to continue therapy.

Religion often contains *non-rational* claims (such as the beliefs that God became incarnate in Jesus of Nazareth or that Moses led his followers through the Red Sea by means of splitting the water); religious beliefs and religious experiences, therefore, are often viewed by health professionals with skepticism because they observe the *irrational* (and often religious) nature of psychotic delusions, such as when patients believe themselves to be Jesus Christ.[4] Religious claims and religious experiences, often for good reasons, are viewed with skepticism in mental health settings.

This basic distrust of religious experience among health care professionals can create a distance between patients and their caregivers. Patients like Donald wonder if they are going to be taken seriously. Kehoe writes, "[H]elping a person reframe the narrative of his or her life is the essence of therapy," but, in Donald's case, because no one would listen to his concerns about religion, "the whole story could never be told because no one wanted to listen."[5] Caring for the patient as a whole person, we concur, means acknowledging and witnessing the religious concerns of patients.[6] And in recent years clinicians are taking these concerns more seriously.[7]

Questions, Focus, and Approach of this Chapter

In what ways can we understand the relationships between religious experience and mental health? Are religious experiences really "real"? What is the clinical significance of these experiences? This chapter explores some possible answers to these questions and offers some practical advice as well. In so doing we will not focus on what seem to be obvious religious delusions – as when persons believe themselves to be Jesus Christ – but rather on experiences that blur the line between mental illness and insight.

The purpose of this chapter is not to provide an overview of the scholarship on mental illness in medical humanities, although we do discuss some of this literature in the conclusion of this chapter. The purpose is much more modest; it is to emphasize a particular way of knowing in medical humanities: idiographic inquiry. The approach in the previous chapter was objective-empirical (or quantitative) with a focus on populations rather than a focus on individuals; this chapter, in contrast, focuses on individuals and could be called subjective-empirical (or qualitative).[8] Another difference is that the previous chapter focused on religion and health broadly, while this chapter focuses on religion and mental health. It is worth pointing out that this chapter is most closely related to Chapter 7 ("Narratives of Illness").

This chapter will explore four experiences. The first involves the religious conversion of an American physician; the second involves a mystical experience of a patient; the third involves a near-death experience; and the fourth involves a writer's use of religious language to describe his experience of depression. In exploring these narratives, we will observe different functions and interpretations of religious experience.

A PHYSICIAN'S RELIGIOUS EXPERIENCE: A REDUCTIONISTIC INTERPRETATION

In an essay titled "A Religious Experience," Sigmund Freud (1856–1939) notes that a German-American journalist published an interview with him in the fall of 1927. In the interview with Freud, he made some controversial remarks about religion, including the fact that he gave no thought to the matter of life after death.[9] The interview inspired some readers to write Freud letters, and he relates one such exchange with an American physician. In the letter, the physician relays an experience he had when he was about to graduate from medical school. He writes:

> One afternoon while I was passing through the dissecting-room my attention was attracted to a sweet-faced dear old woman who was being carried to a dissecting-table. This sweet-faced woman made such an impression on me that a thought flashed up in my mind: "There is no God: if there were a God he would not have allowed this dear old woman to be brought into the dissecting-room."

When the physician went home that day, he had the thought that he should stop going to church. He recalled that before this episode he had had some doubts about some Christian doctrines. While he was contemplating not going to church, he heard a voice that told him to consider the step that he was about to take, and he communicated with this voice by saying: "If I knew of a certainty that Christianity was [the] truth and the Bible was the Word of God, then I would accept it." The physician went on to explain that God did in fact reveal this to be true to him, and he encouraged Freud to ask the same of God so that Freud would become religious.

Freud notes that he sent a polite answer. He wrote stating that he was pleased that this experience enabled the doctor to hold onto his faith, but that God, unfortunately, had not done the same for him. Freud added that if God were going to do so, he had better do it soon, because he was now an old man and that if God did not do so it would not be his fault if he remained "an infidel Jew" until his death. The physician wrote back stating that Freud's Judaism should not be a problem and that he and others were praying for God to intervene in Freud's life.

Freud thinks that the physician's experience provides interesting food for thought. There are many horrors of modern life, so why did *this* particular experience cause the physician to doubt the existence of God? Freud offers a psychoanalytic interpretation to answer this question. He suggests that this woman reminds the physician of his mother. This is why he describes her in such affectionate terms ("sweet-faced dear old woman") and why he addresses Freud as *brother* physician." This woman, possibly around the age of his own mother and either naked or about to be undressed, aroused in the doctor a longing for his own mother and also inspired in him an indignation toward his father for having to share his mother. These emotional conflicts were then displaced onto the religious sphere. In other words, the indignation that he felt toward his father was displaced onto Father God in the form of doubt. The man could have left religion altogether, but the conflict was resolved in another way: a religious (hallucinatory) experience leading to submission to the will of the (F)ather.

Was this religious experience "real"? For Freud the answer is clearly "no." Religious experience can often be explained – and explained away – in terms of psychological conflicts. Freud attributed this experience to an Oedipal conflict within the man that became expressed symbolically in religious experience. Freud's basic hope, as articulated in *The Future of an Illusion*,[10] was that human beings would grow up and let go of religion to be able to live without a protective parent in the sky. Clinical advice from this orientation would suggest that health care professionals should not collude with patients in their religious beliefs.

PRESENCE WITHOUT SHAPE, VOICE WITHOUT WORDS: A SYMPATHETIC INTERPRETATION

This next narrative offers a different perspective. Andrew Sullivan is a British author who self-identifies as a politically conservative Roman Catholic. He is also gay as well as HIV+.

In *Love Undetectable*, Sullivan chronicles his relationship with his friend Patrick and writes about being gay in America during the 1980s and 1990s.[11] He also writes about coming to terms with the fact that he is HIV+ in light of his religious faith. Sullivan prefaces his remarks by noting that the story he is about to convey will sound absurd to some, delusional to others, and self-aggrandizing to still others – yet, he suggests, this is the nature of writing about faith.

One summer night Sullivan went out for dinner. He returned home, and after about an hour, he fell ill with a fever. He assumed it was food poisoning. Sullivan's fever had risen to 104 degrees. It then fell, but then later rose again, and fell again. This went on for a few days. He then assumed it was the flu. One of these days while Sullivan was in bed he felt a presence: "I know where it was on the wall, a space that had no shape, a presence that had no form, something I can only call an intensification of light and space." For a moment he thought that the fever was causing him to hallucinate, but when he checked his temperature it was normal, as was his pulse, skin, and mouth. The presence then "commanded a tone" that was "at once admonitory and intimate, firm and solid but of a kindness I could not even allow myself feel." He insists that it wasn't a hallucination and that it was in some sense real even while incomprehensible. A few weeks later Sullivan encountered the presence again, this time at Mass. It was much less intense but the tone was the same: "the sense of calm and urgency, the sense of warning and intimacy, the sense of judgment, and unimaginable concern." Two weeks later, he learned that he was HIV+. When he told his friends about his infection, Sullivan remembers the tone of one in particular who said, "Andrew, Andrew." He writes, "I recognized at once the voice, instantly and shockingly, and I recognized the tone. Another person, a few days later, responded the same way: "Andrew, Andrew."

A short while after these experiences, Sullivan was reading the Bible and came upon a passage in the Gospel of Luke, the story about Mary and Martha (cf. Luke 10:38–42). They were hosting Jesus for dinner. While Mary and Martha were preparing dinner for Jesus, Martha found herself doing all of the work and therefore asked Jesus: "Lord, do you not care that my sister is leaving me to do the serving all by myself?" Jesus responded: "Martha, Martha." He then went on and said that "you worry and fret about so many things, and yet few are needed, indeed only one. It is Mary who has chosen the better part; it is not to be taken away from her." Sullivan notes that Jesus's tone is loving, admonitory, and intimate, the very tone that he had been previously experiencing: Martha, Martha – Andrew, Andrew. The implication is that Sullivan believes that the presence of Jesus had been visiting him.

Sullivan offers a kind of religious experience that is not fantastic or excessive. He is not claiming to have literally heard or to have seen God or angels – what he is suggesting is that he felt the presence of God and that the presence of God became apparent to him in some rather mundane but curious ways: light on a wall, words and tones of friends, and in devotional reading. This experience could be read as a deep desire or need to experience the presence of God during a crisis. But if God does exist and if God does have a personal relationship with us, are not these precisely the times that God *would* visit us? Sullivan's experience perhaps suggests so.

Religious experience offers people a way of making sense of suffering. If religion is a crutch, as Freud might say, one could counter and suggest that religion, while a crutch, is a *good* crutch and that some of us need it to walk. Why, then, should religion be taken away even if it is a crutch? Clinical advice informed by Sullivan's experience would suggest that health care professionals should recognize that religious beliefs and experiences may be adaptive for patients.

A NEAR-DEATH EXPERIENCE: AN AGNOSTIC INTERPRETATION

The ontological question – are religious experiences "real"? – is often raised in hospital settings. People recovering from car wrecks, heart attacks, strokes, and other medical emergencies often have crises that take them close to death, and many such persons report having had religious experiences during or after such close encounters. Indeed, Fred Frohock (1938–) observes that some recent studies suggest that up to 45 percent of people who have "almost died" have reported some features of a near-death experience.[12]

Frohock has collected a number of narratives of near-death experiences. One involves the case of Helen Thornton. Thornton had a near-death experience where she almost died after surgery. As she lay in the recovery room, still under the effects of the drugs that were used to sedate her, she felt as though she were moving through an aluminum-like tunnel. She saw her son who had died when he was fifteen months old at the end of the tunnel waiting for her and calling out to her, "Mom, Mom." Then Thornton turned and noticed that she was floating above the operating room. As she looked down, she could see doctors and nurses working on her. She disliked the sight of her body and wanted the team to stop working on her so that she could be with her son. When she awoke, she did not remember returning to her body. Her cousin, who was a nurse, greeted her: "What is your name?" Thornton answered, "Don't you know me? Did I die?" At this everyone laughed, apparently because Thornton was confusing a standard clinical question with an experience of the afterlife. Yet later Thornton learned that she *did* almost die. While she is no longer afraid of death, Thornton doesn't know what the experience means. Frohock writes: "[S]he ... acknowledges that the experience could have been an imaginary episode triggered by drugs. That is the unsolvable conflict for her – either explanation fits the experience." She offers a definitive "maybe" to the ontological question.[13]

Like Sullivan, Thornton's religious experience was positive, and the same clinical advice would follow: Religious experiences ought to be judged by their fruits; if they are helpful to patients, health care professionals should not challenge them.

The study of anomalous experience is not new. Indeed, Frederic Myers (1843–1901) recounts many such experiences in his *Human Personality and Its Survival after Bodily Death*[14] (Myers also founded the Society for Psychical Research to provide a venue for exploring such experiences). It may be surprising to the reader that a major mainstream study (i.e., grant-funded research) of these experiences has been ongoing in recent years with the results being published in peer-reviewed journals.[15] For example, in 2008 Sam Parnia of the University of Southampton in the United Kingdom launched a large study (which is called AWARE) in which Parnia and his colleagues have placed postcards that are only viewable from the ceiling in cardiac resuscitation rooms in twenty-five hospitals in the United Kingdom and the United States,[16] because many persons, such as Thornton, have claimed to have floated to the ceiling during operations. One newspaper article referred to this study as looking for "postcards from heaven."[17] It goes without saying that, if Thornton's experience is "real" in the sense that her out-of-body experience was literal, a radical alteration our current understanding of human consciousness would have to occur.

CHRONICLING THE IRREDUCIBILITY OF HUMAN EXPERIENCE: A METAPHORICAL INTERPRETATION

The previous experiences presented in this chapter may or may not be examples of acute mental illness (i.e., psychosis). This ambiguity is what makes them interesting and difficult to interpret. This next experience deals directly with mental illness but does not address the ontological question; it takes an entirely different angle on the relationship between mental illness and religious experience.

William Styron (1925–2006), as noted in a previous chapter, was a widely acclaimed and award-winning American novelist and essayist. We noted that Styron suffered from severe bouts of clinical depression, which he wrote about in his memoir titled *Darkness Visible*.[18] Our previous discussion of this book focused on it as a "pathography." This chapter draws attention to the role of religion in the book.

While religion is not a major focus of the memoir – *Darkness Visible* is not a spiritual autobiography – there are several significant places where religion appears. The first such place is the epigram:

> For the thing which
> I greatly feared is come upon me,
> and that which I was afraid of
> Is come unto me.
> I was not in safety, neither
> had I rest, neither was I quiet;
> yet trouble came.[19]

This epigram is Job 3:25–26. The Book of Job in the Hebrew Bible is a form of skeptical wisdom that challenges the traditional wisdom of the Hebrew Bible as articulated in the Book of Deuteronomy, which suggests that if the faithful are obedient to God then God will bless the faithful but if the faithful are disobedient then God will punish them (see Deuteronomy 28). The Book of Job challenges this wisdom, as it is about a man who is upright and faithful and yet still suffers, apparently unjustly.

Troubled? What elements of this drawing suggest that this is a troubled man? What might the small figure that appears to be speaking in his ear be saying to him? What could the jagged shapes that surround his head represent?

This picture could represent the physician described in this chapter who heard a voice urging him to reconsider giving up church after he saw the cadaver of a "sweet-faced dear old woman" in the dissecting room. It might also represent the British author who wrote that he felt a presence that he described as "an intensification of light and space." What feelings does the picture evoke in you? Do you want to study it closely, or does it make you uncomfortable?

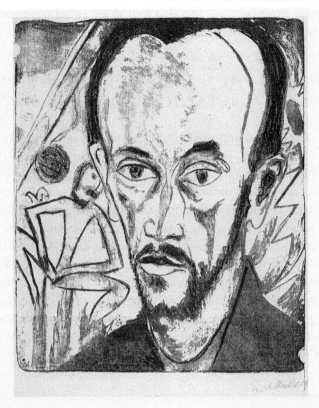

Figure 21. *Männliches Bildnis (Selbstbildnis) (Portrait of a Man (Self Portrait)),* 1919, Erich Heckel, 1883–1970. Museum of Fine Arts, Houston. Museum purchase with funds provided by the Marjorie G. and Evan C. Horning Print Fund © 2013 Artists Rights Society (ARS), New York/VG Bild-Kunst, Bonn.

The style of this work, called "expressionism," arose in the early twentieth century, in Germany, where artists began to respond to industrialism, urbanism, and the horrors of the First World War and to create subjective, highly emotional images. Visual artists continue to employ the expressionist style, and you will find many examples – more than in literature or film – if you search for them on the Internet. Try to understand the subjective, emotional qualities of the images you find.

Styron writes, "Since antiquity – in the tortured lament of Job, in the choruses of Sophocles and Aeschylus – chroniclers of the human spirit have been wrestling with a vocabulary that might give proper expression to melancholia." The value of religious language, for Styron, is not its ontological validity but rather its descriptive prowess. He also notes that Shakespeare (1564–1616), Dickinson (1830–1886), Van Gogh (1853–1890), and Beethoven (1770–1827) have all given us ways to express the human suffering of depression. In his view, however, no one has done better than Dante (1265–1321):

In the middle of the journey of our life
I found myself in a dark wood,
For I had lost the right path.

Styron writes, "To most of those who have experienced it, the horror of depression is so overwhelming as to be quite beyond expression, hence the frustrated sense of inadequacy found in the work of even the greatest artists." What religion and the arts have to offer is *metaphor* (e.g., being depressed is being lost in a dark wood). Clinical language such as the checklists found in the *Diagnostic and Statistical Manual of Mental Disorders* simply does not do justice to the richness of human experience.

Styron argues that the experience of depression is "irreducible." This is another connection to religion in that discussions of irreducibility are common in theological circles.[20] What does irreducible mean? Things such as the color red are irreducible; red cannot be described or understood in terms other than itself. "Redness" is something that stop signs and blood do share and that lipstick and dresses can share. Yet the color red cannot be reduced to something other than itself – it is what it is. Theologians and religious studies scholars also often make similar claims about religion, that, for example, religious experience cannot always be reduced to or explained by, say, psychological phenomena. For instance, a reductionistic explanation of a feeling of oneness during a mystical experience might be that it is really a re-experiencing of experiences in the womb (as Freud might insist), whereas a theological interpretation of the experience might insist that the experience is "real" (as a mystic – or Sullivan – might insist).[21] The mystic's claim is that reality is more complicated than philosophical and scientific materialism imagines and that one must have had a mystical experience in order to understand mysticism. For example, in his classic study of mystical experience titled *The Idea of the Holy* Rodolf Otto (1869–1937) argues that the religious experiences that he is writing about are *sui generis* (i.e., they are not reducible to any other kind of experience). Near the beginning of the book, Otto asks his readers to reflect on their own such experiences so that they can understand his argument, and, if his readers have had no such experiences, he requests them to read no further.[22]

EXERCISE: LISTENING

Listen to the song "Hurt" by Nine Inch Nails. Now listen to the song again, this time covered by Johnny Cash. The lyrics are the same, but the song feels differently depending on who is singing it. Why? What are the differences between the two versions? How do you think age factors into the listener's experience of the song? Do you think this is a song about depression? Is this a modern day lament, as found in, say, the Book of Lamentations in the Hebrew Bible? What might the relationship between pain and art be?

What is striking about Styron is that he makes the similar claim that depression cannot be reduced to something else. He suggests that depression is:

> nearly incomprehensible to those who have not experienced it in its extreme mode, although the gloom, "the blues," which people go through occasionally and associate with the general hassle of everyday existence are of such prevalence that they do give many individuals a hint of the illness in its catastrophic form.[23]

In other words, unless you have had the experience of severe depression, you cannot really understand it. Red is red. Mystical experiences are mystical experiences. And depression is depression.

Perhaps it would be most helpful for patients suffering from mental and emotional disorders to be cared for by a health professional who has some personal experience with mental and emotional disorders – Steven Miles (1950–), a physician, and Kay Jamison (1946–), a psychologist, are both health professionals who have risked writing about their own struggles with mental illness and are gifts to the clinical community.[24] In any case, clinical advice following from Styron's insights would suggest that health care professionals who have not experienced mental illness should recognize the limitations of their perspective when caring for persons with mental illness.

CONCLUSION

This chapter focused on the relationship between mental illness and religious experience. We noted clinical lessons that can be derived from looking at this relationship as well as epistemological questions that can be raised. As noted, the previous chapter presented an overview of some research on religion and health, and the approach there was objective-empirical with a focus on populations and large sample sizes. This chapter presented brief case studies or observations about individual persons; the approach was subjective-empirical and textual. The major limitation of population studies is that they do not, by necessity, provide much context. A subjective-empirical approach provides a means for thicker description.[25] The major limitation of subjective-empirical approaches, however, is that one cannot make any claims for generalizablity. There are, then, strengths and weaknesses to both approaches, and we have presented both in these chapters to demonstrate two ways of knowing in medical humanities.

Mental Illness and Medical Humanities: Sample Literature and Further Reading

Recently, topics related to mental illness have been receiving more attention in medical humanities. Indeed, some of this scholarship is practical in nature by focusing on writing as a means of recovery from serious mental illness[26] or by exploring how studying literature might enhance the education of psychiatry students.[27] Other scholarship is critical in nature, focusing on the marketing of mental illness in consumer depression manuals[28] or by applying Michel Foucault's (1926–1984) insights as articulated in *Madness and Civilization*[29] to destabilize the various power relationships related to conceptions of mental illness.[30] And still other scholarship uses the humanities broadly to explore representations of mental illness, as in constructions of psychopathy in literature and in film[31] as well as to examine the experience of mental illness for individuals and their loved ones and families.[32]

Two key essays in this body of literature should be noted: Anne Hawkins's (1944–) "Pathography: Patient Narratives of Illness" and Anne Jones's (1944–) "Literature and Medicine: Narratives of Mental Illness."[33] These essays are important because they are written for clinical audiences in major journals. A recent noteworthy monograph in medical humanities is Jonathan Metzl's *The Protest Psychosis: How Schizophrenia Became a Black Disease* – this book is of significance because Metzl is both a certified psychiatrist and a trained humanities scholar.[34]

In closing, we note that some scholarship that fits all four components of our definition of medical humanities as attending to context, experience, formation, and conceptual analysis related to medicine – in this case, mental illness. This body of literature will likely continue to grow.

SUMMATION

This chapter explored the relationship between religious experience and mental health. Beginning with a discussion of the general distrust of religious experience among health care professionals, it examined Sigmund Freud's reductionistic interpretation of a physician's religious experience; Andrew Sullivan's sympathetic interpretation of his own religious experience in the wake of learning that he was HIV+; Fred Frohock's agnostic interpretation of Helen Thornton's near-death experience; and William Styron's metaphorical interpretation of his depression. Then, with a focus on recent scholarship, it suggested some other ways of studying the intersections of religious experience and mental health. Overall, though, this chapter attempted to emphasize that a subjective-empirical and textual approach to the study of religion and mental health can provide us with thick, contextual descriptions that quantitative (or objective-empirical) approaches lack.

EXERCISES FOR CRITICAL THINKING AND CHARACTER FORMATION

QUESTIONS FOR DISCUSSION

1. Do you have a family member who suffers from mental illness? If so, what has this been like? Do you have any stories or special insights to share?
2. To what extent should health care professionals talk to mental health patients about religion and spirituality? What are the potentials and pitfalls of such conversations?
3. To what extent can religious, spiritual, and anomalous experiences inform our understanding of reality?
4. Discuss the limitations of both clinical and metaphorical descriptions of mental illness.

SUGGESTED WRITING EXERCISE

Spend ten minutes thinking about the time that you felt the lowest during your life. Why do you think you felt so low? What happened? How long did these feelings last? Was God or religion or spirituality relevant to this experience in any way? Looking back on the experience, write a narrative of this account.

SUGGESTED VIEWING

A Beautiful Mind (2001)
One Flew Over the Cuckoo Nest (1975)

Silver Linings Playbook (2012)

SUGGESTED LISTENING

"Can You Hear Them?" by Ozzy Osbourne
"Lithium" by Nirvana

"Manic Depression" by Jimi Hendrix

FURTHER READING

Nick Flynn, *Another Bullshit Night in Suck City*
Kay Jamison, *Touched with Fire*
Susanna Kaysen, *Girl, Interrupted*

Elyn Saks, *The Center Cannot Hold*
Alexandra Styron, *Reading My Father*
William Styron, *Darkness Visible*

ADVANCED READING

Carol Aneshensel, Jo Phelna, and Alex Bierman, eds., *Handbook of the Sociology of Mental Health*
Donald Capps, *Fragile Connections*
Donald Capps, *Understanding Psychosis*
Michel Foucault, *Madness and Civilization*
David Goldberg and Peter Huxley, *Mental Illness in the Community*
Nancy Kehoe, *Wrestling with Our Inner Angels*

Harold Koenig, *Handbook of Religion and Mental Health*
Kenneth Pargament, *The Psychology of Religion and Coping*
Rosemary Radford Ruether, *Many Forms of Madness*
Thomas Szasz, *The Myth of Mental Illness*

ONLINE RESOURCES

Elyn Saks TED Talk
http://www.ted.com/talks/elyn_saks_seeing_mental_
illness.html
Georgetown Bioethics Library: Mental Health
http://bioethics.georgetown.edu/resources/topics/
mentalhealth/index.html
John Campbell on Schizophrenia
http://philosophybites.com/2013/01/john-campbell-on-
schizophrenia.html
National Alliance on Mental Illness Website

http://www.nami.org/Content/NavigationMenu/Inform_
Yourself/About_Mental_Illness/About_Mental_Illness.
htm
This American Life, "Edge of Sanity"
http://www.thisamericanlife.org/radio-archives/
episode/52/edge-of-sanity
Thomas Insel TED Talk
http://www.ted.com/talks/thomas_insel_toward_a_new_
understanding_of_mental_illness.html

22 Religion and Bioethics

Why is it that the intellectual engine of bioethics seems to be driven by legal or medical theorists rather than theologians?

– Laurie Zoloth[1]

Bioethics began in religion, but religion has faded from bioethics.

– Albert Jonsen[2]

ABSTRACT

This chapter explores the brief history of religion and bioethics. Beginning with a discussion of the religious roots of the field, it examines the key contributions of early figures such as James Gustafson, Paul Ramsey, Joseph Fletcher, Karen Lebacqz, William May, H. Tristram Engelhardt Jr., and Daniel Callahan. Then, with a focus on contemporary debates surrounding religion and bioethics, it notes some recent developments in the field, including the "conservative turn" and the emergence of non-Christian perspectives.

INTRODUCTION

The purpose of this chapter is to introduce the reader to the role that religious thinkers have played, and, to a lesser extent, still do play, in bioethics. This chapter is historical and thematic and has three parts. In part one, we provide a brief overview of the history of religion and bioethics. In part two, we explore some of the writings and themes of key thinkers in this history. And in part three, we outline some current debates and discussion.

PART 1: AN OVERVIEW OF THE HISTORY OF RELIGION AND BIOETHICS

As noted previously in this book, the American Society for Bioethics and Humanities (ASBH) is the flagship organization for bioethics in the United

States. This organization was formed in 1998 by merging the Society for Bioethics Consultation (SBC), the Society for Health and Human Values (SHHV), and the American Association of Bioethics (AAB). The SHHV was formed in 1969 from the Committee on Medical Education and Theology, a group created by Methodists and Presbyterians in 1965. So bioethics, at least organizationally speaking, had strong roots in religion.[3]

Albert Jonsen (1931–), a Roman Catholic Jesuit priest, is one of the "founders" of bioethics. He is well known for his book *The Birth of Bioethics*[4] and his coauthored book – with Stephen Toulmin (1922–2009) – *The Abuse of Casuistry*.[5] Jonsen has recently written an essay titled "A History of Religion and Bioethics,"[6] which is helpful for gaining a sense of the history of religion and bioethics.

In the essay, Jonsen discusses a number of early theological thinkers in bioethics. One is Richard McCormick (1922–2000), who taught at Georgetown University and the University of Notre Dame. He was considered "moderately liberal" for arguing, for example, that patients should be allowed to die if their medical outlook were futile (he defined "futile" as cases where there does not seem to be any chance of reasonable success and where the burdens of treatment outweigh the benefits). He drew on Roman Catholic natural law theory to ground his arguments.[7]

Another thinker whom Jonsen discusses is Joseph Fletcher (1905–1991). Fletcher was ordained as an Episcopal priest and taught at various schools, including Harvard Divinity School and the University of Virginia. Jonsen describes Fletcher as "an unusual moral theologian" in that he "had the heart not of [a] scholar but of a social activist."[8] He adds: "His goal was to convert the church to its Jesus-given mission of serving the poor and oppressed."[9] Fletcher was unusual because (1) very few Protestant theologians addressed medical ethics in those days; and (2) he consistently argued for a patient's right to choose, even for medical procedures such as euthanasia and artificial insemination (these were radically liberal positions for a theological thinker to take in the 1950s). Many of his views were articulated in *Morals and Medicine*,[10] published in 1954, but Fletcher's most influential book was *Situation Ethics*,[11] published in 1966. Fletcher described himself as a utilitarian.

Yet another theological thinker whom Jonsen discusses is Paul Ramsey (1913–1988), arguably the most influential theologian of early – or of *all* – bioethics. Ramsey, a Methodist, taught Christian ethics at Princeton University and was well known for his book *Basic Christian Ethics*.[12] Ramsey argued against Fletcher (and situation ethics) on virtually every issue. He rejected utilitarianism and took a conservative view on all of the major debates in bioethics of the day, such as genetic manipulation, reproduction, and preserving life. He grounded his arguments in the idea of covenant, which Jonsen describes in this way: "God's steadfast love endows human life ... with sanctity and [God] expects [a] faithful response of obedience."[13] He also drew on the methods of casuistry and natural law theory. Ramsey's major contribution to bioethics is *The Patient as Person*,[14] published in 1970, which Jonsen sees as "the first major contribution to bioethics as a discipline."[15]

McCormick, Fletcher, and Ramsey, then, are the three theological thinkers whom Jonsen highlights. All three were Christian – a Roman Catholic and two Protestants – and all three were founders of bioethics. They represented a spectrum of views: McCormick as a moderate, Fletcher as a liberal, and Ramsey as a conservative. Jonsen notes other major theological thinkers of early bioethics as well, but he does not discuss them in any detail. Key points include the fact that James Gustafson (1925–), who taught at Yale University, the University of Chicago, and Emory University, trained the first generation of bioethicists, including James Childress (1940–), LeRoy Walters (1940–), and Stanley Hauerwaus (1940–); that Robert Veatch (1939–), who, as a young man, wanted to become a medical missionary but shifted his interests to secular bioethics, received the first doctoral degree from Harvard University in medical ethics (in the religion and society track) in 1971; and that Kenneth Vaux (1939–) hosted one of the earliest conferences on bioethics at the Institute of Religion (now called the Institute for Spirituality and Health) in Houston, Texas.[16]

Today bioethics is known as a secular enterprise.[17] This raises the question: If the most important voices in the early years of bioethics were theological, how did bioethics become secular? Jonsen asserts that many religious thinkers in bioethics voluntarily shed their theology to be able to speak on rational, secular, and neutral grounds (he cites himself as a case in point) and describes the shift in bioethics this way:

> During the first two decades of bioethics, many scholars from outside the theological disciplines entered the conversation. Philosophers such as Hans Jonas, Samuel Gorovitz, Sissela Bok, and Dan Callahan, physicians such as Edmund Pellegrino, Willard Gaylin, Eric Cassel, lawyers such as Jay Katz, George Annas, and Alex Capron collaborated to create a field of questions and arguments that merited the name bioethics. The initial theologians moved easily into this collaboration and, as they did, lost their distinctive mode of discourse. Bioethics was not, and has never been, a unitary discipline. It is an amalgam of many modes of discovery and discourse.[18]

Thus, while bioethics may have begun in religion, religion faded from bioethics as it became established. The exception that proves the rule is that Karen Lebacqz (1945–), whom Jonsen also identifies as a major early contributor to bioethics, was one of the few theological thinkers in bioethics who retained a strong theological voice in her writing.

Jonsen concludes his essay by pointing out that while the beginning of bioethics was largely a Christian story there were a few influential non-Christian voices. He notes that, while there were no significant Muslim, Buddhist, or Hindu voices during the first decade of bioethics, there were Jewish voices, such as Immanuel Jacobovits (1921–1999),[19] J. David Bleich (1936–),[20] and, later,

Baruch Brody (1943–).[21] He also emphasizes the fact that Brody adopted secular means of arguing.[22]

In "The Tension between Progressive Bioethics and Religion," John Evans offers a slightly different take on how bioethics became secular.[23] He suggests that major religious thinkers in bioethics, such as Gustafson, voluntarily left the field once the "big questions" about the ends of bioethics were solved. The ends of bioethics were determined and codified in a mode of secular ethics that came to be called "principlism."[24] This mode of ethics, for better or for worse, transcends all particular traditions – both religious (e.g., Christian or Jewish) and secular (e.g., deontological or utilitarian) – and attends to the following four principles as they apply to medical settings and situations: autonomy, beneficence, non-maleficence, and justice (see Chapter 16). Bioethicists once asked big questions (e.g., what does it mean to be a human being?), but, since these kinds of questions are not helpful in solving clinical dilemmas in real time (e.g., under what circumstances should physicians involuntarily hospitalize a person with psychoses for their own good?), the big questions – and those who were interested in them – slowly became marginalized. Theologians became less interested in bioethics because, at least from the point of view of theologians, bioethics became reduced to working out the answers to little questions according to the logic of an authorized system (principlism). Evans quotes a somewhat arrogant quip by Gustafson on what became of bioethics:

> Should one cut the power source to a respirator for patient y whose circumstances are a, b, and c? [This] is not utterly dissimilar to asking whether $8.20 an hour or $8.55 an hour ought to be paid to carpenter's helpers in Kansas City.[25]

These questions were simply not interesting to theologians, and so, Evans argues, they gradually left bioethics. But, as we will see, some observe that religion and bioethics is undergoing a rebirth.[26]

There is merit in both Jonsen's traditional narrative and Evans's revised history on the secularization of bioethics. Their interpretations are not mutually exclusive. But we would emphasize that it seems likely that other factors such as the slow development of a body of technical knowledge in bioethics meant that it became harder for young theologians to enter into a developed field without additional training. In the early days of bioethics, when no such training existed, theologians moved easily into bioethics, but now it is more difficult to do so.[27]

PART 2: SOME THEOLOGICAL FOUNDERS OF BIOETHICS ON SELECTED TOPICS

Having provided a brief overview of the origins of bioethics, paying special attention to the role of theologians in founding the field, we now turn to the thinkers (not all of whom are primarily theologians) themselves, offering snapshots of their views. The thinkers selected here are James Gustafson, Paul Ramsey, Joseph Fletcher, Karen Lebacqz, William May, H. Tristram Engelhardt Jr., and Daniel Callahan.

James Gustafson on the Contributions of Theology to Medical Ethics

James Gustafson (1925–) taught theological ethics at various institutions, including Yale University, the University of Chicago, and Emory University. In *The Contributions of Theology to Medical Ethics*, Gustafson begins by defining theology as reflection upon the religious dimension of human experience and ethics as reflection upon the moral dimension of human experience.[28] Thus, he defines theological ethics as reflection on moral experience from a point of view that is informed by religious beliefs or spiritual experiences: "Stories and symbols of God and his activities," he writes, "have been used to interpret the religious and moral significance of events and circumstances in such a way that a particular course of human moral action 'follows' from such interpretation."[29] Three theological assertions inform his medical ethics:

1. God intends the well-being of creation;
2. God sustains the well-being of creation and creates new possibilities for well-being; and
3. Human beings are finite and sinful agents whose actions can in part determine the well-being of creation.[30]

Gustafson notes that he does not defend these theological assertions but that all of his particular moral stances follow from them.

Perhaps an example will clarify Gustafson's theological method. Gustafson's second theological assertion (God sustains the well-being of creation and creates new possibilities for well-being) provides a theological rationale for pursuing medical and scientific research that on the one hand is risky and potentially harmful (such as the side effects of experimental cancer research), yet on the other hand yields possibilities for greater well-being and the relief of suffering (such as a cure for cancer). This research can be theologically justified if God is viewed as working through physicians and scientists to create new possibilities for well-being (such as a world without cancer).

Gustafson concluded by noting that he has not sought to judge the significance of the contributions of theology to medical ethics: "For most persons involved in medical care and practice, the contribution of theology is likely to be of minimal importance, for the moral principles and values needed can be justified without reference to God, and the attitudes that religious belief ground can be grounded in other ways."[31] He adds, "The significance of theology's contribution to medical ethics is likely to be greatest to those who share in that religious consciousness, who have an experience of the reality of God."[32] Gustafson's deductive approach – the articulation and application of theological assertions to questions in medical ethics – is consistent, and it can lead to original insights for religious persons. But theology, if it is to be of genuine significance for medical ethics, needs to strive to offer insights that cannot be, or at least are not, offered by other means.

Paul Ramsey on End-of-Life Issues

As noted, Paul Ramsey (1913–1988) taught Christian ethics at Princeton University. In retirement, he resided in the Center for Theological Inquiry, affiliated with Princeton Theological Seminary. In order to prepare for his writing on medical ethics, he took a sabbatical at Georgetown University where he observed patient care in the university's hospitals. In "On (Only) Caring for the Dying," a selection of passages from *The Patient as Person*, Ramsey discusses ethical issues related to caring at the end-of-life.[33] He notes three common distinctions made in these discussions:

1. The distinction between "ordinary" and "extraordinary" treatment;
2. The distinction between prolonging life and prolonging death; and
3. The distinction between direct killing and allowing to die.

Ramsey argues against medical overtreatment – that is, he argues against "extraordinary" treatment and against the prolonging of death. However, he also argues against direct killing. He contrasts his position with two other common views in these debates. One is the position that life must be saved at all costs, and the other is the position that life can be taken "for the sake of some earthly good to come."[34] Ramsey draws on the thought of theologian Karl Barth (1886–1968) to suggest, in contrast to the two views just noted, that (1) death must not be seen as an absolute enemy, because, for the Christian, death, just like life, is a gift from God, but that (2) life must not been taken or death allowed arbitrarily. Ramsey also argues against direct killing or euthanasia on the grounds that it is the moral equivalent of murder. Death may be willed as an end, but not all means to this end are acceptable. This point of view became widely accepted in secular bioethics.[35]

This patient is appealing to us, the viewers, but why? What can we do to help him? How can we interpret his dilemma? The human-like figure in the clouds may represent an angel in Heaven. The skeleton, pointing to the cross and grave, is usually associated with death. The Devil is often depicted with horns, like the creature at the foot of the patient's bed. How might the certainty of death and the promise of eternal salvation or perpetual damnation affect the care he receives? How would the picture be different if any of those figures stood between the patient in the bed and the viewer? Would the patient's fate be decided? How might the patient's end-of-life care be affected by his religious beliefs, or those of the medical staff or the hospital administration? How might you use this drawing, by the Mexican artist José Guadalupe Posada, who died in 1913, to explore the relationship between religion and bioethics? You can find more of Posada's satirical and political cartoons, many of which depict death's skeleton in the midst of daily life, on the Internet.

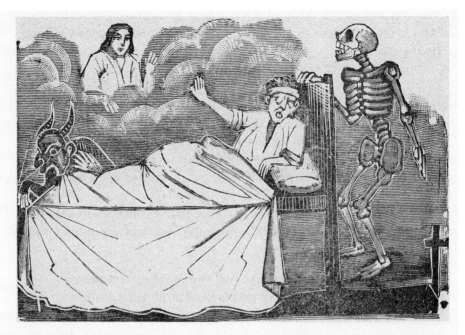

Figure 22. *Separacion del Cuerpo y del Alma (Separation of the Body and the Soul)*, no date, José Guadalupe Posada 1852–1913. The Museum of Fine Arts, Houston. Gift of the Friends of Freda Radoff.

In "The Indignity of 'Death with Dignity,'" an essay published in *The Hastings Center Studies* (later renamed as *The Hastings Center Report*) in 1974, four years after the publication of *The Patient as Person*, Ramsey qualified his earlier views.[36] Because he considered himself a "controversialist" in ethics, he noted that he was led to change his previous views because he felt that too many people were agreeing with him! So he made his views more conservative. Specifically, if he previously argued that death ought not to be considered the enemy (death, like life, is a gift from God), he was now arguing that death *should* be considered the enemy. He still did not believe that life must be saved at all costs in that he inveighed against philosophies of life and death that attempt to see death as "a part of life" and philosophies of life and death that attempt to see death as "good" or "beautiful." In this piece, Ramsey grounds his argument in various biblical passages (such as 1 John) and theological writers (such as St. Augustine) to make the point that death is, in fact, the enemy and that there is nothing dignifying about it.

In both selections from Ramsey's writings offered here, he distinguishes his views, in very critical ways, from the views of Fletcher. The fact that Ramsey could so easily reverse his previous position demonstrates both a strength (flexibility) and a weakness (arbitrariness) of his method.

Joseph Fletcher on Personhood

Joscph Fletcher (1905–1991), as noted, was ordained as an Episcopal priest and taught at various schools, including Harvard Divinity School and the University of Virginia. In his 1975 essay, titled "Four Indicators of Humanhood," Fletcher writes about the debate concerning what constitutes humanhood and expands on an essay that he had previously published in *The Hastings Center Report* in 1972 where he argued that neocortical function (the neocortex is a part of the brain of mammals that has evolved recently and is involved with higher-level functioning such as conscious thought) is "the cardinal or hominizing trait upon which all the other human traits hinge."[37] He notes that the point of his 1972 essay was to keep the debate moving forward and that since its publication three other traits have emerged as potential indicators: Michael Tooley argues for self-consciousness; Richard McCormick argues for relationality; and an unnamed pediatrician at the Texas Medical Center in Houston, Texas, argues for capacity for happiness. Fletcher stands by his original position, arguing that neocortical function is a prerequisite for all other traits. And he points out problems with self-consciousness and relationality as indicators – namely, that persons with dementia or schizophrenia may lose their ability to relate to others and thus could be viewed as losing their status as persons. According to Fletcher's defini-tion, such human beings would still be persons because they have some ability to think, even if their thinking is false or misguided.

There is nothing explicitly theological about this essay, although Fletcher engages various religious thinkers and leading theologians of his day who were writing in bioethics. His view of what constitutes humanhood is a secular one that reduces to neocortical function. But a Christian anthropology could be grounded in a different understanding of relationships, such as God's relation-ship to us even when we do not have the capacity – that is, the neocortical func-tion – to be in relationship with God, that God is in relationship with *all* of creation, including inanimate objects, not simply the beings in creation that hap-pen to have neocortical function.

Karen Lebacqz on the Theological Implications of Justice

Karen Lebacqz (1945–) has taught at various institutions, including the Pacific School of Religion and McGill University, and she is an ordained minister in the United Church of Christ. She is one of the most interesting theological thinkers in bioethics because she was one of the "founders" of bioethics who contributed to the drafting of "The Belmont Report"[38] and because, as noted, she is one of the few founders who never parted with theology.

In an essay titled "Philosophy, Theology, and the Claims of Justice," Lebacqz argues that (1) a biblically based understanding of justice both "implodes" and "explodes" articulations of justice in mainstream bioethics, thereby expanding the scope of justice; (2) the categories of "oppression" and "liberation" ought to be central in discussions of justice; and (3) the principle of justice should be "first," that, in other words, questions of justice should have priority over other principles such as autonomy and beneficence (autonomy often has priority in practice over beneficence, non-maleficence, and justice in mainstream bioethics[39]).[40] Her understanding of justice is informed by liberation theology (a kind of political theology, first developed within Roman Catholic circles, that interprets the teachings of Jesus in light of unjust economic and social practices and attempts to provide justice for the oppressed).

The primary difference between her understanding of justice and articulations of justice in mainstream bioethics is that mainstream bioethics, by and large, focuses on abstract questions of distribution and allocation, whereas her understanding of justice focuses on systems of oppression and structures of power – this is what she means by "exploding" articulations of justice in bioethics. By "implosion," she means recovering more traditional understandings of justice by focusing on character formation, a notion that has reemerged in medical education in recent decades under the rubric of "professional identity formation" or "professional formation."[41]

By placing justice first among the traditional four principles of bioethics (i.e., autonomy, non-maleficence, beneficence, and justice), Lebacqz aims to refocus some major discussions among policymakers. A practical example might be the choice between, on the one hand, building a new neonatal intensive care unit in an urban city in North America or, on the other hand, dedicating resources to improve nutrition and sanitation in an underdeveloped region in Africa. The basis for such a decision would not come from an abstract reasoning about doing the greatest good for the greatest number but from listening to the voices of the oppressed – which, in liberation theology, is called "the epistemological privilege of the oppressed."[42] All knowledge comes from some point of view, and Lebacqz is arguing that the point of view of the oppressed ought to take priority in discussions of justice in bioethics because power distorts one's vision.

Lebacqz notes that her conclusions can be reached by other methods and on secular grounds, but she points out that it was theologians who first made this kind of a contribution to bioethics and that "the field ... might yet benefit from attention to categories that are not uniquely theological but have received more emphasis and attention in theological circles than in mainstream philosophical bioethics."[43]

William May on the Basis of Professional Ethics

William May (1928–) was affiliated with Georgetown University in Washington, DC. In "Code and Covenant or Philanthropy and Contract?" he writes about conceptions of the doctor-patient relationship and their implications for professional ethics.[44] May notes that codes are concerned with style and that medical ethics, when rooted in codes, becomes a matter of aesthetics where physicians are apprenticed into the "art" of medicine. Various bodies, such as the American Medical Association, determine what is expected of physicians in terms of technical competence and personal behavior – that is, they determine what medicine should look like in terms of aesthetics – so an ethics rooted in codes is not so much about internal states as it is about external behavior. Codes establish what physicians must be able to do and how they must behave.

A covenant is different from a code. Covenants involve a gift, an exchange of promises, and a change in identity. In the Judeo-Christian tradition, the covenant *par excellence* is God's covenant with Israel: God liberated the Jewish people from Egypt (the gift); He promised to be their God, so long as they obeyed His Law (the promises); and they became God's people (the change in identity). May invokes covenant language here to contrast it with the language not only of codes but also of contracts. Contracts are legalistic and minimalist – they only specify what is required and what is owed if a party violates the contract – while covenants are responsive in nature. As May puts it, covenants "require a fidelity that exceeds any specification."[45]

In what sense can the profession of medicine be understood in light of the idea of covenant? Where, in other words, is the gift, the exchange of promises, and the change of identity? May identifies several gifts that are sometimes unrecognized by the profession. The first is the gift of being able to study medicine at all. Not everyone has this opportunity, and these opportunities to some extent arise out of the social conditions in which persons are born. Another gift is that every physician has been trained by some other group (e.g., medical students are taught by residents, residents by junior attendings, junior attendings by senior attendings), and so all physicians are indebted to the work of others. And yet another gift is clinical access, the gift of having patients. Without patients, medical students and residents could not learn. Certain rituals in medical education – such as reciting the Hippocratic Oath at graduation ceremonies (which can be viewed as a declaration of a promise relating to the covenant between physicians and society) and the white coat ceremony at the beginning of the clinical years and/or the beginning of medical school (which marks a change in professional identity) – speak to the covenantal nature of medicine. May wants to ground professional identity in indebtedness such that physicians know and appreciate how much has been given to them. His hope is that they will want to give back to the community in various ways, such as working for just policies, doing clinical research, volunteering their time, being generous with their money, and so forth. May wants to contrast the kind of giving that he is advocating with regard to philanthropy because philanthropy assumes a kind of superior position while May wants physicians to give out of a sense of gratitude.

May's ideas seem compelling. It seems to us that his ideas can be fruitfully supplemented with research and inquiry as well as teaching and learning regarding social and economic determinants of advantage and disadvantage.

H. Tristram Engelhardt Jr. on Pluralism

We now turn to a thinker who is not a theologian but a philosopher. H. Tristram Engelhardt Jr. (1941–), who became a deeply committed Christian later in his professional life, holds degrees in both philosophy and medicine and has taught at both Rice University and Baylor College of Medicine. He is one of the most well-known and controversial thinkers in mainstream secular bioethics due to his lively presentation style and his procedural approach in bioethics, articulated most thoroughly in *The Foundations of Bioethics*.[46] This approach, and especially its implications for religion and bioethics, is succinctly outlined in his "Bioethics in Pluralistic Societies."[47]

Engelhardt has a vision of medicine as a secular profession that "focuses more on procedures such as free and informed consent than on content."[48] He writes:

Increasingly, physicians see their primary moral charge to be that of explaining to patients the geography of possible outcomes of therapeutic interventions and their consequences and allowing patients to choose among those possibilities.[49]

The medical profession, as Engelhardt observes, is similar to that of the mail carrier who "delivers with equal reliability the *New England Journal of Medicine*, *Playboy*, and the *Journal of Medicine and Philosophy*."[50] Just as it is not the mail carrier's job to judge the morality of what his or her patrons read but to deliver the mail, a physician should not judge the morality of a given medical procedure such as abortion. It is his or her job to perform medical procedures, not assess their moral meaning. Physicians do have the right to a conscientious objection (if, say, they are morally opposed to abortion), but this does not absolve them from their professional obligation for referral.[51]

Engelhardt is skeptical that any particular vision of the moral life – such as utilitarian, deontological, Christian, Marxist, feminist, and so forth – can be justified on rational grounds, for all such visions beg the question, *Why do ethics from this point of view?* Engelhardt argues that the most secular bioethics can offer is guidance in matters of bureaucratic procedure (i.e., how to maximize the freedom of free and consenting adults) and intellectual clarification (i.e., how to realize the implications of a given perspective or decision). He concludes his essay by suggesting a distinction between public ethics and private morality. He notes that procedure must always be given particular moral content from particular moral traditions:

The development of secular bioethics will force us to live within two moral viewpoints: that of our particular communities and that of secular public morality. There will be unavoidable moral schizophrenia. Truthfulness of heart will force us always to embrace more than one moral stance. One cannot choose one or the other. One must embrace both.[52]

Surely bioethics should be able to offer more than recommendations on bureaucratic procedure and insights regarding intellectual clarification. Engelhardt's position is minimalist and inadequate for clinical practice.[53]

Daniel Callahan on the Need for Religion in Bioethics

Daniel Callahan (1930–), who also is not a theologian but a philosopher, cofounded (with Willard Gaylin) the Hastings Center in New York in 1969. The Hastings Center has become the premier independent research institute for bioethics in the world.

In "Religion and the Secularization of Bioethics," published in 1990, Callahan observes that "The most striking change over the past two decades or so has been the secularization of bioethics," as "[t]he field has moved from one dominated by religious and medical traditions to one now increasingly shaped by philosophical and legal concepts."[54] He notes three dangers that bioethics faces with regard to the marginalization of religion, and he makes these points as a self-confessed unbeliever (specifically, as an ex-Roman Catholic). First, without religion, bioethics could be tempted to turn to the law for moral guidance. The problem with this, as Callahan sees it, is that law is better at pointing out forbidden actions rather than inspiring admirable ones. Second, without religion, bioethics ignores centuries of moral reflections from a wide variety of traditions. He notes that one does not need to be a Jew to appreciate the wisdom of the rabbis or a Roman Catholic to appreciate the Pope's point of view. Third, bioethics, in its search for a common and neutral language, neglects the fact that all moral thought is the product of particular communities. By excluding religion in the name of pluralism, bioethics becomes a restrictive rather than an expansive voice.

The case that Callahan makes here marks a transition for the field or area of religion and bioethics and sets the stage for a rebirth of religion in bioethics. As Courtney Campbell observes, theologians and persons of faith have every reason to be interested in bioethics:

> [F]aith traditions and religious communities have direct responsibilities to their members to provide practical guidance for situations in clinical medical practice. Thus, theologians addressing age-old questions of abortion, contraception, euthanasia, or suicide, as well as more recent issues of reproductive technology, genetic screening, or organ procurement, must be responsive and answerable to the pastoral needs of a faith-informed audience. By contrast, there is no such similar constituency addressed by philosophical writers in bioethics.[55]

Pastoral theologians in particular should play a prominent role in the rebirth of religion in bioethics, given the centrality of lived experience in these age-old questions and contemporary quandaries.[56]

PART 3: CONTEMPORARY DISCUSSIONS

We now want to move to contemporary discussions of religion and bioethics. The most substantial contribution in recent years is an edited volume by David Guinn, titled *Handbook of Bioethics and Religion*.[57] In the introduction to the volume, Guinn lays out some of the basic issues and current debates. We highlight major issues that he identifies and note some other recent developments.

What Role Should Religion Play in Public Policy?

The most fundamental question for religion and bioethics, as Guinn sees it, is this one: "In a liberal, religiously pluralistic country like the United States, what role should religion play in the formation and development of public policies and practices regarding health care?"[58] Based on the First Amendment to the Constitution of the United States, some think that religion should not play any role in public policy. But Guinn notes that it is not clear what the First Amendment means, as it has both an establishment clause and a free exercise cause: "Congress shall make no law respecting an establishment of religion [the establishment clause] or prohibiting the free exercise thereof [the free exercise clause]."[59] Some, such as Thomas Jefferson, have argued for the neutrality standard that establishes "a wall of separation between Church and State."[60] Yet in practice it is unclear and ambiguous what this wall would (or should) look like, because a person of faith, just like any other person, has every right to express his or her views, and this includes perspectives grounded in faith. Should state governors, as persons of faith, be allowed to make, say, prolife arguments that are based on doctrinal statements? Is it realistic to expect them to separate their personal beliefs from their public leadership?

Common Objections to Religious Arguments in Public Discourse

Guinn notes some common reasons offered to exclude religious points of view from public discourse:

1. Religion is not shared by everyone;
2. Religion separates people and groups, sometimes creating factions;
3. Religion has been violent in the past and continues to inspire violence today;
4. Religious arguments subvert rational discussion because people often get too emotional and heated.[61]

Guinn offers some rebuttals to each of these arguments and notes that more substantial engagements with these criticisms are included in his edited volume. But his basic response to these criticisms can be put this way: These critiques fail to see that religion is not a monolith and that many of these critiques apply to secular ways of thinking as well. Some of the most violent, authoritarian, divisive, and exclusive movements in history have been secular (e.g., Stalinism), and some of the greatest modern tragedies (e.g., the Vietnam War) have been carried out by democracies and inspired by ideals such as freedom. Secular ideologies, like religious ideologies, have blood on their hands.[62] Without denying the problems of religion, Guinn suggests that one must also consider what religion has to offer.

Are Secular Arguments Neutral?

Guinn suggests that secular language is not neutral. On this point, he quotes Michael McConnell with approval:

> In the marketplace of ideas, secular viewpoints and ideologies are in competition with religious viewpoints and ideologies. It is no more neutral to favor the secular over the religious than it is to favor the religious over the secular.[63]

Guinn argues that "all worldviews rest upon certain unprovable assumptions."[64] He continues: "For religious worldviews these foundational assumptions may be identified with beliefs *about the transcendent or the ultimate reality*. Philosophically or empirically based worldviews rest upon certain assumptions *about the nature of the world*."[65] Guinn points out that utilitarians assume, but cannot prove, that happiness or utility is good and that empiricists assume, but cannot prove, that the universe is a closed system. Why should the unprovable assumptions of utilitarianism or empiricism – worldviews that influence political philosophies, both conservative and liberal – be allowed to influence public policy while the unprovable assumptions of Christianity and Buddhism be not allowed to do so?[66]

Should Religious Arguments be Translated into Secular Reasoning?

Should the conclusions of religious perspectives be translated into secular language? Guinn notes that requiring religious believers to translate their arguments so that they are convincing on secular grounds is offensive to religious believers: "Those people of faith feel discriminated against in the same way that many feminists feel discriminated against by the grammatical rule that masculine pronouns are neutral and represent any person."[67] "Hiding the religious justification for a policy," Guinn notes, "has the same effect," as "[i]t conveys the message that religious justification is not legitimate."[68]

The Conservative Turn

Another important development in recent discussions of religion and bioethics is what might be called the "conservative turn" (e.g., traditional Roman

Catholic voices, Eastern Orthodox voices, evangelical Christian voices, and fundamentalist Christian voices – perspectives that are typically prolife and against the withdrawal of treatment). We noted John Evans's "The Tension between Progressive Bioethics and Religion" above. Evans points out that all of the religious thinkers in early bioethics would be considered liberal or progressive today. Even Ramsey, who was once considered a conservative voice, would be considered liberal by today's standards. So Evans's point is that the secularization of bioethics meant, in effect, the exodus of liberal and progressive religious voices from bioethics. What is distinctive about religion and bioethics today is that the rebirth of religion in bioethics is largely an introduction of conservative voices. Evans points out that the way that religious conservatives have made their voices heard and their point of view recognized in bioethics and in public policy has involved media campaigns over cases such as the Terri Schiavo case.[69] With the election of George W. Bush in 2000, conservative voices gained a substantial amount of political weight with the formation of the President's Council on Bioethics, chaired by Leon Kass from 2001–2005 and Edmund Pellegrino from 2005–2009.

CASE STUDY: TERRI SCHIAVO

Teresa Marie "Terri" Schiavo (1963–2005) suffered a cardiac arrest in 1990 from which she sustained massive brain injury from a lack of oxygen. She spent a couple of months in a coma and was subsequently given the diagnosis of persistent vegetative state (PVS). Comas are states in which patients lack both awareness and wakefulness. PVS patients, in contrast, sometimes demonstrate wakefulness but apparently not awareness (though some studies in recent years seem to have suggested that it is possible to communicate with PVS patients who are minimally conscious). In the Schiavo case, her husband wished to withdraw life support measures but her parents refused. This disagreement led to legal battles and the case drew national attention, even attention from the White House. The courts eventually sided with Schiavo's husband, granting his wish to allow her to die fifteen years after her cardiac arrest.

How long should PVS patients receive life support? Is withdrawing life support murder, or is it allowing death to occur – or is it something else? How should disagreements among family members be handled? To what extent, if any, should religious beliefs play a role in these debates? If it is possible to communicate with PVS patients, does this affect your views? If so, how?

Also of interest is a recent shift in Engelhardt's thinking. In 1995, he launched a new journal, *Christian Bioethics*, which is committed to content-full understandings of bioethics from the perspective of traditional Christianity:

[This journal] will examine the traditional content-full commitments of the Christian faiths with regard to the meaning of life, sexuality, suffering, illness, and death within the context of medicine and health care. The Journal seeks to break new ground by taking the content of Christianity seriously while critically assessing the extent to which the different Christian faiths and their different health care policies authentically realize that content with respect to bioethical issues.[70]

The emergence of journals such as these seems to indicate a resurgence of religion and bioethics.

Non-Christian Perspectives in Bioethics

The vast majority of religious thinking with regard to bioethics remains Christian and Jewish. However, scholarship outside of these traditions has begun to be developed in recent decades. Some examples are listed in exercises at the end of the chapter.

CONCLUSION

Did bioethics begin in religion, and then fade away? Jonsen suggests that he does not think the bioethics began "in religion" but that "[i]ndividuals from quite different denominational backgrounds with very different training addressed the issues of the day."[71] And to make their arguments understandable, theological thinkers in bioethics, by and large, did not appeal to doctrine or to scripture but to reasons and arguments that everyone could understand. This view of the history of religion and bioethics has been qualified further in recent decades. Also, religious voices in bioethics have reemerged in bioethics, with the conservative turn in religion and bioethics being one of the most substantial developments in this regard as well as the emergence and development of non-Christian perspectives.

SUMMATION

This chapter explored the brief history of religion and bioethics. Beginning with a discussion of the religious roots of the field, it examined the key contributions of early figures such as James Gustafson, Paul Ramsey, Joseph Fletcher, Karen Lebacqz, William May, H. Tristram Engelhardt Jr., and Daniel Callahan. Then, with a focus on contemporary debates surrounding religion and bioethics, it noted some recent developments in the field, including the "conservative turn" and the emergence of non-Christian perspectives. Overall, though, this chapter attempted to emphasize the strong, yet often unacknowledged, historical relationship between religion and bioethics.

EXERCISES FOR CRITICAL THINKING AND CHARACTER FORMATION

QUESTIONS FOR DISCUSSION

1. To what extent does faith or religion influence your own private morality?
2. If you are religious, what does your religion teach about abortion?
3. If you are religious, what does your religion teach about caring for the poor?

4. What role, if any, should religion play in public policy and in clinical practice? Should the practice of medicine be a secular enterprise, functioning like the mail carrier, as Engelhardt suggested in "Bioethics and Pluralist Societies"?

SUGGESTED WRITING EXERCISE

List three "gifts" that enabled you to go to college and/or to pursue medicine (e.g., being born into a family with relative affluence, being born into a family that values education, being born with a certain level of intellectual ability, and having good mentors). Write a letter of gratitude to someone responsible for giving you this gift. The letter can be to a mentor, a family member, God, or anyone else. You can also write a personal letter to something impersonal, like chance or fate.

SUGGESTED VIEWING

Hold Your Breath (2007)
The Terri Schiavo Story (2009)

ADVANCED READING

Major Works in Judaism
Elliot Dorff, *Matters of Life and Death: A Jewish Approach to Modern Medical Ethics*
Benjamin Freedman, *Duty and Healing: Foundations of a Jewish Bioethic*
Immanuel Jakobovits, *Jewish Medical Ethics*
Fred Rosner, *Modern Medicine and Jewish Ethics*
Major Works in Christianity
Joseph Fletcher, *Situation Ethics: The New Morality*
James Gustafson, *The Contributions of Theology to Medical Ethics*
William Werpehowski and Stephen Crocco, eds., *The Essential Paul Ramsey: A Collection*
Major Works in Islam

Dariusch Atighetchi, *Islamic Bioethics: Problems and Perspectives*
Jonathan Brockopp and Thomas Eich, eds., *Muslim Medical Ethics: From Theory to Practice*
Abdulaziz Abdulhussein Sachedina, *Islamic Biomedical Ethics: Principles and Application*
Major Works in Hinduism and Buddhism
S. Cromwell Crawford, *Hindu Bioethics for the Twenty-First Century*
Kazumasa Hoshino, ed., *Japanese and Western Bioethics: Studies in Moral Diversity*
Damien Keown, *Buddhism and Bioethics*

OTHER ADVANCED READING

The American Journal of Bioethics, December 2012: "In Defense of Irreligious Bioethics"

Curlin, Farr, Lawrence, Ryan, Chin, Marshall, and John Lantos. "Religion, Conscience, and Controversial Clinical Practices." *The New England Journal of Medicine*. 356 (2007): 593–600.

Dena Davis and Laurie Zoloth, eds., *Notes from a Narrow Ridge: Religion and Bioethics*

David Guinn, ed., *Handbook of Bioethics and Religion*

Jack Hanford, *Bioethics from a Faith Perspective: Ethics in Healthcare for the Twenty First Century*

Stephen Lammers and Allen Verhey, eds., *On Moral Medicine: Theological Perspectives in Medical Ethics*

Gilbert Meilaender, *Body, Soul, and Bioethics*

Post, Stephen. "Interacting with Other Worlds: A Review of Books from the Park Ridge Center." *Medical Humanities Review*. 4 (1990): 45–54.

David Smith, ed., *Caring Well: Religion, Narrative, and Health Care Ethics*

JOURNALS

Christian Bioethics

Linacre Quarterly

The National Catholic Bioethics Quarterly

Second Opinion: Health, Faith, and Ethics (1986–1995)

ONLINE RESOURCES

American Academy of Religion – Bioethics and Religion Group
http://www.aarweb.org/meetings/annual_meeting/program_units/PUinformation.asp?PUNum=AARPU052

Bioethics.Net – Religion and Bioethics
http://bioethics.net/resources/index.php?&cat=5&t=sub_pages

Leon Kass Lecture on Immorality
http://www.youtube.com/watch?v=3Wq6DI4XMwc

National Catholic Bioethics Center
http://www.ncbcenter.org/NetCommunity/

The Park Ridge Center for the Study of Health, Faith, and Ethics

http://www.parkridgecenter.org/

Peter Sinter TED Talk on Altruism
http://www.ted.com/talks/peter_singer_the_why_and_how_of_effective_altruism.html

PEW Forum
http://pewforum.org/Topics/Issues/Science-and-Bioethics/

The President's Council on Bioethics (chaired by Leon Kass and Edmund Pellegrino)
http://bioethics.georgetown.edu/pcbe/index.html

Presidential Commission for the Study of Bioethical Issues (chaired by Amy Gutmann)
http://www.bioethics.gov/

23 Suffering and Hope

Pandora, the first mortal woman, received from Zeus a box that she was forbidden to open. The box contained all human blessings and all human curses. Temptation overcame restraint, and Pandora opened it. In a moment, all the curses were released into the world, and all the blessings escaped and were lost – except one: hope. Without hope, mortals could not endure.[1]

– Greek Mythology

Providence does not mean a divine planning by which everything is predetermined . . . . Rather, Providence means that there is a creative and saving possibility implied in every situation.[2]

– Paul Tillich

ABSTRACT

This chapter explores suffering and hope in the context of medicine. Beginning with a discussion of Eric Cassell's claim that physicians should attend to pain and suffering, it examines possible religious answers to patients' existential struggles to find meaning in their illnesses; the practical theodicies that health care professionals often construct or hold onto to help them deal with suffering; and the nature and role of hope in patients' lives and clinical practice. Then, with a focus on the inevitability of suffering, it suggests that we should do our best to create the conditions for hope.

INTRODUCTION

In this Pulitzer Prize-winning photograph, Kevin Carter images a young girl in Africa collapsing from starvation and exhaustion. Being leered at by a hungry vulture, this girl without food could become food.

Arthur Kleinman (1941–) and Joan Kleinman (1939–2011) note that this photograph has been used to mobilize social action and has functioned as a force for good. They also note that the photograph originally appeared with an accompanying news story about political violence in southern Sudan. Once the image

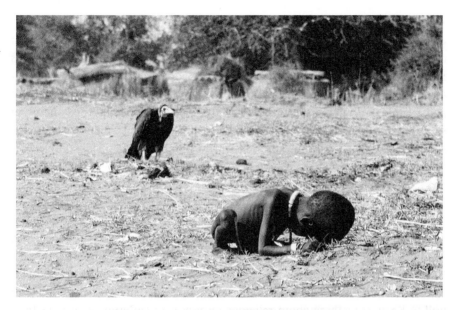

Figure 23. *Famine in Sudan,* 1993, Kevin Carter 1960–1994 © Kevin Carter/Corbis.

is put in the context of civil war, it becomes all the more powerful, as the "real" forces of evil are not in the world of nature – that is, the vulture – but in the world of politics, because in southern Sudan famine has been used as "a political strategy."[3]

Kleinman and Kleinman also raise some standard questions in the ethics of photography: Why did Carter allow the vulture to get this close? Did he help the little girl after taking this photograph? Does not the girl's physical condition demand immediate attention? How long did he spend trying to get this shot?

The moral ambiguity of photography was not lost on Carter, who committed suicide at the young age of thirty-three. His suicide note stated that he was being haunted by the images of suffering he had witnessed over the years, perhaps suggesting some feelings of guilt and shame for making a living based on the suffering of others. But Kleinman and Kleinman note that, while it is easy to moralize about Carter and other such photographers, to do so would fail to see their courage. Indeed, many journalists and photographers lose their lives each year as they go to do their work in war zones. Moreover, such journalism often inspires worldwide collective action to alleviate suffering, as this photograph did.

Nevertheless, Kleinman and Kleinman offer their own critiques of this photograph. One is that the photograph could be taken to imply that Africans cannot take care of themselves (and therefore require foreign intervention); another is that it could imply that Africans cannot represent themselves (and therefore require foreign journalists to represent them). These implications seem to encourage the racist assumption that Western societies are superior to African societies.

Another critique is that witnessing suffering in the media has become a form of entertainment in the West (suffering, like sex, "sells"). Still another problem with exploring suffering on the other side of the world, and witnessing it so often, is that this could have the effect of desensitizing people to suffering and encouraging apathy. Yet while exploring suffering has such moral ambiguities, Kleinman and Kleinman do not suggest that we ought not to explore suffering – ignoring suffering would seem to be worse – but they do suggest that, when one does, one should attend to the various and multivalent political and ethical complexities and ambiguities of such exploration.

The Layout of This Chapter

The purpose of this chapter is to explore suffering in the context of medicine. Because the vast majority of the people in the world are religious and/or spiritual,[4] and because persons often turn to religious traditions in order to cope with suffering,[5] we suggest that clinicians and those interested in health care would do well to know something about religious responses to suffering, as well as their limits.

This chapter has three parts. Part one deals with the nature of suffering in the context of the goals of medicine. Part two deals religious responses to suffering by exploring (1) traditional theological responses from Christianity, Hinduism, and Buddhism, and (2) religious critiques, especially from chaplaincy, of these responses. Part three deals with the nature of hope as well as hope in clinical practice.

PART 1: SUFFERING

If there are canonical texts in medical humanities, Eric Cassell's (1928–) *The Nature of Suffering and the Goals of Medicine* would certainly qualify as one.[6] Cassell's basic argument is that physicians should attend to persons as well as bodies and to suffering as well as pain. Pain is easy to understand; it is what we feel when, for example, we stub our toe. But what is "suffering"? "Suffering," Cassell writes, "is an affliction of the *person*, not the body."[7] What does he mean by "person"? He defines a person as having: a past; a family; a culture; roles; relationships with others; a relationship with oneself; political interests; activities that they do; an inner life; regular behaviors; a body; secrets; a perceived future; and a transcendent dimension.[8] He offers these characteristics of personhood to demonstrate the complexity of suffering, which he defines as a perception of the "impending destruction" of one's personhood. He notes that this "impending destruction" can happen to any aspect of his typology of personhood (e.g., a person can suffer in terms of loss of roles, relationships, activities, and so forth), and he provides this case to illustrate what he means by suffering:

[A] forty-seven-year-old single woman, in whom the sudden appearance of widespread metastatic breast cancer caused her to be hospitalized and near death, suffers. But it is not primarily the weakness, profound anorexia, and generalized swelling, as distressing as these things are, that are the source of her suffering, but the loss of control and inability to prevent the evaporation of her career, whose brilliant promise had finally been realized a few months earlier.[9]

Relieving suffering in this case means attending to the personal concerns of this woman. It is not enough to treat the body, Cassell argues, because one must also care for the person. Cassell suggests that one's caring for the person means attending to the specific *personal* and *individual* nature of suffering, here meaning attending to the patient's concerns about her loss of control and her loss of roles – the evaporation of her career.

How do we know if someone is suffering? Cassell offers a straightforward answer: We ask them. When he asks patients if they are suffering, he notes that patients often initially do not know what they are being asked and so he rephrases the question in various ways:

"I know you have pain, but are there things that are even worse than just the pain?" "Are you frightened by all this?" "What exactly are you frightened of?" "What do you worry (are afraid) is going to happen to you?" "What is the worst thing about all this?"[10]

Simply witnessing suffering in this way, Cassell suggests, will go a long way in meliorating it because in lending an empathic ear we lend strength to patients, helping them to draw on their own natural resiliency. It also is worth pointing out that Cassell suggests that sometimes suffering cannot be meliorated.[11]

Possible Critiques of Cassell

There are at least two straightforward critiques of Cassell from a practical and clinical standpoint:

1. Do physicians have time to attend to "suffering"?
2. Is it the role of physicians to address "suffering"? Would these issues be best left to those who have specifically studied human personality extensively, like psychologists?

There are possible substantive and philosophical critiques of Cassell as well. One involves his list of dimensions that constitute personhood. How did he come up with this list? What assumptions about personhood are being made here that advance certain power relationships? Is an infant, for example, somehow less of a person because it has less of a past than, say, a working adult? Are persons with mental disabilities somehow less of a person if they are not able to reflect on their inner life? We are not suggesting that Cassell makes either of these assumptions; we are simply pointing out potential problems with his model. Also, why doesn't his list include gender? Another critique is that his list is not integrated in any way. He notes that suffering involves the "impending destruction" of the person, but what is it that holds the person together?

Despite these critiques, we believe that Cassell's notion of suffering is a useful one. Whether one finds the details of his model convincing or not, his work simply cannot be ignored because it is so widely read and cited. For the remaining part of the chapter, we want to emphasize one dimension of his model of personhood – the transcendent dimension – because this section of the textbook focuses on religions.

PART 2: WHY?

In "Discussing Religious and Spiritual Issues at the End of Life," Bernard Lo and his colleagues write about two meanings of the question of "why" in clinical practice.[12] They point out that patients could be asking "why" in a biomedical sense: *What caused this cancer – bad genes, bad habits?* But patients could also be asking "why" an existential sense: *Why would God allow me to suffer like this?* The authors suggest that when patients ask existential questions health professionals should not go beyond their professional expertise (and should therefore refer such patients to chaplains). While we agree that physicians should not step beyond their roles, we also endorse Cassell's position that it *is* the role of physicians to attend to suffering, and so we hope that physicians would make some effort in this regard. Perhaps a middle ground would be for physicians to take spiritual histories and then refer patients to chaplains if significant existential questions arise (it seems that such a strategy would work better in inpatient rather than outpatient settings). How to take a spiritual history will be discussed later in the Exercises for Critical Thinking and Character Formation.

What follows are some responses that patients often give when trying to explain the "why" of their suffering. We explore common responses given in monotheistic religions such as Christianity as well as common responses given in non-monotheistic traditions such as Hinduism and Buddhism. This presentation is necessarily selective.

Monotheistic Responses

In monotheistic religions such as Christianity, the existence of suffering causes a problem. If God is good and powerful, why does suffering exist?[13] Because suffering exists, it would seem that God is not good and/or not powerful. Since this conclusion is unacceptable to most theologians, they try to come up with alternative reasons for why suffering exists. The term "theodicy" refers to this type of theological reflection (i.e., theological inquiry attempting to address the problem of evil and/or suffering).

CASE STUDY: THE BOOK OF JOB

In the Hebrew Bible, the Book of Job tells the story of a man who suffered for no apparent reason. In the Book of Deuteronomy, also in the Hebrew Bible, it states that God will reward those who are good and punish those who are bad. But Job was a man without sin and yet suffered. The Book of Job, then, attempts to provide a kind of answer to suffering. As Job makes his case to God – that is, as he pleads with God to tell him why he is suffering because he knows that he is an upright and blameless man – God eventually responds to Job. The passage below is an excerpt of God's response.

"Then the LORD answered Job out of the whirlwind:

Who is this that darkens counsel by words without knowledge? Gird up your loins like a man, I will question you, and you shall declare to me. Where were you when I laid the foundation of the earth? Tell me, if you have understanding. Who determined its measurements – surely you know! Or who stretched the line upon it? On what were its bases sunk, or who laid its cornerstone when the morning stars sang together and all the heavenly beings shouted for joy?

Or who shut in the sea with doors when it burst out from the womb? – when I made the clouds its garment, and thick darkness its swaddling band, and prescribed bounds for it, and set bars and doors, and said, Thus far shall you come, and no farther, and here shall your proud waves be stopped?

Have you commanded the morning since your days began, and caused the dawn to know its place, so that it might take hold of the skirts of the earth, and the wicked be shaken out of it? It is changed like clay under the seal, and it is dyed like a garment. Light is withheld from the wicked, and their uplifted arm is broken. Have you entered into the springs of the sea, or walked in the recesses of the deep? Have the gates of death been revealed to you, or have you seen the gates of deep darkness? Have you comprehended the expanse of the earth? Declare, if you know all this." – The Book of Job, 38:1–18

What do you make of God's response here? What kind of answer is this? Do you think this answer is "true"? Is it helpful? Can a message be both true and unhelpful?

In *When Faith Is Tested*, Jeffry Zurheide notes some classic so-called "answers" to the problem of suffering.[14] The *deterministic answer* refers to such statements as "It is a part of God's plan." What may appear to human beings as unfair is in reality a part of a larger plan known only by God, and what does not make sense now will make sense when we when we see God face-to-face. The *didactic answer* refers to statements such as "God is teaching me something." This answer holds that God uses pain and suffering to teach us. Pain and suffering have a way of focusing our attention, causing us to be introspective, helping us to achieve insights that we would not otherwise achieve. The *athletic answer* refers to statements such as "God only gives you things you can handle." This interpretation of suffering emphasizes the fact that suffering can not only teach us something but also can enable us to grow. Just like an athlete needs to fatigue a muscle for that muscle to grow, we need to go through certain experiences to achieve spiritual maturity. The *disciplinarian answer* refers to statements such as "I am suffering because of my sins." Here suffering is conceived as a punishment from God. God is imagined to be like a parent, putting us back on track when we have gone wayward. This response to suffering has been very important to Jews, as they have struggled to make sense of their collective suffering as a people during, for example, the Babylonian exile.

Non-Monotheistic Responses

From the religions of India, two key ideas related to suffering are especially noteworthy: reincarnation and karma (discussed previously in Chapter 19). These traditions suggest that all of life is suffering and that the only way to escape suffering is to be released from life.[15] This does not mean, however, that suicide or death is the answer; the goal, rather, is liberation. The claim here is that human beings and other beings are caught in an endless cycle of birth, death, and rebirth (reincarnation), and, depending on how one acted in one's previous life, one accrues karma, which prevents one from attaining liberation. But there are methods of becoming free of karma; these basically involve living a moral life and practicing spiritual disciplines such as various forms of yoga. Over many lives – sometimes over thousands of years – a soul is able to exit the cycle and therefore cease to suffer.

Because Hinduism and Buddhism are not monotheistic religions, they do not face the same theological problems that monotheistic religions face with regard to suffering. There is no God whose goodness or power is somehow in doubt because of the reality of suffering. Rather, suffering in this life is understood to be a result of accrued karma in a previous life. In some traditions, one's caste is determined by a previous life (one's soul travels through all of the stations of life[16]); one's gender is determined by a previous life (one moves closer to liberation by being born as a male[17]); and if one is born with a birth defect, this, too, can be the result of karma. As one scholar of Buddhism explains, "If bad actions are not serious enough to lead to a lower birth, they can affect the nature of a human rebirth: stinginess leads to being poor, injuring beings leads to frequent illnesses, and anger leads to being ugly."[18]

The relationship between suffering and desire deserves special attention. Siddartha Gautama, or the Buddha, observed suffering in four aspects of life: birth, aging, disease, and death. While he concluded that some pain is unavoidable, he also observed that suffering seems to be caused unnecessarily by desire. One contemporary Tibetan Lama speaks about the Buddha's insights in this way:

> When you begin to desire something, by definition that means you haven't got it yet. While you are chasing that desire, there is a constant feeling of being unfulfilled. You are waiting

and hoping for something that has yet to happen. And when you finally attain what you want, it is typically not as satisfying as you had hoped .... This continuous cycle of desire and dissatisfaction makes people unhappy.[19]

Desire, then, is another explanation for suffering, so controlling desire is key in mitigating suffering.

Practical Theodicies

When reading the religious responses to suffering offered above – both from Christianity and from Hinduism and Buddhism – we expect that many of our readers will have been dissatisfied with these "answers." These traditional responses to us seem too detached from human experience to be satisfying. While each explanation may have some truth to it, they each risk exacerbating suffering. It would seem offensive to say "The reason you have cancer is because God is punishing you for the sins of your youth" or "The reason your child is autistic is on account of accrued karma from a previous life." What is needed, it seems to us, is theological reflection from the ground up as opposed to theological reflection from the top down. We now turn to such perspectives.

In *Partnership with the Dying*, David Smith (1939–) writes about interviews that he conducted with some thirty health care professionals in the early 2000s.[20] Health care professionals face traumatic and acute suffering on a routine basis, and in his interviews he discovered that this suffering sometimes proves to be problematic for their religious beliefs. Smith argues that these kinds of experiences lead chaplains and other health care professionals to construct practical theodicies, or "fragments of beliefs," because many of them find the common responses to suffering articulated in their traditions to be unsatisfying. Smith has found that health care professionals tend to hold onto three "fragments of belief" of their tradition:

1. God is in charge;
2. God identifies with us; and
3. There is some kind of life after death.

These "fragments of belief" reflect the fact that Smith's sample was overwhelmingly Christian. It is unclear, from Smith's analysis, what the "practical theodicies" of Hindus or Buddhists (or others) would look like. In any case, he found that the idea that "God is in charge" for his sample of health care professionals presumes that God is powerful and good, but not much more is claimed to be known. He notes that there seems to be a difference between saying that "suffering is God's will" and "God is in charge," and the difference entails a confidence level about how much is known about God. He also notes that his subjects made no attempt to explain suffering in any concrete way – suffering was simply acknowledged and they presumed that God is still in control and that there still is a plan. Also, the idea that "God identifies with us," Smith found, assumes that while we may not know *why* suffering exists we do know *that* God does not abandon us or leave us alone. Similarly, the idea that "there is some kind of life after death" affirms a hope that death is not the final word.

Smith's work on theologies of suffering raises the issue of how chaplains and other religious intellectuals might contribute to medical humanities. We suggest that pastoral theologians are in a unique place to contribute to medical humanities because pastoral theology critiques and revises traditional theology in light of human experience. We now turn to a contemporary pastoral theologian (Robert Dykstra) who has worked as a chaplain in the emergency room setting as an example of how pastoral theologians can contribute (and, in some sense, have already unknowingly contributed) to medical humanities, specifically with regard to suffering. Dykstra's essay is especially important precisely because he was, like Smith's subjects, in danger of losing his faith in the face of so much unceasing suffering and tragic death.

Pastoral Theology

In "The Intimate Stranger" Dykstra draws on his experience as a hospital chaplain in the emergency room to explore the theological significance of crisis situations.[21] He discovered by means of this work that his previous theological language was "flat," meaning that it did not seem to be helpful for others or for himself. However, this did not lead Dykstra to conclude that theological language is unimportant; it had the opposite effect in that he was driven to craft a new theological language.

In crafting this language, Dykstra draws on (1) the Hebrew Bible, specifically Deuteronomy 10:17–19 where God reminds Israel that they were once strangers in the land of Egypt and therefore instructs Israel to show the same love to strangers; and (2) his experiences of intimacy with strangers in the hospital. We experience God, Dykstra discovered in his own experiences, when we are strangers and when we treat strangers with hospitality – thus he suggests the theological metaphor of "the intimate stranger" as an image of and for pastoral care in crisis situations. What does Dykstra mean by this metaphor, and how can it apply to hospital settings? He suggests several possibilities:

1. Chaplains experience *patients as strangers*;
2. Patients experience *chaplains as strangers*; and
3. Patients and chaplains alike sometimes experience themselves as estranged from God in crisis situations (*God as a Stranger*).

In the midst of all of the strangeness and all of the suffering in the emergency room, it was Dykstra's experience that God was somehow there – not unlike how God was with Israel when they were in the land of Egypt. This work felt, to Dykstra, to be intimate, strange, and sacred all at once: "I had the haunting sense that the minutes or hours I would spend with these people would be among the most critical of their lives in terms of at least charting the course for the future integration of, or failure to integrate, this crisis into the fabric of meaning in their lives."[22]

The idea that God is with us when we are strangers, along with the following injunction that we are to treat strangers with hospitality because God treated us with hospitality, becomes the basis for Dykstra's practical recommendations for chaplains. He notes that Israel was instructed to:

1. Advocate for the justice needs of strangers;
2. Attend to the bodily needs of strangers; and
3. Take theological responsibility and risk.

One way chaplains can be hospitable is by passing through hospital doors in order to take information back-and-forth from health care professionals to families, thereby helping to preserve patient autonomy in specific situations. (It is occurs to us that this is may be more easily accomplished with chaplains than bioethicists because bioethicists are, in many hospitals, called in only when an ethical problem arises.) Another way chaplains can be hospitable is by attending to the bodily needs of families, showing them where to get food and where to go to the bathroom. Yet another way chaplains can be hospitable is by attending to the spiritual and religious needs of patients and their families. Chaplains are experts at listening and can help patients and their families articulate the meaning, or lack thereof, of their suffering. Dykstra also notes that chaplains (unlike a person's pastor, priest, rabbi, guru, imam, or other religious official) can hear doubts and laments in ways that people may not be comfortable expressing with, say, their parish priest whom they see on a regular basis. Chaplains can provide a certain kind of (sacred) intimacy precisely because they are strangers.

PART 3: HOPE

In the epigram for the chapter that tells the story of Pandora, we are told that hope is the only blessing that humanity has left and that without hope the suffering entailed in living would be too much to bear. Hope, in other words, is the answer to suffering. But what is hope? And, if physicians are to cultivate hope, what should this look like in clinical practice? To answer these questions, we turn to a pastoral theologian and to a medical humanist.

The Nature of Hope

In "The Agent of Hope," Donald Capps (1939–) offers a definition of hope. He makes a distinction between "hoping" and "hopes." Hoping is "the perception that what one wants to happen will happen, a perception that is fueled by desire and in response to felt deprivation."[23] Hoping, therefore, is not an emotion; it is a way of seeing the world. Hopes are "projections that envision the realizable and thus involve risk."[24] So hoping, in others words, is a process or an activity fueled by desire, and hopes provide the content of our desires. Capps also points out that our hopes change over time. When we see that some of our hopes are not realizable (or after we achieve certain hopes), we create new ones.

It is important to note that Capps does not use the word "realistic" to describe hopes (he uses the word "realizable"). It does not make sense, for Capps, to speak of "false hope," because hope, by definition, is perceived to be realizable. Yet, Capps writes, "To say that hope envisions the realizable does not mean that it is bound by the practical, the sensible, the proven, or the tried and true," and, moreover, "the adoption of a realistic approach [to life] can erode a hopeful approach to life, as it may cause us to settle for a less full and vital life than would in fact be accessible to us."[25] He observes that, when parents or other authority figures tell us to be "realistic," they are, in effect, telling us to give up our hopes. While this advice has good intentions, Capps observes that we often resent such guidance because we feel as though the person offering it does not fully understand our unique situation, and, if they did understand us as individuals, they would not be asking us to give up our hopes because they would understand why we perceive them to be realizable. A difficulty for medical humanities and clinical practice is that the line between realistic and realizable is sometimes hard to locate.

Hope in Clinical Practice

In "Hope and the Cancer Patient," a chapter in *How We Die*, surgeon Sherwin Nuland (1930–2014) writes that "[a] young doctor learns no more important lesson than the admonition that he must never allow his patients to lose hope, even when they are obviously dying."[26] In fleshing out what hope should look like in clinical practice, he writes about two patients: Harvey Nuland and Robert DeMatteis. We will present some lessons Nuland learned from both of these patients.

Harvey Nuland is Sherwin Nuland's brother. For the sake of clarity we will refer to Harvey Nuland as "Harvey" and Sherwin Nuland as "Nuland." Nuland notes that his brother began experiencing pains in his bowels at age sixty-two. Nuland knew immediately that this was an ominous sign. As it turned out, his intuitions were right:

> Harvey was found to have a very large intestinal cancer that had invaded the tissues around his right colon and virtually all the draining lymph nodes. The tumor had deposited clumps of itself on numerous surfaces and tissues within the abdominal cavity, metastasized to at least half a dozen sites in the liver, and bathed the whole murderous outburst in a bellyful of fluid loaded with malignant cells – the findings could not have been worse.[27]

But even after the diagnosis was confirmed, Nuland chose not to explain the implications of the condition to his brother. Harvey's doctors, hiding behind medical jargon, did not explain the situation to Harvey either. Despite decades of experience that indicated to him that he should do otherwise, Nuland did something that he knew in his heart was wrong: He gave his brother hope for a cure.

And so they chose treatment. The result was that they inflicted a great deal of pain and suffering on Harvey with no real medical benefit. "Had I been wiser, or consulted disinterested colleagues who knew me well," Nuland writes, "I might have understood that my way of giving Harvey the hope he asked for was not only a deception but, given what we know about the toxicity of the experimental drugs, an almost certain source of added anguish for all of us."[28] And so one of Nuland's main points in this chapter is that there is a difference between denial and hope. In a sense, Nuland and his doctors did not give Harvey a chance to hope because they did not let him know all of the facts.

Nuland also tells the story of Robert DeMatteis, a forty-nine-year-old attorney, in this chapter to illustrate the varieties of hope. One day Bob's internist called Nuland to tell him that Bob had been having pains in his abdomen, that he had blood in his stool, and that the odor of his stool had changed – all ominous signs. After a number of tests, a tumor was found. It was suggested to Bob that he have an operation but Bob initially refuses though later reluctantly agreed. The operation revealed a:

> poorly differentiated adenosquamous carcinoma arising in cecum adjacent to ileocecal valve, exhibiting transmural [through the wall] invasion into peri-colic fat, extensive lymphatic and vascular involvement and metastases to 8 to 17 lymph nodes.[29]

Nuland also adds that the center of the tumor was "necrotic" and "deeply ulcerated." More tests were needed, but Nuland knew that Bob's prognosis was very poor.

Bob was the kind of patient who wanted to know all of the details. And so, unlike with his brother, Nuland did share all of the details. Bob concluded that he did not want to go through chemotherapy and/or radiation and was determined to accept his fate. Nuland agreed with his decision. But at the prodding of his wife, Bob decided to pursue treatment. However, within a couple of weeks chemotherapy had to be stopped because of various complications. The cancer kept spreading; his condition kept getting worse; it was clear that Bob was dying – and so the course of treatment was changed in order to focus on managing his pain.

Nuland notes that Bob was a man who loved Christmas. He threw a big party every year with lots of food and lots of laughter. As he was dying, his wish more than anything was to host one more Christmas party. He got his wish. And the party, by all accounts, was a huge success – everyone had a wonderful time. He described it as one of the best that he had ever hosted.

After the party, Bob said to his wife that one has to live before one dies. Nuland comments: "[I]n the short amount of time left to him, Bob was able to see a form of hope that was his alone. It was the hope that he would be Bob DeMatteis to his last breath, and that he would be remembered for the way he lived."[30] Shortly after Christmas, Bob entered hospice care – first with a home-care program, and then with an inpatient-care program, and he died about a month after Christmas. Nuland notes that his gravestone reads: "And it was always said of him that he knew how to keep Christmas well."[31] "He had taught me," Nuland writes, "that hope can still exist even when rescue is impossible."[32]

CONCLUSION

The causes of suffering – the curses from Pandora's box – are many, but the relief of suffering – the blessing retained from Pandora's box – is singular: hope. The purpose of this chapter has been to introduce the reader to the category of suffering (as distinguished from pain) and to explore suffering from various religious viewpoints. We have seen that religious traditions have various responses to the "why" of suffering but that these responses are often found to be unsatisfying, leading chaplains and others to advocate for and to produce theological reflection that is informed by actual human suffering. While it is not possible to relieve all of the causes of suffering, we can do our best to create the conditions for hope.

What, finally, about the suffering of the little girl in Kevin Carter's photograph? Why is she suffering? We cannot, in the end, claim to know. We find ourselves endorsing those religious intellectuals, like Paul Tillich (1886–1965) and the Buddha, who believe that suffering is a part of human existence. What gives us hope, however, is the social activism that was inspired by this photograph. Perhaps one day this form of suffering – a form of suffering that is inflicted by social forces – will cease to exist if we all do our part. But even if suffering will always exist so long as this world exists, it still gives us hope to know that we can nevertheless pick one another up when one of us falls down, protecting each another from the various vultures of life.

SUMMATION

This chapter explored suffering and hope in the context of medicine. Beginning with a discussion of Eric Cassell's claim that physicians should attend to pain and suffering, it examined possible religious answers to patients' existential struggles to find meaning in their illnesses; the practical theodicies that health care professionals often construct or hold onto to help them deal with suffering;

and the nature and role of hope in patients' lives and clinical practice. Overall, though, this chapter attempted to emphasize that while the causes of suffering are many, the relief of suffering, which often comes in the form of religious explanation, is singular: hope.

EXERCISES FOR CRITICAL THINKING AND CHARACTER FORMATION

QUESTIONS FOR DISCUSSION

1. What do you hope for now? How have your hopes changed over the years?
2. Describe a time when you witnessed someone else's suffering.
3. To what extent is it the role of physicians to address suffering in the way that Cassell uses the term?
4. If you think that physicians should attend to suffering, how would you respond to the claim that physicians have no time to do so?

SUGGESTED WRITING EXERCISE

This writing exercise is divided into two parts. First, think about your worst physical injury, and write about it in as much detail as possible. How did it happen? How old were you? Did it leave a scar? How do you feel about it now? Second, think about your most profound experience of suffering, and write about it in as much detail as possible. How did it happen? Did this experience involve a physical injury? Or was it purely an emotional experience (such as going through a breakup or experiencing the death of a parent)? How old were you? How do you feel about it now? After writing about these experiences, share them, and also compare and contrast pain and suffering in light of your own personal experience.

SUGGESTED VIEWING

The Diving Bell and the Butterfly (2007)
Hope Floats (1998)

How to Die in Oregon (2011)
Philadelphia (1993)

FURTHER READING

The Book of Job
Phillip Moffitt, *Dancing with Life: Buddhists Insights for Finding Meaning and Joy in the Face of Suffering*
Nicholas Wolterstorff, *Lament for a Son*

ADVANCED READING

Reuven Bulka, *Judaism on Illness and Suffering*
Wendy Cadge, *Paging God: Religion in the Halls of Medicine*
John Douglass Hall, *God and Human Suffering*
Stanley Hauerwas, *God, Medicine, and Suffering*

W. S. F. Pickering and Massimo Rosati, eds., *Suffering and Evil: The Durkheimian Legacy*
Dorothee Soelle, *Suffering*

JOURNALS

Journal of Hospice and Palliative Nursing
American Journal of Hospice and Palliative Medicine

ONLINE RESOURCES

The American Academy of Pain Medicine
http://www.painmed.org/patientcenter/facts_on_pain.
aspx
Christina Puchalski at Chautauqua Institute
http://www.youtube.com/watch?v=vQtbk1x0SB0
Harvard Business Review Blog, "A Framework for
Reducing Suffering in Health Care"
http://blogs.hbr.org/2013/11/a-framework-for-reducing-
suffering-in-health-care/

Peter Sinter on Life and Death Decision-Making
http://hwcdn.libsyn.com/p/c/d/d/cddd007e51b31c8e/
Peter_Singer_on_Life_and_Death_Decision-Making.
mp3?c_id=4491373&expiration=1385853926&hwt=5bb9
b0de65fd845bfd141f6a031f4143
Ray Barfield Lecture, "God, Medicine, and Suffering"
http://www.youtube.com/watch?v=N8IP9V49JBQ

Epilogue

Out of the crooked timber of humanity, no straight thing was ever made.[1]

                                                      – Immanuel Kant

Medical humanities is a field for undergraduate and premed students, medical students and students in other health professions, as well as practicing physicians and health care practitioners. Medical humanities asks the most important questions. It asks existential questions about suffering and hope, life and death, the goals of medicine, the nature of disease, the experience of illness, the distinctions between curing and caring. And it asks moral questions about power in medicine, poverty and illness, just health care, and ethical issues in care of the dying. It uses the tools and methods of the humanities to engage these questions. As we articulate in the Introduction, medical humanities is *an inter- and multidisciplinary field that explores contexts, experiences, and critical and conceptual issues in medicine and health care, while supporting professional identity formation.*

Character development and critical thinking are complementary goals of medical humanities. This flows, to repeat our point in the Introduction, from our view that medical humanities is – or should be – fueled by the pursuit of *humanitas,* that compassionate stance toward others that ideally emerges from education in the liberal arts. This humanist educational ideal, whose origins lie in ancient Greece, was formulated by Cicero (104–43 BCE), refashioned in the Renaissance,[2] and shaped again into the idea of a "liberal education" in Europe and the United States.[3] Despite sharp criticism,[4] it lives in strong form today, for example, in the work of Martha Nussbaum (1947–).[5] The purpose of this ideal is to help form individuals who take charge of their own minds, who are free from narrow and unreflective forms of thought, who are compassionate and knowledgeable, and who act in the public or professional world.

The humanistic educational ideal applies to all students – whether one is a medical student or a student in another health profession, whether she is an undergraduate student in the liberal arts or sciences, or engineering, or premed, or in some other form of preprofessional education. Knowledge, humane feeling and action – these things are acquired slowly, individually, and they are brought together within a person over a long period of time. Hence, we designed this introductory text with a long view that is not simply to bring the humanities to students but also to evoke the humanity *of* students by encouraging ongoing, active engagement in interpretation of texts and visual images, role playing, reflective writing, and discussion of moral and ethical problems.

Yet "humanity," as Kant (1724–1804) reminds us, is ever a crooked timber. And students, patients and families, physicians, and other health care professionals are not cut from a single tree. Individuals are internally divided, shaped by conflicting values and social forces, and constrained by varieties of class, gender, race, and age. Societies and cultures are divided as well; they are constrained by historical circumstances of science, technology, religion, economic development, epidemiology, and – we now have special reason to know – climate and environment. Many human problems, in other words, cannot be "straightened out." They are intractable, not amenable to scientific or technological solutions. Intractable problems lead us to ask the most important questions. Medical humanities helps us address them with intelligence and humility, as we see in the following brief examples of death; suffering; and power and the pursuit of justice.

Take the problem of death, which despite the stunning accomplishments of modern medicine, remains perhaps the defining characteristic of humanity. Everyone who has ever lived – or will live – has died or will die. Yet in spite of its universality, the meanings and experiences of death and care of the dying are by no means universal. They vary according to individuals, historical and religious contexts, conditions of public health, climate, social class, and other factors.

The Greeks taught that death was what separated "man" from "the gods." For them, acknowledging and contemplating one's mortality is the beginning of self-knowledge. For medieval Christians, what happens after death was more important than life in this world. Christian belief and conduct could make the difference between an eternal life in heaven or one in hell. Until the eighteenth century, doctors stepped aside in favor of clergy in care of the dying. By the nineteenth century, medicine came to see its obligation as comforting and easing the pain of the dying. In the 1960s, doctors and hospitals came to see their new intensive care units as a means of rescuing patients from death, which led to the view of death as a failure of medicine and ironically undercut humane care of those who were irreversibly dying.

The history of death is also represented in art, literature, religion, and popular culture. As we paraphrased Frank Kermode (1919–2010) earlier, death is a fact of imagination as well as a fact of life. Despite our efforts to deny or avoid it, the brute reality of death has always stimulated the kind of moral and spiritual reflection made possible by the humanities. There are many responses to death – acceptance, love, struggle, faith, care – that shape its meaning rather than deny its reality.

Take the problem of suffering – in this context the suffering of individuals and families who suffer from accidents, infectious or chronic disease, or terminal illness. Suffering, we learned from Eric Cassell (1928–), "is an affliction of the person, not the body." Suffering is an intense form of illness, a personal experience of disease that threatens the whole fabric of an individual's life. Suffering is a loss of identity, a loss of a sense of wholeness due to pain, debilitating disease, or impending death. In Leo Tolstoy's (1828–1910) classic novella, *The Death of Ivan Ilych*, Ivan suffers from the loss of his career, from realization that he has lived a superficial life, and from the failure of his physicians to tell him that he is dying. His intense suffering is partly ameliorated by his faithful caregiver Gerasim. It is alleviated only at the very end of his life through an experience of religious transcendence (and perhaps a kind of reconciliation with his family).

Suffering is inherent in human existence. It is rooted in the ineradicable conflict between our infinite dreams and aspirations and our fragile, mortal bodies, between our limited human capacities and forces beyond our control. In Chapter 23, we learn about a classic example of undeserved suffering in the west, which comes from the Book of Job in the Hebrew Bible. Job is a man without sin, an upright and righteous man who suffers greatly. He comes to question his view that the righteous are rewarded and the evil are punished. He pleads with God to explain his suffering, to no avail. In the end, however, Job's faith is rewarded.

Religion can be a source of suffering as well as of healing. Some religious people feel that they are being punished by God. Or that there is no explanation for their illness. Supporting hope is an essential element in relief of suffering. For believers and nonbelievers alike, as we learned from Robert Dykstra, the work of hospital chaplains can be crucial to relief of suffering. Sometimes suffering cannot be ameliorated; it can only be witnessed.

Finally, take the perennial problems of the imbalance of power and the pursuit of justice. Medical humanities, we argue in the Introduction, is not only a scholarly and educational enterprise. It also involves moral critique and political aspiration: among its goals are respect for individuals, protection of the vulnerable, tolerance of difference, care of the needy, and pursuit of justice in promoting health and providing care. In Chapter 5, we learned that poverty has always been the primary reason why some populations are sicker and live shorter lives than others. This is true both within nations and, speaking globally, between developed countries of the North and developing, impoverished countries of the South. Medicine cannot be expected to eliminate poverty or various forms of social pathology. But physicians in urban hospitals and emergency rooms all over the United States and elsewhere must nevertheless respond to the patients whose bodies and minds bear the brunt of social problems. And advocacy for the medically indigent is one of the moral responsibilities of those in the health professions.

Medical humanities points to the connections between health and society. It asks, Why do the poor lead shorter lives than the wealthy and what can be done about it? It asks what prevents American health policy from providing adequate care for all poor and uninsured individuals? What is fairness in the distribution of health care resources? It asks, globally, do the wealthier, developed countries have an obligation to help eliminate life-threatening diseases in poorer countries? Or to ameliorate the drastic health effects of climate change?

The impact of the powerful over the vulnerable is particularly expressed along the lines of gender and race (although we have noted its effects on age, ethnicity, or sexual orientation). One index of health disparity between men and women, we learned from Amartya Sen's (1933–) essay "More than 100 Million Women Are Missing," is the artificially low ratio of women to men in certain parts of Asia and Africa, where access to health care favors men, and birth and abortion policies reflect a preference for male babies. We also know that until recently, medicine has been a predominantly male profession, which not only denied opportunity to women but has also affected their health care in negative ways.

Racism and prejudice toward African Americans and people of color have a grim history which continues, though in less severe form, today. We learned about nineteenth-century experiments on black women, conducted without their consent, which led to advances in gynecological surgery; and about the more infamous Tuskegee study of syphilis in African American males, which failed to treat them when penicillin became available. As if to confirm Walter Benjamin's (1892–1940) notion that every act of civilization is also an act of barbarism, new biomedical knowledge has often been obtained from other populations considered less than fully human – the subjugated or enslaved, prisoners of war, those institutionalized in prisons, the hospitalized indigent, and patients in asylums and mental hospitals. While personal responsibility is now seen as a key factor in health status, the health and longevity of African Americans compared to Caucasians has long suffered from poverty, discrimination, and lack of access to health care. In the 1990s, blacks lived on average six fewer years than whites and enjoyed eight fewer years of healthy life.

Suffering, death, and injustice – medical humanities does not have singular answers or solutions to these and other intractable questions and problems. It equips students with stories, insights, angles of vision, images, critical thinking skills and knowledge with which to respond. Medical humanities asks students to learn about the history of biomedical progress and to understand the existential and ethical problems it poses. It teaches students to read literature closely, in order to better understand themselves, improve their narrative competence, expand the range of their empathy, and strengthen their capacity to care. Medical humanities teaches students how to think about the goals of medicine. It shows them the historical context of ethical problems, and demonstrates the sometimes ambiguous power of religion and spirituality in suffering and patient care.

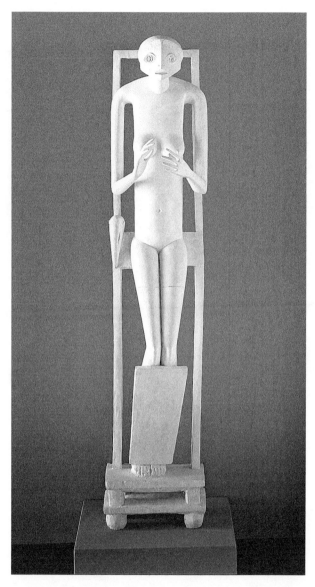

Figure 24. *Hands Holding the Void,* Alberto Giacometti. Yale University Art Gallery, New Haven, Connecticut, Anonymous gift. © 2013 Alberto Giacometti Estate/Licensed by VAGA and ARS, New York, NY.

Medical humanities will never straighten out the crooked timber of humanity. Instead, it cultivates awareness of limits and respect for difference in health care. It also opposes abuse of power and aspires to justice in medicine and health policy. Above all, it engages students in their own learning and in the development of their own humanity. It helps prepare them for a life of reflective practice and action in the professional and public worlds.

NOTES

INTRODUCING MEDICAL HUMANITIES

1 Cited in Laurence McCullough, "The Discourses of Practitioners in Eighteenth-Century Britain," in *The Cambridge World History of Medical Ethics*, eds. Robert Baker and Laurence McCullough (New York: Cambridge University Press, 2009), 409.

2 Steven G. Hsi, *Closing the Chart: A Dying Physician Examines Family, Faith, and Medicine* (Albuquerque: University of New Mexico Press, 2008), 3.

3 Ibid.

4 Ibid., 6–7.

5 Ibid., 4.

6 For more on this topic, see Thomas Cole and Nathan Carlin, "Faculty Health and the Crisis of Meaning: Humanistic Diagnosis and Treatment," in *Faculty Heath in Academic Medicine: Physicians, Scientists, and the Pressures of Success*, eds. Thomas Cole, Thelma Jean Goodrich, and Ellen Gritz (New York: Springer, 2008), 147–156.

7 Ronald A. Carson, "Introduction," in *Practicing the Medical Humanities: Engaging Physicians and Patients*, eds. Ronald A. Carson, Chester R. Burns, and Thomas R. Cole (Hagerstown, MD: University Publishing Group, 2003), 1.

8 See David Barnard, "The Coevolution of Bioethics and the Medical Humanities with Palliative Medicine, 1967–1997," *Journal of Palliative Medicine* 1(1998): 187–193.

9 Brian Hurwitz, "Textual Practices in Crafting Bioethics Cases," *Journal of Bioethical Inquiry* 9 (2012): 395–401.

10 For example, see Jack Coulehan, "Viewpoint: Today's Professionalism: Engaging the Mind but Not the Heart," *Academic Medicine* 80 (2005): 892–898. Also see Mary Beach, et al., "Relationship-Centered Care: A Constructive Reframing," *Journal of General Internal Medicine* 21 (2006): S3-S8. See, too, Harold Koenig, *Spirituality in Patient Care* (Philadelphia and London: Templeton Foundation Press, 2007); and Rita Charon, *Narrative Medicine: Honoring the Stories of Illness* (Oxford: Oxford University Press, 2006).

11 John Stephens, *The Italian Renaissance: The Origins of Intellectual and Artistic Change before the Reformation* (London: Longman, 1990), chs. 3–5; Robert Proctor, *Education's Great Amnesia: Reconsidering the Humanities from Petrarch to Freud* (Bloomington: Indiana University Press, 1988), part 1.

12 Lionel Trilling, "The Uncertain Future of the Humanistic Educational Ideal," *The American Scholar* 44 (1974–1975): 52–67. Reprinted as Lionel Trilling, "The Uncertain Future of the Humanistic Educational Ideal," in *The Last Decade: Essays and Reviews 1965–75*, ed. Diana Trilling (Harcourt Brace Jovanovich, 1981), 160–176.

13 Martha Nussbaum, *Cultivating Humanity: A Classical Defense of Reform in Liberal Education* (Cambridge, MA: Harvard University Press, 1998); also see Martha Nussbaum, *Not for Profit: Why Democracy Needs the Humanities* (Princeton, NJ: Princeton University Press, 2010).

14 Commission on the Humanities, *The Humanities in American Life* (Berkeley: University of California Press, 1980), 1.

15 Ronald S. Crane, *The Idea of the Humanities and Other Essays* (Chicago: University of Chicago Press, 1967).
16 Cathy Davidson and David Goldberg, "Engaging the Humanities," *Profession* (2004): 42–62; see also Immanuel Wallerstein and Richard Lee, *Overcoming the Two Cultures: Science versus the Humanities in the Modern World-System* (Boulder: Paradigm Press, 2004).
17 Frank Huisman and John Harley Warner, "Medical Histories," in *Medical Histories: The Stories and Their Meanings*, eds. Frank Huisman and John Harley Warner (Baltimore, MD: Johns Hopkins University Press, 2004), 4.
18 Cited in J. Warner, "The Humanizing Power of Medical History: Responses to Biomedicine in the 20th Century United States," *Medical Humanities* 37 (2011): 93.
19 See The American Osler Society: www.americanosler.org.
20 See Michel Foucault, *Power/Knowledge: Selected Interviews and Other Writings, 1972–1977*, ed. Colin Gordon (New York: Pantheon Books, 1980); Jean-Francois Lyotard, *The Postmodern Condition: A Report on Knowledge*, trans. Geoff Bennington (Minneapolis: University of Minnesota Press, 1984); and Luce Irigaray, *Speculum of the Other Woman*, trans. Gillian C. Gill (Ithaca, NY: Cornell University Press, 1985). Also see Cary Wolfe, *What is Posthumanism?* (Minneapolis: University of Minnesota Press, 2010).
21 Thomas R. Cole and Faith Lagay, "How the Medical Humanities Can Help Revitalize Humanism and How a Reconfigured Humanism Can Help Nourish the Medical Humanities," in *Practicing the Medical Humanities*, eds. Ronald A. Carson, Chester R. Burns, and Thomas R. Cole (Hagerstown, MD: University Publishing Group, 2003), ch. 5. Also see Allan Bloom, *The Closing of the American Mind* (New York: Simon and Schuster, 1987).
22 Edmund Pellegrino, "Medical Humanism and Technologic Anxiety," in *Humanism and the Physician*, ed. Edmund Pellegrino (Knoxville: University of Tennessee Press, 1979), 9.
23 Ibid., 10.
24 Ibid., 3.
25 H. Martyn Evans and David Greaves, "Medical Humanities – What's in a Name?" *Medical Humanities* 28 (2002): 1–2.
26 See, for example, H. Martyn Evans and Jane MacNaughton, "Should Medical Humanities Be a Multidisciplinary or an Interdisciplinary Study?" *Medical Humanities* 30 (2004): 1–4.
27 Cf. David Smith, "Quality, not Mercy: Some Reflections on Recent Work in Medical Ethics," *Medical Humanities Review* 5 (1991): 9–18.
28 David Greaves and H. Martyn Evans, "Coming of Age? Association for Medical Humanities Holds First Annual Conference," *Medical Humanities* 29 (2003): 57–8; Joanna Rogers, "Being Skeptical about the Medical Humanities," *Journal of Medical Humanities* 16 (1995): 265–277; Delese Wear, "The Medical Humanities: Toward A Renewed Praxis," *Journal of Medical Humanities* 30 (2009): 209–220.
29 See www.healthhumanities.org.
30 Therese Jones, Delese Wear, and Lester D. Friedman, eds., *The Health Humanities Reader* (New Brunswick, NJ: Rutgers University Press, 2014).
31 See, for example, in our own work, Jeffrey P. Spike, Thomas R. Cole, and Richard Buday, *The Brewsters: An Interactive Adventure in Ethics for the Health Professions* (Houston, TX: University of Texas Health Science Center, 2011). Also see Nathan Carlin et al., "The Health Professional Ethics Rubric: Practical Assessment in Ethics Education for Health Professional Schools," *Journal of Academic Ethics* 9 (2011): 277–290; and Nathan Carlin, "Bioethics and Pastoral Concern," *Pastoral Psychology* 62 (2013): 129–138.
32 Anne Hudson Jones, "Reflections, Projections, and the Future of Literature and Medicine," in *Literature and Medicine: A Claim for a Discipline*, eds. Delese Wear, Martin Kohn, and Susan Stocker (Society for Health and Human Values, 1987): 29–39.
33 Jeffrey Bishop, "Rejecting Medical Humanism: Medical Humanities and the Metaphysics of Medicine," *Journal of Medical Humanities* 29 (2008): 15–25.
34 Jones, Wear, and Friedman, *The Health Humanities Reader*, 5.

35 Raimo Puustinen, Mikael Leiman, and Anna Maria Viljanen, "Medicine and the Humanities: Theoretical and Methodological Issues," *Medical Humanities* 29 (2003): 77.

36 George L. Engel, "The Clinical Application of the Biopsychosocial Model," *American Journal of Psychiatry* 137 (1980): 535–544.

37 Eric J. Cassell, *The Nature of Suffering and the Goals of Medicine* (New York: Oxford University Press, 2004).

38 Edmund Pellegrino and David Thomasma, *A Philosophical Basis of Medical Practice: Toward a Philosophy and Ethic of the Healing Professions* (New York: Oxford University Press, 1981).

39 Christina M. Pulchalski and Betty Ferrell, *Making Health Care Whole* (West Conshohocken, PA: Templeton Press, 2010); Christina M. Pulchalski, *A Time for Listening and Caring* (New York: Oxford University Press, 2006).

40 Puustinen, Leiman, and Viljanen, "Medicine and the Humanities," 77–8.

41 Ibid., 78.

42 Engel, "The Clinical Application of the Biopsychosocial Model," 535–544.

43 Cassell, *The Nature of Suffering*.

44 Puustinen, Leiman, and Viljanen, "Medicine and the Humanities," 78.

45 See Leon Eisenberg, "Disease and Illness: Distinctions between Professional and Popular Ideas of Sickness," *Culture, Medicine, and Psychiatry* 1 (1977): 11. Also see Arthur Kleinman, *Patients and Healers in the Context of Culture: An Exploration of the Borderland between Anthropology, Medicine, and Psychiatry* (Berkeley: University of California Press, 1980), 72.

46 See Charon, *Narrative Medicine*.

47 See P. Rancour, "Guided Imagery: Healing When Curing is Out of the Question," *Perspectives in Psychiatric Care* 27 (1991), 30–33.

48 Howard Brody, *Stories of Sickness* (New York: Oxford University Press, 2002); Arthur Kleinman, *The Illness Narratives: Suffering, Healing, and the Human Condition* (New York: Basic Books, 1989).

49 Thomas R. Cole and Sharon Ostwald, *Living after Stroke: Conversations with Couples* (Chicago, Terra Nova Films, 2006).

50 Elaine Scarry, *The Body in Pain: The Making and Unmaking of the World* (New York: Oxford University Press, 1987); Deborah Padfield, Brian Hurwitz, and Charles Pither, *Perceptions of Pain* (Stockport, UK: Dewi Lewis Publishing, 2003).

51 David Greaves and Martyn Evans, editors of the journal *Medical Humanities*, note that medical humanities developed for many years in the United States but that only in recent years – they were writing in the year 2000 – has medical humanities developed in Great Britain. They offer two competing definitions of the field, each with its own goal. One is that medical humanities *adds to* the curricula of medical school, introducing humanistic education to medical education that is rooted in basic science. Another approach, a more political approach, is that all of medical education needs to be reformulated in light of medical humanities, so that technical knowledge and humanistic knowledge are *integrated* throughout the curricula and forming the knowledge base of medicine. See David Greaves and Martyn Evans, "Conceptions of Medical Humanities," *Medical Humanities* 26 (2000): 65.

52 Coulehan, "Viewpoint," 895.

53 K. Danner Clouser, "Humanities in Medical Education: Some Contributions," *Journal of Medical Philosophy* 15 (1990): 289–301.

54 See Robert Coombs, *Surviving Medical School* (London and New Delhi: Sage Publications, 1998); also see Allan Peterkin, *Staying Human during Residency Training* (Toronto, ON: University of Toronto Press, 2008).

55 Edmund D. Pellegrino, "Educating the Humanist Physician," *JAMA* 227 (1974): 1288.

56 Ibid.

57 Ibid., our emphasis.

58 Ronald A. Carson, "Engaged Humanities: Moral Work in the Precincts of Medicine," *Perspectives in Biology and Medicine* 80 (2007): 321–333.

59 See Nathan Carlin, Thomas Cole, and Henry Strobel, "Guidance from the Humanities for Professional Formation," in *Oxford Textbook of Spirituality in Healthcare*, eds. Mark Cobb, Christina Puchalski, and Bruce Rumbold (Oxford: Oxford University Press, 2012), 443–450.

60 Mohammadreza Hojat, Salvatore Mangione, Thomas Nasca, Susan Rattner, James Erdmann, Joseph Gonnella, and Mike Magee, "An Empirical Study of Decline in Empathy in Medical School," *Medical Education* 38 (2004): 934–941.

61 Carlin, Cole, and Strobel, "Guidance from the Humanities for Professional Formation."

62 See Thomas Cole and Nathan Carlin, "The Suffering of Physicians," *The Lancet* 374 (2009): 1414–1415.

PART I HISTORY AND MEDICINE

1 The following discussion of the history of medicine in the twentieth-century United States relies on John Harley Warner, "The Humanizing Power of Medical History: Responses to Biomedicine in the 20th century United States," *Medical Humanities* 37 (2011): 91–96.

2 Susan M. Reverby and David Rosner, "'Beyond the Great Doctors' Revisited: A Generation of the "New Social History of Medicine," in *Locating Medical History*, eds. Frank Huisman and John Harley Warner (Baltimore, MD: Johns Hopkins University Press, 2004), 167–193; see also David Rosner and Gerald Markowitz, eds., *Dying for Work: Workers' Safety and Health in 20th-Century America* (Bloomington: Indiana University Press, 1987); David Rothman and Sheila Rothman, *The Willowbrook Wars* (New York: Harper and Row, 1974); Howard Markel, *Six Major Epidemics That Have Invaded America since 1900 and the Fears They Have Unleashed* (New York: Pantheon Books, 2004).

3 See Jacalyn Duffin (ed.), *Clio in the Clinic: History in Medical Practice* (New York: Oxford University Press, 2005).

4 Cited in Warner, "The Humanizing Power of Medical History," 93.

5 Ibid.

6 Henry Sigerist, *The Great Doctors: A Biographical History of Medicine* (New York: W. W. Norton, 1933); *American Medicine* (New York: W. W. Norton, 1934); *Socialized Medicine in the Soviet Union* (New York: W. W. Norton, 1937); *Primitive and Archaic Medicine* (New York: Oxford University Press, 1951); and *Early Greek, Hindu, and Persian Medicine* (New York: Oxford University Press, 1961).

7 Erwin H. Ackerknecht, *Therapeutics from the Primitives to the 20th Century* (Ann Arbor, MI: Hafner Press, 1973); *Rudolph Virchow (The Development of Science)* (North Stratford, NH: Ayer Company Publishing, 1953); *A Short History of Medicine* (Baltimore, MD: Johns Hopkins University Press, 1982); *Malaria in the Upper Mississippi Valley, 1760–1900* (Ann Arbor, MI: Arno Press, 1977).

8 George Rosen, *The History of Miners' Diseases* (New York: Henry Schuman, 1943); and *A History of Public Health* (New York: MD Publications, 1958).

9 Warner, "The Humanizing Power of Medical History," 94.

10 Howard Markel, *When Germs Travel: Six Major Epidemics That Have Invaded America Since 1900 and the Fears They Have Unleashed* (New York: Pantheon Books, 2004).

11 Edmund D. Pellegrino, ed., *Humanism and the Physician* (Knoxville: University of Tennessee Press, 1979).

12 Susan Reverby and David Rosner, eds., *Health Care in America: Essays in Social History* (Philadelphia: Temple University Press, 1979).

13 Howard I Kushner, "Medical Historians and the History of Medicine," *The Lancet,* 372, n. 9640 (30 August 2008): 710–711.

14 Roy Porter, *The Greatest Benefit to Mankind* (New York: Norton Press, 1997). See also Sheldon Watts, *Disease and Medicine in World History* (New York: Routledge, 2003); Lois Magner, *A History of Medicine* (New York: M. Dekker, 1992); Paul Strathern, *A Brief History of*

Medicine: From Hippocrates to Gene Therapy (London: Robinson, 2005); and Philip Rhodes, *An Outline History of Medicine* (London: Butterworths, 1985).

15 Jacalyn Duffin, *A History of Medicine: A Scandalously Short Introduction*, 2nd ed. (Toronto, ON: University of Toronto Press, 2010).

16 Charles Rosenberg, *The Care of Strangers: The Rise of America's Hospital System* (New York: Basic Books, 1987); *The Cholera Years: The United States in 1832, 1849, and 1866* (Chicago: Chicago University Press, 1987); *Our Present Complaint: American Medicine, Then and Now* (Baltimore, MD: Johns Hopkins University Press, 2007); *Explaining Epidemics and other Studies in the History of Medicine* (Cambridge: Cambridge University Press, 1992); and *Framing Disease: Studies in Cultural History* (Rutgers, NJ: Rutgers University Press, 1992).

17 Mark Jackson, *The Oxford Handbook of the History of Medicine* (Oxford and New York: Oxford University Press, 2011).

18 Robert Baker and Laurence McCullough, *The Cambridge World History of Medical Ethics* (Cambridge: Cambridge University Press, 2008).

19 Guenter Risse, *Mending Bodies, Saving Souls: A History of Hospitals* (New York: Oxford University Press, 1999).

20 Charles Rosenberg, *The Care of Strangers*.

21 Ellen S. More, Elizabeth Fee, and Manon Parry, eds., *Women Physicians and the Cultures of Medicine* (Baltimore, MD: Johns Hopkins University Press, 2009); and Ellen S. More, *Restoring the Balance: Women Physicians and the Profession of Medicine, 1850–1995* (Cambridge, MA: Harvard University Press, 1999).

22 Thomas Bonner, *Becoming a Physician: Medical Education in Britain, France, Germany, and the United States, 1750–1945* (New York: Oxford University Press, 1995).

23 Kenneth Ludmerer, *Learning to Heal: The Development of American Medical Education* (New York: Basic Books, 1985); and *A Time to Heal: American Medical Education from the Turn of the Century to the Era of Managed Care* (New York: Oxford University Press, 1999).

24 Stanley Reiser, *Medicine and the Reign of Technology* (Cambridge: Cambridge University Press, 1978); and *Technological Medicine: The Changing World of Doctors and Patients* (Cambridge: Cambridge University Press, 2009).

25 John Harley Warner, *The Therapeutic Perspective: Medical Practice, Knowledge, and Identity in America, 1820–1885* (Cambridge, MA: Harvard University Press, 1986).

26 Paul Starr, *The Social Transformation of American Medicine* (New York: Basic Books, 1982).

27 David Rothman, *Strangers at the Bedside: A History of how Law and Bioethics Transformed Medical Decision Making* (New York: Basic Books, 1991).

28 William McNeill, *Plagues and Peoples* (New York: Anchor Press, 1976).

29 J.N. Hays, *The Burdens of Disease: Epidemics and Human Response in Western History* (New Brunswick, NJ and London: Rutgers University Press, 1998).

30 Dorothy Porter, *Health, Civilization and the State: A History of Public Health from Ancient to Modern Times* (London and New York: Routledge, 1999).

31 Philippe Ariès, *Western Attitudes Toward Death: From the Middle Ages to the Present* (Baltimore, MD: Johns Hopkins University Press, 1974); and Philippe Ariès, *The Hour of Our Death* (New York: Alfred E. Knopf, 1981).

32 Emily Abel, *The Inevitable Hour: A History of Caring for Dying Patients in America* (Baltimore, MD: Johns Hopkins University Press, 2013).

1 THE DOCTOR-PATIENT RELATIONSHIP

1 Francis Peabody, "The Care of the Patient," *The Journal of the American Medical Association* 88, no. 12 (March 1927): 877–882.

2 Stanley J. Reiser, A. J. Dyck, and W. J. Curran, "Hippocrates, Precepts VI," in *Ethics in Medicine: Historical Perspectives and Contemporary Concerns*, eds. Stanley J. Reiser, A. J. Dyck, and W. J. Curran (Cambridge, MA: MIT Press, 1977), 5.

3 Tom Beauchamp and James Childress, *Principles of Biomedical Ethics* (Oxford: Oxford University Press, 2001).

4 Quoted in Jay Katz, *The Silent World of Doctor and Patient* (Baltimore: Johns Hopkins University Press), 6.

5 Ibid.

6 See Owsei Temkin, "What Does the Hippocratic Oath Say?" in *On Second Thought: Essays on the History of Medicine* (Baltimore: The Johns Hopkins University Press, 2002), 21–28; and Steven Miles, *The Hippocratic Oath and the Ethics of Medicine* (New York: Oxford University Press, 2004).

7 *The Hippocratic Oath*, trans. Michael North, National Library of Medicine, 2002:http://nlm. nih.gov/hmd/greek/greek_oath.html.

8 According to one translation, Galen declares that "The physician must aim above all at helping the sick; if he cannot, he should not harm them." Quoted in Steven Miles, *The Hippocratic Oath and the Ethics of Medicine*, 143.

9 Roy Porter, *The Greatest Benefit to Mankind: A Medical History of Humanity from Antiquity to the Present* (London: HarperCollins, 1997), 110.

10 Col. 4:14.

11 Darrel Amundsen, "The Discourses of Early Christian Medical Ethics," in *The Cambridge World History of Medical Ethics*, eds. Robert Baker and Laurence McCoullough (Cambridge and New York: Cambridge University Press, 2008), 209.

12 Faye Marie Getz, *Healing and Society in the Middle Ages* (Madison: Wisconsin University Press, 1991), 19.

13 For more on female mystics, see Monica Green, *Women's Healthcare in the Medieval West: Texts and Contexts* (Aldershot, UK: Ashgate, 2000).

14 Quoted in Gianna Pomata, *Contracting a Cure: Patients, Healers, and the Law in Early Modern Bologna* (Baltimore and London: Johns Hopkins University Press, 2001), 120.

15 J. N. Hays, *The Burdens of Disease: Epidemics and Human Response in Western History* (New Brunswick, NJ: Rutgers University Press), 91.

16 Roy Porter, *Greatest Benefit*, 171.

17 Dorothy Porter and Roy Porter, *Patient's Progress: Doctors and Doctoring in Eighteenth-Century England* (Stanford, CA: Stanford University Press 1989), 6.

18 Ibid., 117.

19 Quoted in Robert Baker, "Discourses of Practitioners in Nineteenth- and Twentieth-Century Britain and the United States," in *The Cambridge World History of Medical Ethics*, eds. Robert Baker and Laurence McCullough (Cambridge: Cambridge University Press, 2008), 447.

20 Ibid., 448–449.

21 Ibid., 447–453.

22 Lawrence Jonson, *A Life-Centered Approach to Bioethics: Biocentric Ethics* (Cambridge: Cambridge University Press, 2011).

23 According to one survey, the average patient in the United States saw a doctor 2.9 times per year in 1930; the average number of visits doubled by 1990. Porter, *Greatest Benefit*, 685.

24 George Bernard Shaw, *The Doctor's Dilemma* (New York: The Trow Press, 1911), lxxxi.

25 Porter, *Greatest Benefit*, 685.

26 Edward Shorter, *Doctors and Their Patients: A Social History* (New Brunswick, NJ: Transaction Books, 1991), 86.

27 Christopher Crenner, *Private Practice in the Early Twentieth-Century Medical Office of Dr. Richard Cabot* (Baltimore: The Johns Hopkins University Press, 2005), 245; see also James Schafer, *The Business of Private Medical Practice* (New Brunswick, NJ: Rutgers University Press, 2014).

28 Ibid., 246.

29 For literary portraits, see William Carlos Williams's "Face of Stone" (1938) or "The Use of Force" (1938).

30 Arthur Hertzler, *The Horse and Buggy Doctor* (New York and London: HarperCollins, 1938).

31 Quoted in Porter, *Greatest Benefit*, 675.

32 Charles Rosenberg, *The Care of Strangers* (New York: Basic Books, 1987), 341.

33 Ibid.

34 Joel Howell, *Technology in the Hospital: Transforming Patient Care in the Early Twentieth Century* (Baltimore: Johns Hopkins University Press, 1995), 62.

35 Christopher Crenner, *Private Practice*, 30–42.

36 Quoted in Porter, *Greatest Benefit*, 682.

37 Peabody, "The Care of the Patient," 882.

38 Aaron Wildavsky, "Doing Better and Feeling Worse: The Political Pathology of Health Policy," *Daedalus* 106, no. 1 (Winter 1977), 105.

39 See Charles Rosenberg, *The Care of Strangers*, 311; and Porter, *Greatest Benefit*, 682–683.

40 Paul Starr, *The Social Transformation of American Medicine* (New York: Basic Books, 1982), 362–363; see also, Paul Starr, "Social Transformation Twenty Years On," *Journal of Health Politics, Policy and Law* 29, no. 4–5, (August–October 2004), 1005–1119.

41 Roughly one-third of physicians were solo practitioners in 2005, according to the Center for Studying Health System Change (HSC): http://www.hschange.org/CONTENT/941/.

42 See, for instance, Atul Gawande, "The Cost Conundrum: What a Texas Town Can Teach Us about Health Care," *The New Yorker*, June 1, 2009.

43 See Thomas R. Cole, T. Goodrich, and Ellen Gritz, eds., *Faculty Health in Academic Medicine: Physicians, Scientists and the Pressures of Success* (Totowa, NJ: Humana Press, 2009); and Thomas R. Cole and Nathan Carlin, "The Suffering of Physicians," *The Lancet* 374 (October 2009): 1414–1415.

44 See, for instance, the monthly patient satisfaction surveys conducted by the Hospital Care Quality Information from the Consumer Perspective (HCAHPS): http://www.hcahpsonline.org/files/September%202010%20State%20Summary%20of%20HCAHPS%20Results.pdf.

45 Louise Lemieux-Charles and Wendy L. McGuire, "What do We Know about Health Care Team Effectiveness? A Review of the Literature," *Medical Care Research and Review* 63, no. 3 (2006): 263–300.

2 CONSTRUCTING DISEASE

1 Lewis Carroll, *Through the Looking Glass* (New York: Norton, 1992), 163.

2 Roy Porter, *The Greatest Benefit to Mankind: A Medical History of Humanity from Antiquity to the Present* (London: HarperCollins, 1997), 158.

3 J. N. Hays, *The Burdens of Disease: Epidemics and Human Response in Western History* (New Brunswick, NJ: Rutgers University Press, 1998), 10.

4 Quoted in Stephen Miles, *The Hippocratic Oath and the Ethics of Medicine* (New York: Oxford University Press, 2004), 20.

5 Hippocrates, "Airs, Waters, Places," in *Hippocratic Writings*, trans. J. Chadwick and W. N. Mann, ed. G. E. R. Lloyd (New York: Penguin, 1978), 148.

6 In Mirko Grmek's opinion, tuberculosis had "flourished" since the Neolithic Age. Mirko Grmek, *Diseases in the Ancient Greek World* (Baltimore, MD: Johns Hopkins University Press, 1989), 133.

7 Ibid., 184–190.

8 Ryuji Ishitawa, "On the Moral Aspect of Chronic Illness from the Viewpoint of Comparative Medical Thought," *Journal of Philosophy and Ethics in Health Care and Medicine* 1 (July 2006): 56–58.

9 Owsei Temkin, *Galenism; Rise and Decline of a Medical Philosophy* (Ithaca, NY: Cornell University Press, 1979), 39.

10 Ibid., 12.

11 Porter, *Greatest Benefit*, 84.

12 Hays, *Burdens of Disease*, 78–79.

13 "Three Byzantine Saints; Contemporary Biographies Translated from the Greek," trans. Elizabeth Dawes and Norman H. Baynes, in *Medieval Medicine: A Reader*, ed. Faith Wallis (Toronto: University of Toronto Press, 2010), 50.

14 Hays, *Burdens of Disease*, 22.

15 Roy Porter, *Greatest Benefit*, 26.

16 Kenneth Kiple, *The Cambridge World History of Disease*, (Cambridge: Cambridge University Press, 1993),18.

17 Mark Harrison, *Disease and the Modern World* (Cambridge, UK: Polity Press, 2004), 23.

18 Porter, *Greatest Benefit*, 168.

19 Kiple, *The Cambridge World History of Disease,* 15.

20 Hays, *Burdens of Disease*, 63–64.

21 Gerald Grob, *The Deadly Truth: A History of Disease in America* (Cambridge, MA: Harvard University Press, 2002), 20.

22 Harrison, *Disease and the Modern World*, 33.

23 Hays, *Burdens of Disease*, 66–67.

24 Charles C. Mann, *1493: Uncovering the New World Columbus Created* (New York: Alfred A. Knopf, 2011).

25 Porter, *Greatest Benefit*, 167.

26 Quoted in Porter, *Greatest Benefit*, 246.

27 Jason E. Glenn, "Dehumanization, the Symbolic Gaze and the Production of Biomedical Knowledge," in *Black Knowledges/Black Struggles: Essays in Critical Epistemology*, eds. Jason Ambroise and Sabine Broeck (London: Liverpool University Press, 2013), 6.

28 Harrison, *Disease and the Modern World*, 53–56.

29 Charles Rosenberg, "The Therapeutic Revolution: Medicine, Meaning, and Social Change in Nineteenth-Century America," in *The Therapeutic Revolution: Essays in the History of American Medicine*, eds. Morris J. Vogel and Charles E. Rosenberg (Philadelphia, University of Pennsylvania Press), 3–25.

30 John Harley Warner, *The Therapeutic Perspective: Medical Practice, Knowledge, and Identity in America, 1820–1885* (Cambridge, MA: Harvard University Press, 1986), 587.

31 Kiple, *The Cambridge World History of Disease*, 16.

32 Hays, *Burdens of Disease*, 219.

33 Michel Foucault, *The Birth of the Clinic: An Archaeology of Medical Perception*, trans. A. M. Sheridan (London: Tavistock Publication Limited, 1973).

34 Walter Benjamin, *Illuminations,* trans. Harry Zohn (New York: Schocken Books, 1985), 256.

35 Glenn, "Dehumanization," 1.

36 Quoted in Todd L. Savitt, "The Use of Blacks for Medical Experimentation and Demonstration in the Old South," *The Journal of Southern History* 48, no. 3 (1982): 331–348.

37 Porter, *Greatest Benefit*, 432.

38 Harrison, *Disease and the Modern World*, 119.

39 Kiple, *The Cambridge World History of Disease*, 19.

40 Porter, *Greatest Benefit*, 441.

41 See James Jones, *Bad Blood: The Tuskegee Syphilis Experiment* (New York: The Free Press, 1981).

42 National Commission for the Protection of Human Subjects of Biomedical and Behavioral Research, *The Belmont Report: Ethical Principles and Guidelines for the Protection of Human Subjects*, April 18th, 1979. Accessed May 13, 2013: http://www.hhs.gov/ohrp/humansubjects/guidance/belmont.html.

43 Abdel Omran, "The Epidemiologic Transition: A Theory of the Epidemiology of Population Change," *The Milbank Memorial Fund Quarterly* 49, no. 4 (1971): 509–538.

44 Laura B. Shrestha, "CRS Report for Congress: Life Expectancy in the United States." Congressional Research Serve, August 16, 2006. Accessed May 16, 2013: http://www.fas.org/sgp/crs/misc/RL32701.pdf.

45 Arno Karlen, *Man and Microbes: Diseases and Plagues in History and Modern Times* (New York: Putnam, 1995).

46 Kiple, *The Cambridge World History of Disease*, 6.

47 The President's Council on Bioethics, *Beyond Therapy: Biotechnology and the Pursuit of Happiness* (New York: Regan Books, 2003).

48 Peter Conrad, *The Medicalization of Society: On the Transformation of Human Conditions into Treatable Disorders* (Baltimore, MD: The Johns Hopkins University Press, 2007), 1.

49 American Psychiatric Association, *Diagnostic and Statistical Manual of Mental Disorders II*, 2nd ed. (Washington, DC: American Psychiatric Association, 1974).

50 Allen Frances, *Saving Normal: An Insider's Revolt Against Out-of-Control Psychiatric Diagnosis, DSM-5, Big Pharma, and the Medicalization of Ordinary Life* (New York: William Morrow, 2013).

51 Conrad, *The Medicalization of Society*, 4.

3 EDUCATING DOCTORS

1 William Osler, *The Quotable Osler*, eds. Mark E. Silverman, T. Jock Murray, and Charles S. Bryan (Philadelphia: The American College of Physicians, 2008), xiii.

2 Theodore Puschmann, *A History of Medical Education from the Most Remote to the Most Recent Times* (1891), trans. and ed. Evan Hare (Whitefish, MT: Kissinger Publishing, 2010), 8.

3 Ibid., 19.

4 Quoted in Fridolf Kudlien, "Medical Education in Classical Antiquity," in *The History of Medical Education*, ed. C. D. O'Malley (Berkeley: University of California Press, 1970), 5–7.

5 Ibid., 13, 17.

6 Ibid., 18, 20.

7 Roy Porter, *The Greatest Benefit To Mankind: A Medical History of Humanity From Antiquity to the Present* (London: Harpercollins, 1997), 95, 102.

8 Charles Talbot, "Medical Education in the Middle Ages," in *The History of Medical Education*, ed. C. D. O'Malley (Berkeley: University of California Press, 1970), 76.

9 Ibid.

10 Rubin Erikkson, *Andreas Vesalius' First Public Anatomy at Bologna, 1540: An Eyewitness Report* (Uppsala, SE: Almquist & Wiskell, 1959).

11 Quoted in Roy Porter, *Greatest Benefit*, 229.

12 Jeffrey Bishop, *The Anticipatory Corpse* (Notre Dame, IN: University of Notre Dame Press, 2011).

13 Thomas Bonner, *Becoming a Physician: Medical Education in Britain, France, Germany, and the United States, 1750–1945* (New York: Oxford University Press, 1995), 24.

14 Ibid., 21.

15 John Harley Warner, *Against the Spirit of the System: The French Impulse in Nineteenth-Century American Medicine* (Princeton, NJ: Princeton University Press, 1998).

16 Quoted in Whitfield Jenks Bell, *The Colonial Physician and Other Essays* (Science History Publications, 1975), 8.

17 Quoted in William Rothstein, *American Physicians in the Nineteenth Century: From Sects to Science* (Baltimore, MD: Johns Hopkins University Press, 1985), 36.

18 Bonner, *Becoming a Physician*, 74.

19 Paul Starr, *The Social Transformation of American Medicine* (New York: Basic Books, 1982), 47–50.

20 Kenneth Ludmerer, *Learning to Heal: The Development of American Medical Education* (New York: Basic Books, 1985), 3.

21 Ibid., 9, 10.

22 Erwin Ackerknecht, *Medicine at the Paris Hospital, 1794–1848* (Baltimore, MD: The Johns Hopkins Press, 1967).
23 Quoted in Porter, *Greatest Benefit*, 528.
24 Ludmerer, *Learning to Heal*, 33.
25 Charles W. Eliot, *Charles W. Eliot: The Man and His Beliefs*, ed. William Allan Neilson (New York: Harper, 1926), 6.
26 Quoted in Kenneth Ludmerer, *A Time to Heal: American Medical Education From the Turn of the Century to the Era of Managed Care* (New York: Oxford University Press, 1999), 15.
27 William Osler, *The Quotable Osler*, eds. Mark E. Silverman, T. Jock Murray, and Charles S. Bryan (The American College of Physicians, 2008), 203.
28 Abraham Flexner, "Medical Education in the United States and Canada: A Report to the Carnegie Foundation for the Advancement of Teaching" (New York: The Carnegie Foundation, 1910). Accessed April 14, 2013: http://www.carnegiefoundation.org/sites/default/files/elibrary/Carnegie_Flexner_Report.pdf.
29 See Ellen S. More, *Restoring the Balance: Women Physicians and the Profession of Medicine, 1850–1995* (Cambridge, MA: Harvard University Press, 1999), 4; and Mary Walsh, *"Doctors Wanted, No Women Need Apply": Sexual Barriers in the Medical Profession, 1835–1975* (New Haven, CT: Yale University Press, 1977).
30 Mary Roth Walsh, "Women in Medicine since Flexner," in *Beyond Flexner: Medical Education in the Twentieth Century*, eds. Barbara Barzansky and Norman Gevitz (New York: Greenwood Press, 1987), 51–63.
31 Todd Savitt, "Black Medical Schools," in *Beyond Flexner: Medical Education in the Twentieth Century*, eds. Barbara Barzansky and Norman Gevitz (Westport: Greenwood Press, 1992), 71.
32 Diversity in Medical Education, Facts & Figures 2012, "Current Status of Racial and Ethnic Minorities in *Medical Education*" (Table 24b). Accessed July 3, 2013: https://members.aamc.org/eweb/upload/Diversity%20in%20Medical%20Education_0Facts%20and%20Figures%202012.pdf.
33 See Kenneth Ludmerer, *A Time to Heal*, 79, and Jonathan R. Cole, *The Great American University* (New York: Perseus Books, 2009), 157.
34 Ludmerer, *A Time to Heal*, xxiii.
35 David Blumenthal and Greg S. Meyer, "Academic Health Centers in a Changing Environment," *Health Affairs* 12, no. 2 (1996): 201–215.
36 Ludmerer, *A Time to Heal*, 370.
37 See Thomas Cole, Thelma Jean Goodrich, and Ellen Gritz, eds., *Faculty Health in Academic Medicine: Physicians, Scientists, and the Pressures of Success* (Totowa, NJ: Humana Press), chs. 4, 13, 14, and 17.
38 Takakuwa, Kevin M., Nick Rugashkin, and Karen E. Herzig, *What I Learned in Medical School: Personal Stories of Young Doctors* (Berkeley: University of California Press, 2004), 78–79.
39 Molly Cooke, David M. Irby, and Bridget C. O'Brien, *Educating Physicians: A Call for Reform of Medical School and Residency* (San Francisco: Jossey-Bass, 2010), 223.
40 Ibid.
41 *Core Competencies for Interprofessional Collaborative Practice*, Report of an Expert Panel (May 2011), Sponsored by the Interprofessional Education Collaborative. Accessed November 20, 2013: http://www.aacn.nche.edu/education-resources/ipecreport.pdf.

4 TECHNOLOGY AND MEDICINE

1 Sigmund Freud, Civilization and Its Discontents, in *The Standard Edition of the Complete Psychological Works of Sigmund Freud*, Vol. 21, ed. and trans. James Strachey (London: Vintage Press, 2001), 91–92.

2 Stanley Reiser, *Technological Medicine: The Changing World of Doctors and Patients* (Cambridge: Cambridge University Press, 2009), 187.

3 Roy Porter, *The Cambridge Illustrated History of Medicine* (Cambridge: Cambridge University Press, 1996), 202.

4 Roy Porter, *The Greatest Benefit to Mankind: A Medical History of Humanity from Antiquity to the Present* (London: HarperCollins, 1997), 140.

5 Bruno Halioua and Bernard Ziskind, *Medicine in the Days of the Pharaohs* (Cambridge, MA and London: Harvard University Press, 2005).

6 Guido Majno, *The Healing Hand: Man and Wound in the Ancient World* (Cambridge, MA: Harvard University Press, 1975), 325–424.

7 Porter, *Greatest Benefit*, 116–120.

8 Quoted in A. Earl Walker, *The Genesis of Neuroscience*, eds. Edward R. Laws Jr. and George Udvarhelyi (Chicago: University of Chicago Press, 1998), 66.

9 Stanley Reiser, *Medicine and the Reign of Technology* (Cambridge: Cambridge University Press, 1978), 69.

10 David E. Wolfe, "Sydenham and Locke on the Limits of Anatomy," *Bulletin of the History of Medicine* 25 (1961): 193–200.

11 F. N. L. Poynter and W. J. Bishop, *A Seventeenth-Century Country Doctor and his Patients: John Symcotts, 1592–1662* (Streatley, UK: Bedfordshire Historical Record Society, 1951), 31.

12 Reiser, *Reign of Technology*, 19–22.

13 The following discussion is based on Reiser, *Reign of Technology*, 45–47, 53, 90, 107.

14 Gert H. Brieger, "From Conservative to Radical Surgery in Late Nineteenth-Century America," in *Medical Theory, Surgical Practice*, ed. Christopher Lawrence (London, Routledge, 1992).

15 Martin S. Pernick, *A Calculus of Suffering: Pain, Professionalism, and Anesthesia in Nineteenth-Century America* (New York: Columbia University Press, 1985), 3.

16 Ibid., 58–59.

17 Nicholas L. Tilney, *Invasion of the Body: Revolutions in Surgery* (Cambridge, MA: Harvard University Press, 2011), 71–72.

18 Judith Leavitt, *Brought to Bed: Childbearing in America 1750 to 1950* (New York and Oxford: Oxford University Press, 1986), 59.

19 Ibid., 183.

20 We are grateful to Jason Glenn for his insights in a review of an early draft of this chapter.

21 Reiser, *Reign of Technology*, 68.

22 Thomas Mann, *The Magic Mountain*, trans. by H. T. Lowe-Porter (1924; reprint, New York: Vintage Books, 1969), 348–349.

23 Quoted in Joel D. Howell, *Technology in the Hospital* (Baltimore, MD and London: The Johns Hopkins University Press, 1995), 108.

24 Joel D. Howell, *Technology in the Hospital* (Baltimore, MD and London: The Johns Hopkins University Press, 1995), 69–133.

25 Charles Rosenberg, *The Care of Strangers* (New York: Basic Books, 1987), 341.

26 Howell, *Technology in the Hospital*, 15–16.

27 Florence Nightingale, *Notes on Hospitals* (London: Longman Green, 1863), 175–176.

28 Reiser, *Technological Medicine*, 79.

29 Quoted in Reiser, *Technological Medicine*, 54–55. The following discussion of the iron lung, IPPV, and kidney dialysis is based on Reiser, *Technological Medicine*, chs. 3 and 4.

30 "Health, United States, 2010," *National Center for Health Statistics*. Accessed July 15, 2013: http://www.cdc.gov/nchs/data/hus/hus10.pdf, page 366.

31 We thank Jason Glenn for his insights and comments on the issues of social justice created by modern medical technology.

32 Pope Pius XII, "The Prolongation of Life," *The Pope Speaks* 4, no. 4 (November 1958), 393–398.

33 David Clark and Nanette Pazdernik, *Biotechnology: Applying the Genetic Revolution* (Boston: Elsevier Academic Press, 2009), ix.

34 Huang Xiaohua, Ivan H. El-Sayed, Wei Qian, and Mostafa A. El-Sayed, "Cancer Cell Imaging and Photothermal Therapy in the Near-Infrared Region by Using Gold Nanorods," *Journal of the American Chemical Society* 128 (2006): 2115–2120.

35 Adriano Cavalcanti, "Nanorobot Invention and Linux: The Open Technology Factor – An Open Letter to UNO General Secretary," *CANNXS Project* 1 (2009): 1–4.

36 Ray Kurzweil, *The Singularity is Near: When Humans Transcend Biology* (New York: Viking, 2005), 7.

37 Quoted in Stanley Reiser, *Technological Medicine*, 97.

38 Eric Topol, *The Creative Destruction of Medicine* (New York: Basic Books, 2012).

39 Leon Kass, ed., *Beyond Therapy: Biotechnology and the Pursuit of Happiness: A Report of The President's Council on Bioethics* (March 2003), xvii.

5 THE HEALTH OF POPULATIONS

1 Daniel Defoe, *A Journal of the Plague Year* (Oxford: Oxford University Press, 1990), 166.

2 Marcus Aurelius, *Meditations IX*, trans. Maxwell Staniforth (New York: Penguin, 1964), 21.

3 See George Rosen, *A History of Public Health* (New York: MD Publications, 1958). For an overview of historical approaches to public health, see Dorothy Porter, *The History of Public Health and the Modern State* (Amsterdam: Editions Rodopi, 1994).

4 See Michel Foucault, *Madness and Civilization; A History of Insanity in the Age of Reason* (New York: Vintage Books, 1994); Michel Foucault, *The Birth of the Clinic: An Archaeology of Medical Perception*, trans. A. M. Sheridan (New York: Vintage Books, 1973); and Michel Foucault, *The History of Sexuality, Volume One: An Introduction* (New York: Vintage, 1990).

5 Dorothy Porter, *Health, Civilization and the State: A History of Public Health from Ancient to Modern Times* (Routledge: London and New York, 1999), 4.

6 William McNeill, *Plagues and Peoples* (New York: Anchor Press, 1976), 33.

7 McNeill, *Plagues and Peoples,* 51, 62.

8 Hippocrates, "Airs, Waters, Places," in *Hippocratic Writings*, trans. J. Chadwick and W. N. Mann, ed. G. E. R. Lloyd (New York: Penguin, 1978), 44.

9 Guenter Risse, *Mending Bodies, Saving Souls: A History of Hospitals* (New York: Oxford University Press, 1999).

10 Ibid., 69.

11 Ibid., 126.

12 Porter, *Health, Civilization and the State,* 24.

13 Quoted in Roy Porter, *The Greatest Benefit to Mankind: A Medical History of Humanity from Antiquity to the Present* (London: HarperCollins, 1997), 124.

14 J. N. Hays, *The Burdens of Disease: Epidemics and Human Response in Western History* (New Brunswick, NJ and London: Rutgers University Press, 1998), 44.

15 Frederick Cartwright and Michael Biddiss, *Disease and History* (Stroud, UK: Sutton Publications, 2000), 38.

16 Hays, *Burdens of Disease,* 55.

17 See Gerald Grob, *The Deadly Truth: A History of Disease in America* (Cambridge, MA: Harvard University Press, 2004).

18 McNeill, *Plagues and Peoples*, 2.

19 Hays, *The Burdens of Disease*, 72.

20 Fred Anderson, *Crucible of War: The Seven Years' War and the Fate of Empire in British North America, 1754–1766* (New York: Alfred A. Knopf, 2000), 542.

21 Ibid., 809.

22 Elizabeth Fee, "Public Health and the State: The United States," in *The History of Public Health and the Modern State*, ed. Dorothy Porter (Atlanta, GA: Editions Rodopi, 1994), 226.
23 Porter, *Health, Civilization and the State*, 83.
24 Ibid., 57.
25 Hays, *The Burden of Disease*, 137.
26 Porter, *Health, Civilization and the State*, 113.
27 Thomas Wakley, "Introduction," *The Lancet* 2 (1853): 393.
28 Quoted in Hays, *The Burdens of Disease*, 145. See also Joseph Duffy, *The Sanitarians* (Champaign: University of Illinois Press, 1992).
29 Hays, *The Burdens of Disease*, 146.
30 Quoted in Diane Paul, *Controlling Human Heredity 1865 to the Present* (Atlantic Highlands, NJ: Atlantic Highlands Humanities Press, 1995), 3.
31 Quoted in David Bradshaw, "Eugenics: They Should Certainly Be Killed," in *A Concise Companion to Modernism*, ed. by David Bradshaw (Oxford, UK: Blackwell Publishing, 2003), 39.
32 See Paul Lombardo, *Three Generations, No Imbeciles* (Baltimore, MD: Johns Hopkins University Press, 2008).
33 Rebecca Kluchin, *Fit to be Tied: Sterilization and Reproductive Rights in America, 1950–1980* (New Brunswick, NJ: Rutgers University Press, 2009), 17–20.
34 Roy Porter, *Madness: A Brief History* (Oxford and New York: Oxford University Press, 2000), 186.
35 Porter, *Health, Civilization and the State*, 175.
36 Ibid., 197.
37 Paul Starr, *Remedy and Reaction: The Peculiar American Struggle Over Health Care Reform* (New Haven, CT: Yale University Press, 2011), 5.
38 Abdel Omran, "The Epidemiologic Transition: A Theory of the Epidemiology of Population Change." *The Milbank Memorial Fund Quarterly* 49, no. 4 (1971): 509–538.
39 Fee, "Public Health and the State: The United States," 250.
40 Ibid., 251.
41 American College of Preventive Medicine, accessed June 4, 2012: www.acpm.org.
42 Paul Farmer, *Infections and Inequalities: The Modern Plagues* (Berkeley: University of California Press, 1998), 14.
43 Arno Karlen, *Man and Microbes: Diseases and Plagues in History and Modern Times* (New York: Putnam, 1995), 1–13.
44 Ibid., 6.
45 Susan Sontag, *Illness as Metaphor* (New York: Farrar, Strauss, and Giroux, 1978).
46 *A Human Health Perspective On Climate Change: A Report Outlining the Research Needs on the Human Health Effects of Climate Change* (Research Triangle Park, NC: Environmental Health Perspectives/National Institute of Environmental Health Sciences, April 2010). Accessed November 11, 2013: 3. www.niehs.nih.gov/climatereport.

6 DEATH AND DYING

1 "Code of Medical Ethics," *JAMA* 7, no. 27 (1886): 712.
2 Frank Kermode, *The Sense of an Ending: Studies in the Theory of Fiction* (Oxford and New York: Oxford University Press, 1966), 58.
3 Philippe Ariès, *Western Attitudes Toward Death: From the Middle Ages to the Present* (Baltimore, MD: Johns Hopkins University Press, 1974); and Philippe Ariès, *The Hour of Our Death* (New York: Alfred E. Knopf, 1981).
4 Many critics have pointed to various shortcomings of Aries' work, including its lack of empirical support and reliance on literary sources. For a full account of responses to Ariès, see Roy Porter,

"The Hour of Philippe Aries," *Mortality* 4 (1999): 83–90; and Allan Kellehear, *A Social History of Dying* (Cambridge: Cambridge University Press, 2007), 172–176.

5 E. H. Ackerknecht, "Death in the History of Medicine," *Bulletin of the History of Medicine* 42 (1968), 19–23.

6 Quoted in Paul Strathern, *A Brief History of Medicine: From Hippocrates to Gene Therapy* (New York: Carroll & Graf Publishers, 2005), 15.

7 Roy Porter, *The Greatest Benefit To Mankind: A Medical History of Humanity From Antiquity to the Present* (London: HarperCollins, 1997), 86–87.

8 Ackerneckt, "Death in the History of Medicine," 21.

9 Seneca, *Letters from a Stoic*, trans. by Robin Campell (New York: Penguin, 1969), 161, 183.

10 Peregrine Horden, "What's Wrong with Early Medieval Medicine?" *Social History of Medicine* 24, no.1 (2009): 1.

11 Ibid., 15.

12 Ariès, *The Hour of Our Death*, 23.

13 Quoted in Ariès, *The Hour of Our Death*, 16.

14 John 11:25.

15 Ariès, *The Hour of Our Death*, 107–110.

16 David Stannard, *The Puritan Way of Death* (New York: Oxford University Press, 1977).

17 Quoted in James Farrell, *Inventing the American Way of Death, 1830–1920* (Philadelphia: Temple University Press, 1980), 19.

18 Quoted in Robert B. Baker and Laurence B. McCullough, "Medical Ethics through the Life Cycle in Europe and the Americas," in *The Cambridge World History of Medical Ethics*, eds. Robert Baker and Laurence McCullough (Cambridge: Cambridge University Press, 2008), 149.

19 Ibid., 150.

20 Ibid.

21 Ackerknecht, "Death in the History of Medicine," 22.

22 Roy Porter, "Death and the Doctors in Georgian England," in *Death, Ritual and Bereavement*, ed. Ralph Houlbrooke (London and New York: Routledge), 88.

23 "Code of Medical Ethics," 712.

24 Emily Abel, *The Inevitable Hour: A History of Caring for Dying Patients in America* (Baltimore, MD: Johns Hopkins University Press, 2013), 25.

25 Ibid., 11.

26 Ibid., 14.

27 Joseph Jacobs, "The Dying of Death," *Public Opinion* 27 (August 1899): 241.

28 Porter, *Greatest Benefit*, 85.

29 Leo Tolstoy, The Death of Ivan Ilych, in *The Death of Ivan Ilych and Other Stories*, trans. Aylmer Maude (New York: Penguin Books, 1960), 134–135.

30 Ibid., 154–155.

31 Geoffrey Gorer, The Pornography of Death, in *Death, Grief and Mourning in Contemporary Britain* (Garden City, NY: Doubleday, 1965).

32 Emily K. Abel, "'In the Last Stages of Irremediable Disease': American Hospitals and Dying Patients before World War II," *Bulletin of the History of Medicine* 85 (2011): 32.

33 Quoted in Abel, *The Inevitable Hour*, 51.

34 Quoted. in ibid., 37.

35 See "Facing Death," *Frontline: PBS Houston*, November 10, 2010. Accessed July 16, 2010: www.pbs.org/wgbh/pages/frontline/facing-death/.

36 Stanley Reiser, *Technological Medicine: The Changing World of Doctors and Patients* (Cambridge: Cambridge University Press, 2009), 59–61.

37 See Barney Glaser and Anselm Strauss, *Awareness of Dying* (Chicago: Aldine, 1965); and David Sudnow, *Passing On: the Social Organization of Dying* (Englewood Cliffs, NJ: Prentice Hall, 1967).

38 Quoted in Abel, *The Inevitable Hour*, 167.

39 Cicely Saunders, "Hospice," *Mortality* 1, no. 3 (1996): 317–322.
40 Elizabeth Kübler-Ross, *On Death and Dying* (New York: MacMillan, 1969), 5.
41 Ibid., 6.
42 Marie-Aurèlie Bruno, Didier Ledoux and Steven Laureys, "The Dying Human: A Perspective From Biomedicine," in *The Study of Dying: From Autonomy to Transformation*, ed. Allan Kellehear (New York: Cambridge University Press, 2009), 60–61.
43 Ibid., 53.
44 Robert Veatch, "Defining and Redefining Life and Death," in *The Cambridge World History of Medical Ethics*, eds. Robert Baker and Laurence McCullough (Cambridge: Cambridge University Press, 2008), 684–691.
45 Quoted in ibid., 689.
46 Raymond S. Duff and A. G. M. Campbell, "Moral and Ethical Dilemmas in the Special-Care Nursery," *New England Journal of Medicine* 289 (1973): 890–894; and Richard A. McCormick, "To Save or Let Die: The Dilemma of Modern Medicine," *Journal of the American Medical Association* 229 (1974): 172–176.
47 Sharon Kauffman, *And a Time to Die: How American Hospitals Shape the End of Life* (Chicago: University of Chicago Press, 2005), 65.
48 *How to Die in Oregon* (2011). DVD, directed by Peter Richardson (Clearcut Productions, 2011).
49 James Green, *Beyond the Good Death: The Modern Anthropology of Dying* (Philadelphia: Pennsylvania University Press, 2008), 175–183.

PART II LITERATURE, THE ARTS, AND MEDICINE

1 John Berger, *Ways of Seeing* (London: Penguin Books, 1972), 7–8.
2 Rudolf Arnheim, *Visual Thinking* (Berkeley: University of California Press, 1969).
3 Mary Winkler, "The Visual Arts in Medical Education," *Second Opinion* 19, no. 1 (1993): 65. See also Geri Berg, ed. *The Visual Arts in Medical Education* (Carbondale: Southern Illinois University Press, 1983).
4 This shared insight was a catalyst for the emergence of literature and medicine as a significant field within medical humanities in the 1980s and 1990s. For example, see Joanne Trautmann Banks, "The Wonders of Literature in Medical Education," *Mobius: A Journal for Continuing Education for Professionals in Health Sciences and Health Policy* 2, no. 3 (1982): 23–31; Delese Wear, Martin Kohn, and Susan Stocker, eds., *Literature and Medicine: A Claim for a Discipline* (McLean, VA: Society for Health and Human Values, 1987); Anne Hudson Jones, "Literature and Medicine: Traditions and Innovations," in *The Body and the Text: Comparative Essays in Literature and Medicine*, eds. Bruce Clarke and Wendell Aycock (Lubbock: Texas Tech University Press, 1990); and Rita Charon, Joanne Trautmann Banks, Julia E. Connelly, Anne Hunsaker Hawkins, Kathryn Montgomery Hunter, Anne Hudson Jones, Martha Montello, and Suzanne Poirier, "Literature and Medicine: Contributions to Clinical Practice," *Annals of Internal Medicine* 122, no. 8 (1995): 599–606; M. Faith McLellan and Anne Hudson Jones, "Why Literature and Medicine?" *Lancet* 348 (1996): 109–111.
5 Clifford Geertz, "The Uses of Diversity," *Michigan Quarterly Review* [(XXV) no. 1 (Winter, 1986) 113.] Reprinted in Clifford Geertz, *Available Light: Anthropological Reflections on Philosophical Topics* (Princeton, NJ: Princeton University Press, 2000), 68–88.
6 Lawrence J. Schneiderman, "Empathy and the Literary Imagination," *Annals of Internal Medicine* 137, no. 7 (2002): 627–629.
7 J. M. Cameron, "The Description of Feeling," in *Nuclear Catholics and Other Essays* (Grand Rapids, MI: William B. Eerdmans Publishing Company, 1989), 181.
8 Friedrich Nietzsche, *The Dawn*, in *Werke in drei Bänden*, vol. 1 (München: Carl Hanser Verlag, 1954), 1016. Author's translation.

7 NARRATIVES OF ILLNESS

1 Quoted by Hannah Arendt, "Isak Dinesen: 1885–1963," in *Men in Dark Times* (New York: Harcourt, Brace and Co., 1968), 97.
2 See Anne Hunsaker Hawkins, *Reconstructing Illness: Studies in Pathography* (West Lafayette, IN: Purdue University Press, 1993). Also pertinent is Oliver Sacks, "Clinical Tales," *Literature and Medicine* 5 (1986): 16–23. Note especially: "The delineation of *worlds*, as they may be altered, broken or buffeted by disease; and the relation of altered worlds, disease worlds to *our* world – this seems to me to lie at the heart of any clinical tale, to set it apart from (and beyond) mere case history (though, of course, it will *contain* a case history), and to establish it as an authentic branch of narrative or drama" (p. 18).
3 John Gunther, *Death Be Not Proud* (New York: Pyramid Books, 1949).
4 Lael Tucker Wertenbaker, *Death of a Man* (Boston: Beacon Press, 1957).
5 Stewart Alsop, *Stay of Execution: A Sort of Memoir* (Philadelphia: J. P. Lippincott, 1973).
6 Betty Rollins, *Last Wish* (New York: Linden Press/Simon & Schuster, 1977).
7 Stephen S. Rosenfeld, *The Time of Their Dying* (New York: W. W. Norton, 1977).
8 See Martin Kreiswirth, "Trusting the Tale: The Narrativist Turn in the Human Sciences," *New Literary History* 23, no. 3, (1992): 630: "Narrative and story have come to displace argument and explanation in a whole range of philosophic, theoretical, and cross-disciplinary contexts."
9 Hawkins, *Reconstructing Illness*, 18.
10 Robert Coles, *The Call of Stories: Teaching and the Moral Imagination* (Boston: Houghton Mifflin Company, 1989), 205.
11 Arthur Frank, *The Wounded Storyteller: Body, Illness, and Ethics* (Chicago: University of Chicago Press, 1995), passim.
12 Arthur Frank, "Five Dramas of Illness," *Perspectives in Biology and Medicine* 50, no. 3, (2007): 394.
13 Oliver Sacks, *A Leg to Stand On* (New York: Summit Books/Simon & Schuster, 1984).
14 Ibid., 219.
15 Ibid., 64.
16 Ibid., 72.
17 Ibid., 119.
18 Ibid., 145.
19 Ibid., 150.
20 William Styron, *Darkness Visible: A Memoir of Madness* (New York: Vintage Books, 1990).
21 Lucy Grealy, *Autobiography of a Face* (New York: Harper Perennial, 1994).
22 Aaron Alterra, *The Caregiver: A Life with Alzheimer's* (South Royalton, VT: Steerforth Press, 1999).
23 William Styron, *Darkness Visible*, 63.
24 Ibid., 12.
25 Ibid., 13.
26 Ibid., 45.
27 Ibid., 38.
28 Ibid., 50.
29 Ibid., 7–8, 84.
30 Ibid., 64.
31 Ibid., 69.
32 Ibid., 73.
33 Ibid., 68.
34 Ibid., 76.
35 Ibid., 78.
36 Ibid., 56.
37 Ibid., 81.

38 Lucy Grealy, *Autobiography of a Face*, 13.

39 Ibid., 27.

40 Ibid., 38.

41 Ibid., 43.

42 Ibid., 111–112.

43 Ibid., 219–220.

44 Ibid., 157.

45 Ibid., 223.

46 Ibid., 220.

47 See W. J. T. Mitchell, "Introduction: Pragmatic Theory," in *Against Theory: Literary Studies and the New Pragmatism*, ed. W. J. T. Mitchell (Chicago: University of Chicago Press, 1985), 7: "Theory is monotheistic, in love with simplicity, scope, and coherence. It aspires to explain the many in terms of the one.... Theory places itself at the beginning or the end of thought providing first principles ... and schematizing practice in a general account. It is unhappy with the middle realm of history, practical conduct, and business as usual and so tends to seek a final solution, a utopian perspective, which presents itself as a point of origin."

48 Aaron Alterra, *The Caregiver*, 26.

49 Ibid., 49.

50 Ibid., 79.

51 Ibid., 92–93.

52 Ibid., 158.

53 Ibid., 192.

54 See Rita Charon, "Narrative and Medicine," *New England Journal of Medicine* 350, no. 9 (2004): 862; Martha Montello, "Narrative Competence," in *Stories and Their Limits: Narrative Approaches to Ethics*, ed. Hilde Lindemann Nelson (New York: Routledge, 1997), 185–197; and Rita Charon, *Narrative Medicine: Honoring the Stories of Illness* (New York: Oxford University Press, 2006), especially Part III, "Developing Narrative Competence."

8 AGING IN FILM

1 Sally Chivers, *The Silvering Screen* (Toronto, ON: University of Toronto Press, 2011), 5.

2 Thomas R. Cole and Mary G. Winkler, eds., *The Oxford Book of Aging* (New York: Oxford University Press, 1994), 3.

3 As Amir Cohen-Shalev and Eshter-Lee Marcus put it, "few filmmakers have taken up the challenge of a thorough screen study of the phenomenon of old age, and still fewer social scientists have responded to the demand of an aging society for a serious treatment of its aged via the communication venues so central to its cultural identity." See Amir Cohen-Shalev and Esther-Lee Marcus, "Golden Years and Silver Screen: Cinematic Representations of Old Age," *Journal of Aging, Humanities and the Arts* 1 (2007): 85.

4 Pam Gravagne, *The Becoming of Age: Cinematic Visions of Mind, Body and Identity in Later Life* (Jefferson, NC: MacFarland & Company, 2013).

5 Sally Chivers, *The Silvering Screen* (Toronto, ON: University of Toronto Press, 2011), 5.

6 See Heather Addison, "'Must the Players Keep Young?' Early Hollywood's Cult of Youth," *Cinema Journal* 45, no. 4 (2006): 3–25; and Heather Addison, "Transcending Time: Jean Harlow and Hollywood's Narrative of Decline," *Journal of Film and Video* 57, no.4 (2005): 32–46.

7 Thomas Cole, *The Journey of Life: A Cultural History of Aging in America* (New York: Cambridge University Press, 1992), 232.

8 Addison, "Hollywood's Cult of Youth," 6.

9 Addison, "Hollywood's Narrative of Decline," 33.

10 S. Harvey, "Coming of Age in Film," *American Film* 7, no. 3 (1981): 52–3.

11 See Robert Butler, "The Life Review: An Interpretation of Reminiscence in the Aged," *Psychiatry* 26 (1963): 65–76; and Erik Erikson, "Reflections on Dr. Borg's Life Cycle, *Daedalus* 105, no. 2 (1976): 1–28.

12 Chivers, *The Silvering Screen*, 41–2.

13 Quoted in ibid., xii.

14 Robert Yahnke, "Intergeneration and Regeneration: The Meaning of Old Age in Films and Videos," in *Handbook of the Humanities and Aging*, 2nd ed., eds. Thomas R. Cole, Robert Kastenbaum, and Ruth Ray (New York: Springer Publishing Company, 2000).

15 Robert Yahnke, "The Experience of Aging in Feature-Length Films: A Selected and Annotated Filmography," in *A Guide to Humanistic Studies in Aging*, eds. Thomas R. Cole, Ruth E. Ray, and Robert Kastenbaum (Baltimore, MD: The John Hopkins University Press, 2010).

16 Thomas Cole, "Aging, Home, and Hollywood in the 1980s," *The Gerontologist* 31, no. 3 (1991): 427–30.

17 Yahnke, "Old Age in Films and Videos," 300–301.

18 See Bradley J. Fisher and Sandra Shapshay, "'He Just Got Old:' Aging and Compassionate Care in *Dad*," in *Bioethics at the Movies*, ed. Sandra Shapshay (Baltimore, MD: Johns Hopkins University Press, 2009), 205–224.

19 Elaine Showalter, "An 'Iris' Stripped of Her Brilliance,' *Chronicle of Higher Education* 48, no. 23 (2002): B18.

20 Thomas Waltz, "Crones, Dirty Old Men, Sexy Seniors: Representations of the Sexuality of Older Persons," *Journal of Aging and Identity* 7, no.2 (2002): 99–112.

21 "Westerns insist on this point," writes Jane Tompkins, "by emphasizing the importance of manhood as an ideal. It is not one ideal among many, it is *the* ideal, certainly the only one worth dying for. It doesn't matter whether a man is a sheriff or an outlaw, a rustler or a rancher, a cattleman or a sheepherder, a miner or a gambler. What matters is that he be a *man*." See Jane Tompkins, *West of Everything: The Inner Life of Westerns* (Oxford: Oxford University Press, 1992), 17–18.

22 Chivers, *The Silvering Screen*, 102.

23 Ibid., 112.

24 Munny's comical, bumbling image is further underscored if we contrast the character with Eastwood himself, whose previous, younger cowboy roles – *A Fistful of Dollars* (1964), *The Good, the Bad, and the Ugly* (1966), and *Pale Rider* (1985), among others – epitomize the physically powerful, violent bad-boy hero.

25 This quotation is from Joel and Ethan Coen's film *No Country for Old Men*.

26 Chivers, *The Silvering Screen*, xvi.

9 MEDICINE AND MEDIA

1 Quoted in Jospeh Turow, *Playing Doctor: Television, Storytelling, and Medical Power* (Ann Arbor: University of Michigan Press, 2010), 362.

2 Ibid.

3 Lester Friedman, ed., *Cultural Sutures: Medicine and Media* (Durham, NC: Duke University Press, 2004).

4 Leslie Reagan, Nancy Tomes, and Paula Treichler, eds., *Medicine's Moving Pictures: Medicine, Health, and Bodies in American Film and Television* (Rochester, NY: University of Rochester, 2007).

5 Sandra Shapshay, ed., *Bioethics at the Movies* (Baltimore, MD: Johns Hopkins University Press, 2009).

6 Andrew Holtz, *House, M.D. vs. Reality: Fact and Fiction in the Hit Television Series* (New York: Berkley Publishing Group, 2011).

7 Allan Ross and Harlan Gibbs, *The Medicine of ER: An Insider's Guide to the Medical Science Behind America's #1 TV Drama* (New York: BasicBooks, 1996).

8 Jason Jacobs, *Body Trauma TV: The New Hospital Dramas* (London: BFI Publishing, 2003).

9 Clive Seale, *Media and Health* (London: Sage Publications, 2002).

10 Kirsten Ostherr, *Cinematic Prophylaxis: Globalization and Contagion in the Discourse of World Health* (Durham, NC: Duke University Press, 2005); Kirsten Ostherr, *Medical Visions: Producing the Patient through Film, Television, and Imaging Technologies* (Oxford: Oxford University Press, 2013).

11 See, for example, Timothy Johnson, "Medicine and the Media," *The New England Journal of Medicine* 339 (1998): 87–92.

12 See, for example, Matthew Czarny, Ruth Faden, and Jeremy Sugarman, "Bioethics and Professionalism in Popular Television Medical Dramas," *Journal of Medical Ethics* 36 (2010): 203–206.

13 See, for example, the December 2008 special issue of *The American Journal of Bioethics* on television (Volume 8, Issue 12). Also see Hyunyi Cho, Kari Wilson, and Jounghwa Choi, "Perceived Realism of Television Medical Dramas and Perceptions about Physicians," *Journal of Media Psychology* 23 (2011): 141–148; and Brian Quick, "The Effects of Viewing *Grey's Anatomy* on Perceptions of Doctors and Patient Satisfaction," *Journal of Broadcasting and Electronic Media* 53 (2009): 38–55.

14 Seale, *Media and Health*, 111.

15 Ibid., 113.

16 Matthew Czarny, Ruth Faden, Marie Nolan, Edwin Bodensiek, and Jeremy Sugarman, "Medical and Nursing Students' Television Viewing Habits: Potential Implications for Bioethics," *The American Journal of Bioethics* 8 (2008): 1, emphasis added.

17 Mark Wicclair, "The Pedagogical Value of *House, M.D.*," *The American Journal of Bioethics* 89 (2008): 16.

18 Jeffrey Spike, "Television Viewing and Ethical Reasoning: Why Watching *Scrubs* Does a Better Job than Most Bioethics Classes," *The American Journal of Bioethics* 89 (2008): 11–13.

19 Joseph Turow and Rachel Gans-Boriskin, "From Expert in Action to Existential Angst," in *Medicine's Moving Pictures*, 263–281.

20 Turow, *Playing Doctor*, 10.

21 Ibid., 7–8.

22 Ibid., 51–54. This discussion was largely based on Turow's work.

23 William Regelson, "The Weakening of the Oslerian Tradition," *JAMA* 239 (1978): 317–319.

24 Turow, *Playing Doctor*, 87–109. This discussion was largely based on Turow's work.

25 See James Wittebols, *Watching M*A*S*H, Watching America: A Social History of the 1972–1983 Television Series* (Jefferson, NC: McFarland and Co., 1998).

26 Turow, *Playing Doctor*, 248–271. This discussion was largely based on Turow's work.

27 Ibid., 326–328.

28 Roselyn Epps, "Hats Off to Dr. Huxtable," *JAMA* 254 (1985): 2957.

29 Leslie Inniss and Joe Feagin, "The Cosby Show: The View from the Black Middle Class," *Journal of Black Studies* 25 (1995): 692–711; Sut Jhally and Justin Lewis, *Enlightened Racism: The Cosby Show, Audiences and the Myth of the American Dream* (Boulder, CO: Westview Press, 1992).

30 On this point, see John Hoberman, *Black and Blue: The Origins and Consequences of Medical Racism* (Berkeley: University of California Press, 2012).

31 Jacobs, *Body Trauma TV*, 25.

32 Ibid., 26.

33 Turow, *Playing Doctor*, 343.

34 Ibid., 331–358.

35 Amir Hetsroni, "If You Must Be Hospitalized, Television Is Not the Place," *Communication Research Reports* 26 (2009): 311–322.

36 Holtz, *House, M.D.*, 44.

37 See, e.g., Czarny, Faden, and Sugarman, "Bioethics and Professionalism in Popular Television Medical Dramas."

38 Elena Strauman and Bethany Goodier, "The Doctor(s) in House," *Journal of Medical Humanities* 32 (2011): 43.

39 Ibid.

40 Ibid, 45.

41 Quoted in Turow, *Playing Doctor*, 362.

10 POETRY AND MORAL IMAGINATION

1 Anatole Broyard, *Intoxicated by My Illness and Other Writings on Life and Death* (New York: Fawcett Columbine, 1992), 41.

2 Marianne Moore, "Poetry," in *Collected Poems* (New York: Macmillan, 1935).

3 Cynthia Ozick, "Forewords, Afterwards," *American Poet: The Journal of the American Academy of Poets* (Summer 1997): 9.

4 W. H. Auden, in *The English Auden*, ed. Edward Mendelson (New York: Random House, 1977), 329.

5 W. H. Auden, "A Short Defense of Poetry," *New York Review of Books*, January 30, 1986, 15.

6 Ozick, "Forewords, Afterwards."

7 I offer these readings in the spirit invoked by Lionel Trilling in explaining the purpose of the commentaries he provided on works of literature selected for his anthology, *The Experience of Literature*: "They have one purpose only – to make it more likely that the act of reading will be an experience, having in mind what the word implies of an activity of consciousness and response … and I have tried to have them say no more than might suggest to the reader how he could come into a more active connection with what he has read." See Lionel Trilling, *The Experience of Literature: A Reader with Commentaries* (Garden City, NY: Doubleday & Company, 1967), x and xi.

8 Kenneth Koch, "The Language of Poetry," *New York Review of Books*, May 14, 1998, 47. The same does not apply to objectivist, or formalist, views of poetry which purge the personal and require mastery of some literary-critical apparatus.

9 Alan Shapiro, "The Stroke," *The American Scholar* 52 no. 3 (Summer 1983): 363–364.

10 James Dickey, "The Scarred Girl," in *The Whole Motion: Collected Poems, 1945–1992* (Middletown, CT: Wesleyan University Press, 1992). The rhythm of "The Scarred Girl" is best appreciated when the poem is read aloud, attending especially to the punctuation and taking care to pause after each comma and to stop for a breath following the periods.

11 Robert Cooperman, "What They Don't Know," *The American Poetry Review* 17 no. 2 (March-April 1988): 46.

12 Northrup Frye, *The Educated Imagination* (Bloomington: Indiana University Press, 1964), 135.

13 Mary Warnock, *Imagination* (Berkeley: University of California Press, 1978), 201.

14 Ibid., 196.

15 Stephen Knight, "FROM *The Fascinating Room*," in *Flowering Limbs* (Newcastle upon Tyne, UK: Bloodaxe Books Ltd., 1993), 21–23.

16 Sharon Olds, "The Learner," in *The Unswept Room* (New York: Alfred A. Knopf, 2002), 97–98.

17 John Berger, *And Our Faces, My Heart, Brief as Photos* (New York: Vintage Books, 1984), 97.

11 DOCTOR-WRITERS

1 Anatole Broyard, *Intoxicated by My Illness and Other Writings on Life and Death* (New York: Fawcett Columbine, 1992), 41.

2 William Carlos Williams, *The Doctor Stories*, compiled by Robert Coles (New York: Directions Publishing, 1984), 99.
3 Ibid., 100.
4 Ibid., 101.
5 Ibid.
6 Ibid., 57.
7 Ibid., 58.
8 Ibid., 59–60.
9 Joanne Trautmann, "William Carlos Williams and the Poetry of Medicine," *Ethics in Science & Medicine* 2 (1975): 106.
10 William Carlos Williams, "The Practice," *William Carlos Williams: The Doctor Stories*, compiled by Robert Coles (New York: Directions Publishing, 1984), 123, 126.
11 Richard Selzer, *Letter to a Young Doctor* (New York: Simon & Schuster, 1996), iii.
12 Richard Selzer, *Confessions of a Knife* (New York: Simon & Schuster, 1979), 18–19.
13 Richard Selzer, "A Parable" in *Recognitions: Doctors and their Stories*, eds. Carol Donley and Martin Kohn, (Kent, OH: Kent State University Press, 2002), 171.
14 Ibid., 172.
15 Ibid., 172–173.
16 Ibid., 173.
17 W. H. Auden, *The English Auden: Poems, Essays and Dramatic Writings, 1927–1939*, ed. Edward Mendelsohn (New York: Random House, 1978), 341.
18 David Daiches, "Religion, Poetry, and the 'Dilemma' of the Modern Writer," *Literary Essays* (Chicago: University of Chicago Press, 1968).
19 Kate Scannell, *Death of the Good Doctor: Lessons from the Heart of the AIDS Epidemic* (San Francisco, CA: Cleis Press, 1999), 10–11.
20 Ibid., 12–13.
21 Danielle Ofri, *Incidental Findings: Lessons from My Patients in the Art of Medicine* (Boston: Beacon Press, 2005), 68.
22 Ibid., 70–71.
23 Ibid., 72.
24 Ibid., 73.
25 Ibid., 70.
26 Ibid., 8–9.
27 Pauline Chen, *Final Exam: A Surgeon's Reflections on Mortality* (New York: Alfred A. Knopf, 2007), 6.
28 Ibid., p. 8.
29 Renée C. Fox and Harold I, Lief, "Training for 'Detached Concern' in Medical Students," in *The Psychological Basis of Medical Practice*, eds. Harold I. Lief, et al. (New York: Harper & Row, 1963), 12–35. See also John L. Coulehan, "Tenderness and Steadiness," *Literature and Medicine* 14, no. 2 (1995): 222–236.
30 Chen, *Final Exam*, 46–47.
31 Ibid., 208.
32 Ibid., 209–210.
33 Ibid., 211.
34 Anatole Broyard, *Intoxicated by My Illness*, 41.
35 Carl Elliott observes of doctors who become disheartened by their work that they tend to be those who "expected the practice to carry some deeper significance. They are the ones who thought medicine was a moral calling." See Carl Elliott, "Disillusioned Doctors," in *Lost Virtue: Professional Character Development in Medical Education*, eds. Nuala Kenny and Wayne Shelton (Amsterdam: Elsevier Ltd., 2006), 97.

12 STUDYING MEDICINE

1 Ellen Fox, "Rethinking *Doctor Think*: Reforming Medical Education by Nurturing Neglected Goals," in *The Goals of Medicine: The Forgotten Issues in Health Care Reform*, eds. Mark J. Hanson and Daniel Callahan (Washington, DC: Georgetown University Press, 1999), 196.

2 Abraham Flexner, *Medical Education in the United States and Canada: A Report to the Carnegie Foundation for the Advancement of Teaching*, Bulletin no. 4 (Boston: Updyke, 1910).

3 Leonard D. Eron, "Effect of Medical Education on Medical Students Attitudes," *Journal of Medical Education* 30, no. 10 (1955): 559–556; Renée C. Fox, "Training for Uncertainty," in *The Student Physician*, eds. Robert K. Merton, George Reader, and Patricia Marshall (Cambridge, MA: Harvard University Press, 1957), 207–241; Howard S. Becker and Blanche Geer, "The Fate of Idealism in Medical School," *American Sociological Review* 23 (1958): 50–56; Daniel H. Funkenstein, "Medical Students, Medical Schools, and Society in Three Eras," in *Psychological Aspects of Medical Training*, eds. Robert H. Combs and Clark E. Vincent (Springfield, IL: Charles Thomas, 1971), 229–281.

4 Kenneth Keniston, "The Medical Student," *Yale Journal of Biology and Medicine* 39, no. 6 (1967): 346–58; Daniel H. Funkenstein, "The Learning and Personal Development of Medical Students Reconsidered," *The New Physician* 19 (1970): 229–281.

5 Frederic W. Hafferty and Ronald Franks, "The Hidden Curriculum, Ethics Teaching and the Structure of Medical Education," *Academic Medicine* 69 (1994): 861–871; Frederic W. Hafferty, "In Search of a Lost Cord: Professionalism and Medical Education's Hidden Curriculum," in *Education for Professionalism: Creating a Culture of Humanism in Medical Education*, eds. Delese Wear and Janet Bickel (Iowa City: University of Iowa Press, 2000), 11–34; Delese Wear and Mark G. Kuczewski, "Perspective: Medical Students' Perceptions of the Poor: What Impact Can Medical Education Have?" *Academic Medicine* 83 no. 7 (2008), 639–645.

6 L. Kron, "On Being Poor," *ITIS* 4, no 23 (1970): 1. Cited by Jerrold S. Maxmen in "Medical School as a Radicalizing Experience," *The Pharos* 35 (1972): 27.

7 H. Jack Geiger, "The Causes of Dehumanization in Health Care and Prospects for Humanization," in *Humanizing Health Care*, eds. Jan Howard and Anselm Strauss (New York: John Wiley and Sons, 1975), 16–17.

8 Fitzhugh Mullan, *White Coat, Clenched Fist: The Political Education of American Physician* (Ann Arbor: The University of Michigan Press, 2006), x.

9 Charles E. Lewis and Sharon Winer, "Has Idealism Survived?" *The New Physician* (January 1976): 25–27.

10 Alvin R. Tarlov, quoted in Jean Evangelauf, "Medical Schools Urged to Revamp Curricula," *The Chronicle of Higher Education*, November 18, 1987, 57. Medical school dean Frank N. Miller Jr. captured the sentiment of many in a commencement address at the George Washington School of Medicine: "There is no better preparation than an attentive interest in the humanities and the arts for meeting with wisdom the many situations requiring moral judgments which arise in the practice of medicine." See Franklin N. Miller Jr., "On Sitting Down to Read 'King Lear' Once Again," *The Pharos* 33 no. 1 (January 1970): 7–10.

11 A Rockefeller Foundation study recommended that institutions of higher education actively experiment with ways of integrating the humanities with preprofessional and professional studies (see *The Humanities in American Life*, Report of the Commission on the Humanities, Berkeley: University of California Press, 1980). The Council on Medical Education urged medical schools to encourage applications from undergraduates who have had "a broad exposure to the humanities as well as the physical sciences ... both of which are necessary for the practice of medicine" [see *Future Directions for Medical Education* (American Medical Association, 1982), 6]. And the Association of American Medical Colleges' General Professional Education of the Physician report recommended "that faculties integrate into the common curriculum materials that will provide students with a working knowledge of the ethical dimensions and the social context of medicine ... [and] that each medical school campus

have at least one full-time humanist to lead research in these areas and to act as a catalyst and liaison with other course directors to ensure that humanities materials are integrated into the curriculum" [see *Physicians for the Twenty-First Century*, Report of the Working Group on Personal Qualities, Values, and Attitudes," *Journal of Medical Education* 59, no. 11 (1984): 184–185].

12 Samuel Shem, *The House of God* (New York: Richard Marek Publishers, 1978). See also Howard Markel, "*The House of God* 30 Years Later," *Journal of the American Medical Association* 299, no. 2 (2008): 227–229; Martin Kohn and Carol Donley, eds., *Return to* The House of God*: Medical Resident Education 1978–2008* (Kent, OH: Kent State University Press, 2008); and Susan Dorr Goold and David T. Stern, "Ethics and Professionalism: What Does a Resident Need to Learn?" *American Journal of Bioethics* 6, no. 4 (2004): 9–17.

13 Jack Coulehan and Peter C. Williams, "Vanquishing Virtue: The Impact of Medical Education," *Academic Medicine* vol. 65, no. 6 (2001): 598–605.

14 Edmund D. Pellegrino, "The Humanities in Medicine: Entering the Post-Evangelical Era," in *The Humanities and the Profession of Medicine* (Research Triangle Park, NC: National Humanities Center, 1986), 25–43; Thomas K. McEllhinney and Edmund D. Pellegrino, "The Institute on Human Values in Medicine: Its Role and Influence in the Conception and Evolution of Bioethics," *Theoretical Medicine* 22, no. 4 (2001): 291–317; "The Humanities and Medicine: Reports of 41 U.S., Canadian and International Programs," eds. Lisa R. Dittrich and Anne L. Farmakidis, *Academic Medicine* 78, no. 10 (October 2003). See also Edmund D. Pellegrino, "Educating the Humanist Physician: An Ancient Ideal Reconsidered, "*Journal of the American Medical Association* 227, no. 11 (1974): 1288–1294; Kathryn Montgomery Hunter, "What We Do: The Humanities and the Interpretation of Medicine," *Theoretical Medicine* 8 (1987): 367–378.

15 Maggie Moore-West, Martha Regan-Smith, Allen Dietrich, and Donald O. Kollisch, "Innovations in Medical Education: Enhancing Humanism through the Educational Process," in *Educating Competent and Caring Physicians*, eds. Hugh C. Hendrie and Camille Lloyd (Bloomington: Indiana University Press, 1990), 128–174; Reneé C. Fox, "Training in Caring Competence," 199–216.

16 Manish C. Champaneria and Sara Axtell, "Cultural Competence Training in U.S. Medical Schools," *Journal of the American Medical Association* 291, no. 17 (2004): 2142.

17 Delese Wear, "Professional Development of Medical Students: Problems and Promises," *Academic Medicine* 72 (1997): 1056–1062; Kenneth M. Ludmerer, "Instilling Professionalism in Medical Education," *Journal of the American Medical Association* 282, no. 9 (1999): 881–882; Judith Andre, "The Medical Humanities as Contributing to Moral Growth and Development," in *Practicing the Medical Humanities: Engaging Physicians and Patients*, eds. Ronald A. Carson, Chester R. Burns, and Thomas R. Cole (Hagerstown, MD: University Publishing Group, 2003), 39–69; Jack Coulehan, "Today's Professionalism: Engaging the Mind but Not the Heart," *Academic Medicine* 80, no. 10 (2005): 892–898; Susan Door Goold and David T. Stern, "Ethics and Professionalism: What Does a Resident Need to Learn?" *The American Journal of Bioethics* 6, no. 4 (2006): 9–17; Michael W. Rabow, Rachel N. Remen, Dean X. Parmelee and Thomas S. Inui, "Professional Formation: Extending Medicine's Lineage of Service into the Next Century," *Academic Medicine* 85, no. 2 (2010): 310–317; Nathan Carlin, Thomas R. Cole, and Henry Strobel, "Guidance from the Humanities for Professional Formation," in *Oxford Textbook of Spirituality in Health Care*, eds. Mark Cobb, Christina Puchalski, and Bruce Rumbold (New York: Oxford University Press, 2012), 443–450.

18 "The Human Condition of Health Professionals," a lecture delivered at the University of New Hampshire, November 19, 1979 under the auspices of the James Picker Foundation. See also Diane E. Meier, Anthony L. Back, and R. Sean Morrison, "The Inner Life of Physicians and Care of the Seriously Ill," *Journal of the American Medical Association* 286, no. 23 (2001): 3007–3014; Thomas R. Cole and Nathan Carlin, "The Suffering of Physicians," *The Lancet* 374 (2009): 1414–1415.

19 D. A. Christakis, "Characteristics of the Informal Curriculum on Trainees' Ethical Choices, *Academic Medicine* 71 (1996): 621–642; Joyce M Fried, Michelle Vermillion, Neil H. Parker, and Sebastian Uijtdehaage, "Eradicating Medical Student Mistreatment: A Longitudinal Study of One Institution's Efforts," *Academic Medicine* 87, no. 9 (2012): 1191–1198.

20 Melanie M. Watkins, "Melanie's Story," in *What I Learned in Medical School*, eds. Kevin M. Takakuwe, Nick Rubashkin, and Karen E. Herzig (Berkeley: University of California Press, 2004), 19–22.

21 Karen C. Kim, "Why Am I in Medical School?" in *What I Learned in Medical School*, eds. Kevin M. Takakuwe, Nick Rubashkin, and Karen E. Herzig (Berkeley: University of California Press, 2004), 75–79.

22 Tista Ghosh, "A Case Presentation," in *What I Learned in Medical School*, eds. Kevin M. Takakuwe, Nick Rubashkin, and Karen E. Herzig (Berkeley: University of California Press, 2004), 154–160. See also Florence M. Witte, Terry D. Stratton, and Lois Margaret Nora, "Stories from the Field: Students' Descriptions of Gender, Discrimination during Medical School," *Academic Medicine* 81, no. 7 (2006): 648–654.

23 David Hellerstein, "Touching," in *On Doctoring: Stories, Poems, Essays*, eds. Richard Reynolds and John Stone (New York: Simon & Schuster, 2001), 354–357.

24 John Stone, "My Medical School," in *My Medical School*, ed. Dannie Abse (London: Robson Books, n.d.), 193. On modeling caring behavior, see William T. Branch, "The Ethics of Caring and Medical Education," *Academic Medicine* 75, no. 2, (2000): 127–132.

25 Cortney Davis, "Breathing," *Bellevue Literary Review* 5, no. 2 (2005): 182–191.

26 Ibid., 184.

27 Ibid., 185.

28 Ibid., 186.

29 Ibid., 187.

30 Ibid., 188.

31 Ibid., 189.

32 Ibid., 190.

33 Ibid., 191.

34 Ibid., 191.

35 Eric J. Cassell, "Practice Versus Theory in Academic Medicine: The Conflict Between House Officers and Attending Physicians," *Bulletin of the New York Academy of Medicine* 60, no. 3 (1984): 297–308.

36 Perri Klass, "The Patient Narrative," in *Becoming a Doctor: From Student to Specialist, Doctor-Writers Share Their Experiences*, ed. Lee Gutkind (New York: W. W. Norton, 2010), 47.

37 Ibid., 46–47.

38 Ibid., 44.

39 Ibid., 45.

40 Suzanne Poirier, "Conclusion," in *Doctors in the Making: Memoirs and Medical Education* (Iowa City: University of Iowa Press, 2009). See also Jack Coulehan, "Compassionate Solidarity: Suffering, Poetry, and Medicine, *Perspectives in Biology and Medicine* 52, no. 4 (2009): 585–603; Neeta Jain, Dagan Coppock, and Stephanie Brown Clark, eds., *Body Language: Poems from the Medical Training Experience* (Rochester, NY: BOA Editions, Ltd., 2006); and Daniel Ofri, *What Doctors Feel: How Emotions Affect the Practice of Medicine* (Boston: Beacon Press, 2013).

41 Kenneth M. Ludmerer, *Time to Heal* (New York: Oxford University Press, 1999), ch. 18.

42 Paul Haidet and Howard F. Stein, "The Role of the Student-Teacher Relationship in the Formation of Physicians," *Journal of General Internal Medicine* 21 (2006): S16-S20; Suzanne Poirier, "Relationships," *Doctors in the Making: Memoirs and Medical Education* (Iowa City: University of Iowa Press, 2009), ch. 5.

43 Quoted by Sherwin Nuland in "The Uncertain Art: The True Healers," *American Scholar* 68 (1999): 125–128. See David J. Doukas, Laurence B. McCullough, and Stephen Wear,

"Reforming Medical Education in Ethics and Humanities by Finding Common Ground with Abraham Flexner," *Academic Medicine* 85, no. 2 (2010): 318–323. Also pertinent is Johanna Shapiro, Jack Coulehan, Delease Wear, and Martha Montello, "Medical Humanities and Their Discontents: Definitions, Critiques, and Implications," *Academic Medicine* 84, no. 2 (2009): 192–198.

PART III PHILOSOPHY AND MEDICINE

1 Edmund Pellegrino, "Apologia for a Medical Truant," in *The Philosophy of Medicine Reborn: A Pellegrino Reader*, eds. H. Tristram Engelhardt Jr. and Fabrice Jotterand (Notre Dame, IN: University of Notre Dame Press, 2008), xiv.
2 H. Tristram Engelhardt Jr. and Fabrice Jotterand, "An Introduction: Edmund D. Pellegrino's Project," in *The Philosophy of Medicine Reborn: A Pellegrino Reader*, eds. H. Tristram Engelhardt Jr. and Fabrice Jotterand (Notre Dame, IN: University of Notre Dame Press, 2008), 1.
3 Ibid., 2.

13 WAYS OF KNOWING

1 Stephen Toulmin, "The Marginal Relevance of Theory to the Humanities," *Common Knowledge* 2, no. 1 (1993): 79.
2 On "the clinical core of medical work," see Erik H. Erikson, "The Nature of Clinical Evidence," in *Evidence and Inference: The Hayden Colloquium on Scientific Concept and Method*, ed. Daniel Lerner (Chicago: The Free Press, 1959), 73–95.
3 On "intersubjectivity" see Charles Taylor, "Interpretation and the Sciences of Man," in *Philosophy and the Human Sciences* (Cambridge: Cambridge University Press, 1985), 15–37. This article was originally published in 1971.
4 Stephen Toulmin, *Cosmopolis: The Hidden Agenda of Modernity* (Chicago: The Free Press, 1990).
5 For recent critiques of Cartesianism, see Alasdair MacIntyre, "Epistemological Crises, Dramatic Narrative, and The Philosophy of Science," *The Monist* 60 (1977): 453–472; Richard Rorty, *Philosophy and the Mirror of Nature* (Princeton, NJ: Princeton University Press, 1979); and Charles Taylor, "Overcoming Epistemology," in *Philosophical Arguments* (Cambridge, MA: Harvard University Press, 1995), 1–19.
6 Isaiah Berlin, "A Note on Vico's Concept of Knowledge," in *Giambattista Vico: An International Symposium*, eds. Giorgio Tagliacozzo and Hayden V. White (Baltimore, MD: Johns Hopkins University Press, 1969), 375.
7 See Charles Taylor, "Theories of Meaning," in *Language and Human Agency* (Cambridge: Cambridge University Press, 1985), 248–292 (originally published in 1980); and "The Dialogical Self," in *The Interpretive Turn: Philosophy, Science, Culture*, eds. David R. Hiley, James F. Bohman, and Richard Shusterman (New York: Cornell University Press, 1991), 304–313. See also Richard J. Bernstein, *Beyond Objectivism and Relativism: Science, Hermeneutics, and Praxis* (Philadelphia: University of Pennsylvania Press, 1983), especially part three.
8 Kathryn Montgomery, *How Doctors Think: Clinical Judgment and the Practice of Medicine* (New York: Oxford University Press, 2006), 5–6; see also ch. 2.
9 Kathryn Montgomery Hunter, *Doctors' Stories: The Narrative Structure of Medical Knowledge* (Princeton, NJ: Princeton University Press, 1991), passim.
10 Ellen Singer More, "'Empathy' Enters the Profession of Medicine," in *The Empathic Practitioner: Empathy, Gender, and Medicine*, eds. Ellen S. More and Maureen A. Milligan (New Brunswick, NJ: Rutgers University Press, 1994), 19–39.

11 Isaiah Berlin, *The Sense of Reality: Studies of Ideas and their History* (New York: Farrar, Straus and Giroux, 1996), 23–24.

12 Isaiah Berlin, "The Concept of Scientific History," in *The Proper Study of Mankind* (New York: Farrar, Straus and Giroux, 1998), 52.

13 See Paul Ricoeur, "The Model of the Text: Meaningful Action Considered as a Text," *Social Research* 38 (1971): 529–562; also, Clifford Geertz, "Blurred Genres: The Reconfiguration of Social Thought," in *Local Knowledge: Further Essays in Interpretive Anthropology* (New York: Basic Books, 1983), 19–35.

14 Terry Pringle, *This is the Child* (New York: Alfred A. Knopf, 1983).

15 Ibid., 69.

16 Ibid., 77.

17 Ibid., 136.

18 Ibid., 96.

19 Ibid., 136.

20 Ibid., 177.

21 Martin Buber, "What Is Man?" in *Between Man and Man* (London and Glasgow: The Fontana Library, 1961). This essay was originally published in 1938.

22 Nancy Streuver, *Theory and Practice: Ethical Inquiry in the Renaissance* (Chicago: University of Chicago Press, 1992), 22–23.

23 Richard Weinberg, "Communion," in *On Being a Doctor 2: Voices of Physicians and Patients*, ed. Michael A. LaCombe (Philadelphia: American College of Physicians, 2000), 96–107.

24 Ibid., 96.

25 Ibid., 97.

26 Ibid.

27 Ibid., 98.

28 Ibid., 100.

14 GOALS OF MEDICINE

1 Eric J. Cassell, *The Nature of Suffering and the Goals of Medicine* (New York: Oxford University Press, 2004).

2 Robert Martensen, *A Life Worth Living: A Doctor's Reflections on Illness in a High-Tech Era* (New York: Farrar, Straus and Giroux, 2008), 54–55. See also Arnold Relman, "The New Medical Industrial Complex," *New England Journal of Medicine* 303, no. 17 (1980): 963–970.

3 Martensen, *A Life Worth Living*, xiii.

4 See Robert M. Veatch, "The Impossibility of a Morality Internal to Medicine," *Journal of Medicine and Philosophy* 21, no. 6 (2001): 621–642. This issue of the journal is entirely devoted to discussions of essentialist conceptions of medicine.

5 For example, Edmund D. Pellegrino argues that the proper ends of medicine are derivable "from the concrete realities of the physician-patient relationship .... Moreover, medicine exists because humans become sick. It is an activity conceived to attain the overall end of coping with the individual and social experience of disordered health. Its end is to heal, help, care and cure, to prevent illness, and cultivate health .... The ends of medicine are related to the reasons humans established medicine – that is, as a response to a universal and common experience of illness." See Edmund D. Pellegrino, "The Goals and Ends of Medicine: How Are They to be Defined?" in *The Goals of Medicine: The Forgotten Issues in Health Care Reform*, eds. Mark J. Hanson and Daniel Callahan (Washington, DC: Georgetown University Press, 1999), 58, 62–63; see also Edmund D. Pellegrino and David C. Thomasma, *A Philosophical Basis of Medical Practice: Toward a Philosophy and Ethic of the Healing Professions* (New York: Oxford University Press, 1981), especially ch. 3. Christopher Boorse critically appraises essentialist conceptions of clinical medicine in an unpublished paper titled "Goals of Medicine," August 2012 (draft only – not for quotation), available at www.philosophie.unihamburg.de/Schramme/.

6 Hanson and Callahan, eds., *The Goals of Medicine*, 16–17.

7 See chapters 5 and 15 in Hanson and Callahan, eds., *The Goals of Medicine*.

8 See chapter 23 in ibid.

9 Kathleen M. Foley, "The Treatment of Cancer Pain," in *Palliative Care: Transforming the Care of Serious Illness*, eds. Diane E. Meier, Stephen L. Isaacs, and Robert G. Hughes (San Francisco: Jossey-Bass, 2009), 251–275; also, Joanne Lynn, Joan Harrold, and Janice Lynn Shuster, "Controlling Pain," *Handbook for Mortals: Guidance for People Facing Serious Illness*, rev. ed. (New York: Oxford University Press, 2011), 71–84.

10 See Warren Thomas Reich, "History of the Notion of Care," Historical Dimensions of an Ethic of Care in Health Care," and (with Nancy S. Jecker) "Contemporary Ethics of Care," *Encyclopedia of Bioethics*, ed. Stephen G. Post (New York: Macmillan Reference, 2003), 349–374.

11 Carl Elliott, "The Tyranny of Happiness: Ethics and Cosmetic Pharmacology," in *Enhancing Human Traits: Ethical and Social Implications*, ed. Erik Parens (Washington, DC: Georgetown University Press, 1998), 177–188; also, Carl Elliott and Tod Chambers, eds., *Prozac as a Way of Life* (Chapel Hill: University of North Carolina Press, 2004).

12 See Lauren Slater, "Dr. Daedalus: A Radical Plastic Surgeon Wants to Give You Wings," *Harper's Magazine* (July 2001): 57–67.

13 Wendy Doniger, "The Mythology of the Face-Lift," *Social Research* 67, no.1 (2000): 99–125.

14 As a result of aggressive marketing by self-styled "gender experts," online and elsewhere, prenatal sex selection has become a multimillion dollar industry. See Dr. Daniel Potter's personal website, as well as the websites of clinics promoting prenatal sex selection, such as in-gender.com, genderselection.com, gender-selection.com, gender-select.com, genderselectioncenter.com, among others.

15 See Alisa Von Hagel, "Banking on Infertility," *Hastings Center Report* 43, no. 5 (2013): 1–17.

16 Juengst, "What Does Enhancement Mean?" 29–47.

17 Michael J. Sandel, *The Case Against Perfection: Ethics in the Age of Genetic Engineering* (Cambridge, MA: Belknap/Harvard University Press, 2007), 83. See also Thomas H. Murray, *The Worth of the Child* (Berkeley: University of California, 1996), especially 115–147.

18 Hanson and Callahan, eds., *The Goals of Medicine*, 29.

19 A significant indicator of how widespread public interest in the Quinlan case was at the time is David Rothman's observation about press coverage of the case: "the only cases more prominent were the Supreme Court decisions in *Brown v. the Board of Education* and *Roe v. Wade*." See David J. Rothman, *Strangers at the Bedside: A History of How Law and Bioethics Transformed Medical Decision Making* (New York: Basic Books, 1991), 232.

20 United States Senate, 1978. Congressional Hearings.

21 Albert R. Jonsen, *The Birth of Bioethics* (New York: Oxford University Press, 1998), 113.

22 Tom L. Beauchamp and James F. Childress, *Principles of Biomedical Ethics* (New York: Oxford University Press, 1979); also, see chapter 16 of this volume.

23 See, for example, David Barnard, "The Promise of Intimacy and the Fear of Our Own Undoing," *Journal of Palliative Care* 11, no. 4 (1995): 22–26; David H. Smith, ed., *Caring Well: Religion, Narrative, and Health Care Ethics* (Louisville, KY: Westminster John Knox Press, 2000); Cynthia B. Cohen, "Religious, Spiritual, and Ideological Perspectives on Ethics at the End of Life," in *Ethical Dilemmas at the End of Life*, eds. Kenneth J. Doka, Bruce Jennings, and Charles A. Corr (Washington, DC: Hospice Foundation of America, 2005), 19–40; Daniel P. Sulmasy, "Spiritual Issues in the Care of Dying Patients," *Journal of the American Medical Association* 96, no. 11 (2006): 1385–1392.

24 Daniel Callahan, *The Troubled Dream of Life: Living with Mortality* (New York: Simon & Schuster, 1993).

25 Ibid., 15.

26 Ibid., 126.

27 Paul Ramsey, *The Patient as Person* (New Haven, CT: Yale University Press, 1970), 116.

28 Ibid., 133.

29 Ibid., 133.

30 Ibid., 134. Also see Judith Graham, "When the Doctor Disappears," *New York Times*, November 14, 2013: http://newoldage.blogs.nytimes.com/2013/11/14/when-the-doctor-disappears/?_r=0.

31 C. Saunders, D. H. Summers, N. Teller, *Hospice: The Living Idea* (London: Edward Arnold Publishing, 1981).

32 The dean of the school of nursing at Yale University, Florence Wald, and her colleagues established the first American hospice, the Connecticut Hospice Institute, in 1974.

33 See Carol Levine, "Goldilocks and the Three Hospice Patients," *Bioethics Forum: Diverse Commentary on Issues in Bioethics*, Hastings Center, February 19, 2013.

34 Joan M. Teno and Joanne Lynn, "Putting Advance-Care Planning into Action," *The Journal of Clinical Ethics* 7, no. 3, (1996): 205–206; also Joanne Lynn, "Serving Patients Who May Die Soon: The Role of Hospice and Other Services," *Journal of the American Medical Association* 285, no. 7 (2001): 925–932.

35 J. Andrew Billings, "What Is Palliative Care?" *Journal of Palliative Medicine* 1, no. 1, (1998): 73–81; Diane E. Meier, R. Sean Morrison, and Christine K. Cassel, "Improving Palliative Care," *Annals of Internal Medicine* 127, no. 3 (1997): 225–230. For a comprehensive overview of the evolution and current state of palliative care, see, Diane E. Meier, Stephen Issacs, and Robert Hughes, eds., *Palliative Care: Transforming the Care of Serious Illness* (San Francisco: Jossey-Bass, 2009).

36 The SUPPORT Principal Investigators, "A Controlled Trial to Improve Care for Seriously Ill Hospitalized Patients," *Journal of the American Medical Association* 274, no. 20 (1995): 1511–1598.

37 Marilyn J. Field and Christine J. Cassel, eds., *Approaching Death: Improving Care at the End of Life* (Washington, DC: National Academy Press, 1997).

38 Donald M. Phillips, "JCAHO Pain Management Standards Are Unveiled," *Journal of the American Medical Association* 284, no. 4 (2000): 428–429.

39 Lynn, Harrold and Schuster, eds., *Handbook for Mortals*; Nancy Berlinger, Bruce Jennings, and Susan M. Wolf, eds., *Hastings Center Guidelines for Decisions on Life-Sustaining Treatment and Care Near the End of Life* (New York: Oxford University Press, 2013).

40 See www.thirteen.org/onourownterms.

41 See, for example, Ezekiel Emanuel, Linda Emanuel, Steven Weiss, and Diane Fairclough, "Understanding the Experience of Pain in Terminally Ill Patients," *The Lancet* 357 (2001): 1311–1315, one of a series of eight papers emanating from the Project on the End of Life commissioned by The Commonwealth Fund and the Nathan Cummings Foundation.

15 HEALTH AND DISEASE

1 René Descartes, *Discourse on the Method*, trans. Donald A Cress (Indianapolis: Hackett Publishing, 1998), 18.

2 Christopher Boorse, "Health as a Theoretical Concept," in *Philosophy of Science* 44 (1977): 542.

3 "Constitution of the of the World Health Organization," in *Concepts of Health and Disease: Interdisciplinary Perspectives*, eds. Arthur L. Caplan, H. Tristram Engelhardt, Jr., and James J. McCartney (Reading, PA: Addison-Wesley Publishing Company, 1981), 83.

4 Quoted in David Morris, *Illness and Culture in the Postmodern Age* (Berkeley: University of California Press, 1998), 52.

5 "Preamble to the Constitution of the World Health Organization," in *Concepts of Health and Disease: Interdisciplinary Perspectives*, eds. Arthur Caplan, Tristram Englehardt, Jr., and James McCartney (Reading, PA: Addison-Wesley, 1981).

6 AAMC, *Report* (1999), 3.

7 "What is Health? The Ability to Adapt," *The Lancet* 373 (2009): 781.

8 Daniel Callahan, *The Tyranny of Survival, and Other Pathologies of Life* (New York: Macmillan, 1973).

9 Edmund Pellegrino, "Being Ill and Being Healed: Some Reflections on the Grounding of Medical Morality," in *The Humanity of the Ill: Phenomenological Perspectives*, ed. Victor Kestenbaum (Knoxville: University of Tennessee Press), 157–166.

10 See Howard Brody, *Stories of Sickness* (Oxford: Oxford University Press, 1987); and Eric Cassell, *The Healer's Art* (Cambridge, MA: MIT Press, 1976).

11 Eric Cassell, *The Nature of Suffering and the Goals of Medicine* (New York: Oxford University Press, 1991).

12 Georges Canguilhem, *On the Normal and the Pathological*, trans. Carolyn Fawcett (Boston: D. Reidel Publishing Company, 1978).

13 "What is Health?" 781.

14 Quoted in Jonathan Metzl, "Introduction," in *Against Health: How Health Became the New Morality*, ed. Jonathan Metzl (New York: New York University Press, 2010), 5.

15 Leon Kass, "Regarding The End of Medicine and the Pursuit of Health," in *Concepts of Health and Disease: Interdisciplinary Perspectives*, eds. Arthur L. Caplan, H. Tristram Engelhardt, Jr., and James J. McCartney (Reading, PA: Addison-Wesley Publishing Company, 1981), 4.

16 Metzl, *Against Health*, 1–2.

17 Ibid., 4.

18 Christopher Boorse, "On the Distinction between Disease and Illness," in *Concepts of Health and Disease: Interdisciplinary Perspectives*, eds. Arthur L. Caplan, H. Tristram Engelhardt Jr., and James J. McCartney (Reading, PA: Addison-Wesley Publishing Company, 1981), 550.

19 Christopher Boorse, "A Rebuttal on Health," in *What is Disease?* eds. James M. Humber and Robert F. Almeder (Totowa, NJ: Humana Press, 1997), 1–135.

20 Boorse, "Health as a Theoretical Concept," 546.

21 Ibid., 559.

22 Boorse, "On the Distinction between Disease and Illness," 550.

23 See H. Tristram Englehardt, Jr., "The Concepts of Health and Disease," in *Concepts of Health and Disease: Interdisciplinary Perspectives*, eds. Arthur L. Caplan, H. Tristram Engelhardt, Jr., and James J. McCartney (Reading, PA: Addison-Wesley Publishing Company, 1981), 31–47; and Scott Devito, "On the Value-Neutrality of the Concepts of Health and Disease: Unto the Breach Again," *Journal of Medical Philosophy* 25, no. 5 (2000): 539–567.

24 Englehardt, Jr., "Concepts of Disease," 33.

25 Ibid.

26 Samuel Cartwright, "Report on the Diseases and Physical Peculiarities of the Negro Race," *New Orleans Medical and Surgical Review* 7 (1851): 691–715.

27 Jonathan Metzl, *The Protest Psychosis* (Boston: Beacon Press, 2010).

28 British Medical Association, *Medicine Betrayed: The Participation of Doctors in Human Rights Abuses* (London: Zed Books, 1992), 65.

29 Stephen Post, *The Encyclopedia of Bioethics*, 2nd ed. (New York: MacMillan, 2004), 1079.

30 Quoted in R. E. Kendell, "The Concept of Disease and its Implications for Psychiatry," in *Concepts of Health and Disease: Interdisciplinary Perspectives*, eds. Arthur L. Caplan, H. Tristram Engelhardt, Jr., and James J. McCartney (Reading, PA: Addison-Wesley Publishing Company, 1981), 445.

31 Thomas Szasz, *The Myth of Mental Illness: Foundations of a Theory of Personal Conduct* (New York: Harper & Row, 1974).

32 Kirsten Weir, "The Roots of Mental Illness," *Monitor on Psychology* 43, no. 6 (June 2012): 30.

33 American Psychiatric Association, *Diagnostic and Statistical Manual of Mental Disorders*, 4th ed., text revision (Washington: American Psychiatric Association, 2000), xxx.

34 Kay Jamison, *An Unquiet Mind* (New York: A. A. Knopf, 1995), 6.

35 Kay Jamison, *Touched with Fire: Manic-Depressive Illness and the Artistic Temperament* (New York: The Free Press, 1993).

36 Fyodor Dostoevsky, *The Idiot*, trans. Constance Garnett (New York: Barnes and Noble, 2004), 207–208.
37 Quoted in John Clay, *R. D. Laing: A Divided Self* (London: Hodder and Stoughton, 1997).
38 Leon Eisenberg, "Disease and Illness: Distinctions between Professional and Popular Ideas of Sickness," *Culture, Medicine, and Psychiatry* 1 (1977): 11.
39 George L. Engel, "The Need for a New Medical Model: A Challenge for Biomedicine," in *Health, Disease, and Illness: Concepts in Medicine*, eds. Arthur Leonard Caplan, James J. McCartney, and Dominic A. Sisti (Washington, DC: Georgetown University Press, 2004), 51.
40 Rita Charon, *Narrative Medicine: Honoring the Stories of Illness* (New York: Oxford University Press, 2008).
41 Howard Brody, "'My Story Is Broken, Can You Help Me Fix It?' Medical Ethics and the Joint Construction of Narrative," *Literature and Medicine* 13 (1994): 79–92.

16 MORAL PHILOSOPHY AND BIOETHICS

1 Carl Elliott, *A Philosophical Disease: Bioethics, Culture, and Identity* (New York: Routledge, 1999), xxvi.
2 Shana Alexander, "They Decide Who Lives, Who Dies," *LIFE* 53 (1962): 102–125.
3 Ibid., 108. The passage is in Alexander's own words.
4 Ibid., 110.
5 Henry K. Beecher, "Ethics and Clinical Research," *New England Journal of Medicine* 274 (1966): 1354–1360. See also David J. Rothman, *Strangers at the Bedside: A History of How Law and Bioethics Transformed Medical Decision Making* (New York: Basic Books, 1991), 70–84.
6 Rothman, *Strangers at the Bedside*, 190–203; Raymond S. Duff and A. G. M. Campbell, "Moral and Ethical Dilemmas in the Special-Care Nursery, *New England Journal of Medicine* 289 (1973): 890–894; Richard A. McCormick, "To Save or Let Die: The Dilemma of Modern Medicine," *Journal of the American Medical Association* 229 (1974): 172–176.
7 James H. Jones, *Bad Blood: The Tuskegee Syphilis Experiment*, 2nd ed. (New York: The Free Press, 1993).
8 *The Belmont Report: Ethical Principles and Guidelines for the Protection of Human Subjects of Research* (Washington, DC: Government Printing Office, 1979): http://www.hhs.gov/ohrp/humansubjects/guidance/belmont.html.
    Subsequent related federal commissions and committees and their publications are:

  • President's Commission for the Study of Ethical Problems in Medicine and Biomedical and Behavioral Research (1978–1983), *Defining Death, Splicing Life, The Social and Ethical issues of Genetic Engineering with Human Beings, Deciding to Forego Life-Sustaining Treatment, Screening and Counseling for Genetic Conditions, Securing Access to Health Care, Making Health Care Decisions*;
  • Biomedical Ethical Advisory Committee (1988–1990);
  • Advisory Committee on Human Radiation Experiments (1994–1995);
  • National Bioethics Advisory Commission (1996–2001), *Cloning Human Beings, Ethical Issues in Human Stem Cell Research, Ethics and Policy Issues in Research involving Human Participants, Research Involving Persons with Mental Disorders That May Affect Decision-making Capacity, Research Involving Human Biological Materials: Ethics Issue and Policy Guidance, Ethical and Policy Issues in International Research: Clinical Trials in Developing Countries*;
  • President's Council on Bioethics (2001–2009), *Human Cloning and Human Dignity, Beyond Therapy: Biotechnology and the Pursuit of Happiness, Being Human: Readings from the President's Council on Bioethics, Monitoring Stem Cell Research, Reproduction and Responsibility: The Regulation of New Biotechnologies, White Paper: Alternative Sources of Human Pluripotent Stem Cells, Taking Care: Ethical Caregiving in Our Aging Society,*

Human Dignity and Bioethics Essays Commissioned by the President's Council on Bioethics, The Changing Moral Focus of Newborn Screening: An Ethical Analysis by the President's Council on Bioethics, Controversies in the Determination of Death: A White Paper by the President's Council on Bioethics; and

- Presidential Commission for the Study of Bioethical Issues (2010–).

9 Albert R. Jonsen, *The Birth of Bioethics* (New York: Oxford University Press, 1998), 104.

10 Brand Blanchard, "The Philosophy of Analysis," *Proceedings of the British Academy* 38 (1952): 39–60; Richard J. Bernstein, "The Concept of Action: Analytic Philosophy," in *Praxis and Action: Contemporary Philosophies of Human Activity* (Philadelphia: University of Pennsylvania Press, 1971), 230–304; Alasdair MacIntyre, *A Short History of Ethics: A History of Moral Philosophy from the Homeric Age to the Twentieth Century*, 2nd ed. (London: Routledge, 1998); Mary Warnock, *Ethics Since 1900* (Mount Jackson, VA: Axios Press, 2007).

11 Richard Rorty, "Philosophy in America Today," *The American Scholar* 51, no. 2 (1982): 183–200; Richard Rorty, "Analytic and Conversational Philosophy," in *Philosophy as Cultural Politics* (Cambridge: Cambridge University Press, 2007), 120–130. Bernard Williams writes: "philosophy should get rid of scientistic illusions ... it should not try to behave like an extension of the natural sciences ... it should think of itself as part of a wider humanistic enterprise of making sense of ourselves and our activities." See Bernard Williams, *Philosophy as a Humanistic Discipline* (Princeton, NJ: Princeton University Press, 2006), 197.

12 Hans Jonas, "Technology and Responsibility: Reflections on the New Tasks of Ethics," *Social Research* 40 (1973): 38.

13 Ibid., 31.

14 Ibid., 46.

15 Ibid., 38.

16 Ibid, 50.

17 K. Danner Clouser, "Medical Ethics: Some Uses, Abuses, and Limitations," *New England Journal of Medicine* 293 (1978): 384–387.

18 Daniel Callahan, "Bioethics as a Discipline," *Hastings Center Report* 1 (1973): 66–73; regarding the origins of the term "bioethics," see Warren T. Reich, "The Word 'Bioethics': Its Birth and the Legacies of Those Who Shaped Its Meaning," *Kennedy Institute of Ethics Journal* 4 (1994): 319–336, and "The Word 'Bioethics': The Struggle Over Its Earliest Meanings," *Kennedy Institute of Ethics Journal* 5 (1995): 19–34.

19 Tom L. Beauchamp and James F. Childress, *Principles of Biomedical Ethics* (New York: Oxford University Press, 1979).

20 "W. D. Ross's distinction between *prima facie* and *actual* obligations is basic for our analysis. A *prima facie* obligation must be fulfilled unless it conflicts on a particular occasion with an equal or stronger obligation. This type of obligation is always binding *unless* a competing moral obligation overrides or outweighs it in a particular circumstance.... What agents ought to do is, in the end, determined by what they ought to do *all things considered.*" See ibid., vii.

21 Edmund D. Pincoffs had earlier argued that to reduce ethics to rule responsibility is to overlook elements of character which are central to moral life. See his "Quandary Ethics" (1971) reprinted in *Revisions: Changing Perspectives in Moral Philosophy*, eds. Stanley Hauerwas and Alasdair MacIntyre (Notre Dame, IN: University of Notre Dame Press, 1983), 92–112; see also John Ladd, "Legalism and Medical Ethics," *Journal of Medicine and Philosophy* 4 (1979): 70–80; and in a broader context, "Talk of rules [is] a euphemized form of legalism." See Pierre Bordieu, *Outline of a Theory of Practice* (Cambridge: Cambridge University Press, 1977), 17.

22 Stephen Toulmin, "The Tyranny of Principles," *Hastings Center Report* 11, no. 6 (1981): 31–39; Ronald A. Carson, "Interpretive Bioethics," *Theoretical Medicine* 11 (1990): 51–59; Andrew B. Lustig, "The Method of 'Principlism': A Critique of the Critique," *Journal of Medicine and Philosophy* 17 (1992), 487–510; James F. Childress, "Principles-Oriented Bioethics: An Analysis and Assessment from Within," in *A Matter of Principles? Ferment in U.S. Bioethics*, eds. Edmund R. DuBose, Ron Hamel, and Laurence J. O'Connell (Valley Forge, PA: Trinity Press International, 1994), 72–98; Larry Churchill, "Rejecting Principlism, Affirming Principles: A

Philosopher Reflects on the Ferment in U.S. Bioethics," in *A Matter of Principles? Ferment in U.S. Bioethics*, eds. Edmund R. DuBose, Ron Hamel, and Laurence J. O'Connell (Valley Forge, PA: Trinity Press International, 1994), 321–331; Richard A. McCormick, "Beyond Principlism Is Not Enough: A Theologian Reflects on the Real Challenge for U.S. Biomedical Ethics," in *A Matter of Principles? Ferment in U.S. Bioethics*, eds. Edmund R. DuBose, Ron Hamel, and Laurence J. O'Connell (Valley Forge, PA: Trinity Press International, 1994), 344–361; Tom L. Beauchamp, "The Role of Principles in Practical Ethics," in *Philosophical Perspectives in Bioethics*, eds. L. W. Sumner and Joseph Boyle (Toronto: University of Toronto Press, 1996), 79–95; Onora O'Neill, "Practical Principles and Practical Judgments," *Hastings Center Report* 31, no. 4 (2001): 15–23; Leigh Turner, "Zones of Consensus and Zones of Conflict: Questioning the 'Common Morality' Presumption in Bioethics," *Kennedy Institute of Ethics Journal* 13, no. 3 (2003), 193–218.

23 Robert M. Veatch, *A Theory of Medical Ethics* (New York: Basic Books, 1981); Robert M. Veatch, "Revisiting *A Theory of Medical Ethics*: Main Themes and Anticipated Changes," in *The Story of Bioethics: From Seminal Works to Contemporary Exploration*, eds. Jennifer K. Walter and Evan P. Klein (Washington, DC: Georgetown University Press, 2003), 67–89.

24 William F. May, "Code, Covenant, Contract or Philanthropy," *Hastings Center Report* 5, no. 6 (1975): 29–38; William F. May, "The Medical Covenant: An Ethics of Obligation or Virtue?" in *Theological Analyses of the Clinical Encounter* (Boston: Kluwer Academic Publishers, 1994), 29–44.

25 H. Tristram Engelhardt Jr., *The Foundations of Bioethics*, rev. 2nd ed. (New York: Oxford University Press, 1995), 40 and 382.

26 H. Tristram Engelhardt Jr., "Bioethics in Pluralist Societies," *Perspectives in Biology and Medicine* 26, no. 1 (1982): 70, 76; see also H. Tristram Engelhardt, Jr., "The Physician-Patient Relationship in a Secular, Pluralist Society," in *The Clinical Encounter*, ed. Earl E. Shelp (Dordrecht, Holland: D. Reidel Publishing Company, 1983), 256–266.

27 William F. May, *The Patient's Ordeal*, (Bloomington: Indiana University Press, 1991), 207.

28 Albert R. Jonsen, "Casuistry and Clinical Ethics," *Theoretical Medicine* 7 (1986): 65–74; Eric T. Juengst, "Casuistry and the Locus of Certainty in Ethics," *Medical Humanities Review* 3, no. 1 (1989): 19–27; John Arras, "Getting Down to Cases: The Revival of Casuistry in Bioethics," *Journal of Medicine and Philosophy* 16 (1991): 29–51; James F. Childress, "Ethical Theories, Principles, and Casuistry in Bioethics: An Interpretation and Defense of Principlism," in *Religious Methods and Resources in Bioethics*, ed. Paul F. Camenisch (Boston: Kluwer Academic Publishers, 1994), 181–201; Mark G. Kuczewski, "Casuistry and It Communitarian Critics," *Kennedy Institute of Ethics Journal* 4 (1994): 99–116; Albert R. Jonsen, "Casuistry: An Alternative or Complement to Principles?" *Kennedy Institute of Ethics Journal* 5, no. 3 (1995): 237–251; see also Albert R. Jonsen and Stephen Toulmin, *The Abuse of Casuistry: A History of Moral Reasoning* (Berkeley: University of California Press, 1988); Patricia Beattie Jung, a review of The Abuse of Casuistry, in *Religious Studies Review* 17, no. 4 (1991): 298–302; for a "theory of pluralistic casuistry, see Baruch Brody, *Life and Death Decision Making* (New York: Oxford University Press, 1988).

29 Sally Gadow, "Aging as Death Rehearsal: The Oppressiveness of Reason," *The Journal of Clinical Ethics* 7, no.1 (1996): 35–40; Susan Sherwin, "Feminist and Medical Ethics: Two Different Approaches to Contextual Ethics," in *Feminist Perspectives in Medical Ethics*, eds. Helen Bequaert Holmes and Laura M. Purdy (Bloomington: Indiana University Press, 1992), 18–31 (originally published in *Hypatia* 4, no. 2, Summer 1989); Susan Sherwin, *No Longer Patient: Feminist Ethics and Health Care* (Philadelphia: Temple University Press, 1992); Annette C. Baier, "Alternative Offerings to Asclepius?" *Medical Humanities Review* 6, no. 1 (1992): 9–19; Margaret Urban Walker, "Keeping Moral Space Open: New Images of Ethics Consultancy," *Hastings Center Report* 13, no. 2 (1993): 33–40; Sally Gadow, "Whose Body, Whose Story? The Question about Narrative in Women's Health Care," *Soundings* 73, nos. 3–4 (1994): 295–307; Susan Sherwin, "Feminism and Bioethics," in *Feminism and Bioethics: Beyond Reproduction*, ed. Susan M. Wolf (New York: Oxford University Press, 1996), 47–66; Rosemarie Tong, "Feminist

Approaches to Bioethics," in *Feminism and Bioethics: Beyond Reproduction*, ed. Susan M. Wolf (New York: Oxford University Press, 1996), 67–94; Annette C. Baier, "What Do Women Want in a Moral Theory?" in *Moral Prejudices: Essays in Ethics* (Cambridge, MA: Harvard University Press, 1994), 1–17, 313 [originally published in *Nous*, 19 (March 1985): 53–63].

30 Anne Hudson Jones, "Literary Value: The Lesson of Medical Ethics," *Neohelicon* 14 (1987): 383–392; Suzanne Poirier and Daniel J. Brauner, "Ethics and the Daily Language of Medical Discourse," *Hastings Center Report* 18, no. 4 (1988): 5–9; Anne Hudson Jones, "Literature and Medicine: Illness from the Patient's Point of View," in *Personal Choices and Public Commitments*, ed. William J. Winslade (Galveston, TX: Institute for the Medical Humanities, 1988), 1–15; Howard Brody, "'My Story is Broken: Can You Help Me Fix It?' Medical Ethics and the Joint Construction of Narrative," *Literature and Medicine* 3, no. 1 (1994): 79–92; Anne Hudson Jones, "Reading Patients – Cautions and Concerns," *Literature and Medicine* 13 (1994): 190–200; Anne Hudson Jones, "Darren's Case: Narrative Ethics in Perri Klass's *Other Women's Children*," *Journal of Medicine and Philosophy* 21, no. 3 (1996): 267–286; Anne Hudson Jones, "From Principles to Reflective Practice of Narrative Ethics, Commentary on Carson," in *Philosophy of Medicine and Bioethics: A Twenty Year Retrospective and Critical Appraisal*, eds. Ronald A. Carson and Chester R. Burns (Boston: Kluwer Academic Publishers, 1997), 193–195; Kathryn Montgomery Hunter, *Doctors' Stories: The Narrative Structure of Medical Knowledge* (Princeton, NJ: Princeton University Press, 1991); Tod Chambers, "From the Ethicist's Point of View: The Literary Nature of Ethical Inquiry," *Hastings Center Report* 26, no. 1 (1996): 25–32; Kathryn Montgomery Hunter, "Narrative, Literature, and the Clinical Exercise of Practical Reason," *Journal of Medicine and Philosophy* 21 (1996): 303–320; Kathryn Montgomery, "Medical Ethics: Literature, Literary Studies, and the Question of Interdisciplinarity," in *The Nature and Prospect of Bioethics*, eds. Franklin G. Miller, John C. Fletcher, and James F. Humber (Totowa, NJ: Humana Press, 2003), 141–178; Hilde Lindemann Nelson, ed., *Stories and Their Limits: Narrative Approaches to Bioethics* (London: Routledge, 1997); Rita Charon, "Narrative Contributions to Medical Ethics," in *A Matter of Principles? Ferment in U.S. Bioethics*, eds. Edwin B. DuBose, Ronald P. Hamel, and Laurence J. O'Connell (Valley Forge, PA: Trinity Press International, 1994), 260–283; Rita Charon and Martha Montello, eds., *Stories Matter: The Role of Narrative in Medical Ethics* (London: Routledge, 2002); Ronald A. Carson, "The Hyphenated Space: Liminality in the Doctor-Patient Relationship," in *A Matter of Principles? Ferment in U.S. Bioethics*, eds. Edwin B. DuBose, Ronald P. Hamel, and Laurence J. O'Connell (Valley Forge, PA: Trinity Press International, 1994), 171–182; Rita Charon, *Narrative Medicine: Honoring the Stories of Illness* (New York: Oxford University Press, 2006); Tod Chambers, "Retrodiction and the Histories of Bioethics, *Medical Humanities Review* 12, no. 1 (1998): 9–22.

31 Daniel Callahan, "Religion and the Secularization of Bioethics," *Hastings Center Report* 20, no. 4 (1990): 2–4; Courtney S. Campbell, "Religion and Moral Meaning in Bioethics, *Hastings Center Report* 20, no. 4 (1990): 4–10; William F. May, "The Medical Covenant: An Ethics of Obligation or Virtue?" in *Theological Analyses of the Clinical Encounter*, eds. Gerald F. McKinney and J. R. Sande (Boston: Kluwer Academic Publishers, 1994), 29–44; Courtney S. Campbell, "Bioethics and the Spirit of Secularism," in *Secular Bioethics in Theological Perspective*, ed. Earl E. Shelp (Boston: Kluwer Academic Publishers, 1996), 3–18; Courtney S. Campbell, "Principlism and Religion: The Law and the Prophets," in *A Matter of Principles? Ferment in U.S. Bioethics*, eds. Edwin R. DuBose, Ronald P. Hamel, and Laurence J. O'Connell (Valley Forge, PA: Trinity Press International, 1994), 182–208; Gilbert C. Meilaender, *Body, Soul, and Bioethics* (Notre Dame, IN: University of Notre Dame Press, 1995); Carla M. Messikomer, Renée C. Fox, and Judith P. Swazey, "The Presence and Influence of Religion in American Bioethics," *Perspectives in Biology and Medicine* 44, no. 4 (2001): 485–508; see also Chapter 22 of this textbook, "Religion and Bioethics."

32 George Weisz, ed., *Social Science Perspectives on Medical Ethics* (Boston: Kluwer Academic Publishers, 1990); Patricia A. Marshall, "Anthropology and Bioethics," *Medical Anthropology Quarterly* 6 (1992): 49–73; Barry Hoffmaster, "Can Ethnography Save the Life of Bioethics?"

Social Science and Medicine 35 (1992): 1421–1431; Renee C. Fox, "The Entry of U.S. Bioethics into the 1990s: A Sociological Analysis," *A Matter of Principles: Ferment in U.S. Bioethics*, eds. Edwin R. DuBose, Ron Hamel and Laurence J. O'Connell (Valley Forge, PA: Trinity Press International, 1994), 21–71; Arthur Kleinman, "Anthropology of Bioethics," in *Writing at the Margin: Discourse Between Anthropology and Medicine* (Berkeley: University of California Press, 1995); Daniel F. Chambliss, *Beyond Caring: Hospitals, Nurses, and the Social Organization of Ethics* (Chicago: University of Chicago Press, 1996); "Bioethics and Beyond," *Daedalus: Journal of the American Academy of Arts and Sciences* 128, no. 4, (1999): whole issue; "Quo Vadis? Mapping the Future of Bioethics," *Cambridge Quarterly of Healthcare Ethics* 14, no. 4 (2005): 361–433.

33 Earl E. Shelp, ed., *Beneficence and Health Care* (Dordrecht, NL: D. Reidel Publishing Company, 1982); Gilbert Meilaender, "The Virtues: A Theological Analysis," in *Virtue and Medicine: Explorations in the Character of Medicine*, ed. Earl E. Shelp (Dordrecht, Holland: D. Reidel Publishing Company, 1985), 151–171; Alasdair MacIntyre "The Nature of the Virtues," in *After Virtue: A Study in Moral Theory*, 2nd ed. (Notre Dame, IN: University of Notre Dame Press, 1984), 181–203; Edmund D. Pellegrino and David C. Thomasma, *For the Patient's Good: The Restoration of Beneficence in Health Care* (New York: Oxford University Press, 1988); Susan S. Phillips and Patricia Benner, eds., *The Crisis of Care: Affirming and Restoring Caring Practices in the Helping Professions* (Washington, DC: Georgetown University Press, 1994); Margaret Olivia Little and Robert M. Veatch, issue eds., "The Chaos of Care and Care Theory," *Journal of Medicine and Philosophy* 23, no. 2, (1998); Ruth Groenhout, "The Virtue of Care: Aristotelian Ethics and Contemporary Ethics of Care," in *Feminist Interpretations of Aristotle*, ed. Cynthia A. Freeland (State College: Pennsylvania State University Press, 1998), 171–200; Judith Andre, *Bioethics as Practice* (Chapel Hill: University of North Carolina Press, 2002). See also Philippa Foot, "Virtues and Vices," in *Virtues and Vices and Other Essays in Moral Philosophy* (Berkeley: University of California Press, 1978), 1–18; Ellen S. More, "Empathy as a Hermeneutic Practice," *Medical Humanities Review* 17 (1996): 243–254.

34 Stephen Toulmin, "How Medicine Saved the Life of Ethics," *Perspectives in Biology and Medicine* 5, no. 2 (1991): 9–18.

35 In his memoir, *In Search of the Good: A Life in Bioethics*, Daniel Callahan laments the evident drift away from broad-gauged inquiry into the purposes of science and medicine that animated the pioneers of the bioethics movement.

17 MEDICINE AND POWER

1 Michel Foucault, *The History of Sexuality*, trans., Robert Hurley, vol. 1 (New York: Vintage Books, 1990), 94.

2 Anthony T. Lo Sasso, Michael R. Richards, Chiu-Fang Chou, and Susan E. Gerber, "The $16,819 Pay Gap for Newly Trained Physicians: The Unexplained Trend of Men Earning More than Women," *Health Affairs* 30 (2011): 193–201.

3 Amartya Sen, "More Than 100 Million Women Are Missing," *The New York Review of Books*, December 20, 1990, http://www.nybooks.com/articles/archives/1990/dec/20/more-than-100-million-women-are-missing/?page=1.

4 The Center for Disease Control, "Deaths: Preliminary Data for 2011," *National Vital Statistics Reports* 61/6 (2012): 3.

5 U.S. Census Bureau, "World Population by Age and Sex for 2012," *International Data Base*, http://www.census.gov/cgi-bin/broker.

6 See, for example, Siwan Anderson and Debraj Ray, "Missing Women: Age and Disease," *The Review of Economic Studies* 77 (2010): 1262–1300.

7 Michel Foucault, *The Birth of the Clinic: An Archaeology of Medical Perception*, trans. A. M. Sheridan Smith (New York: Pantheon Books, 1973).

8 Michel Foucault, *Madness and Civilization: A History of Insanity in the Age of Reason*, trans. Richard Howard (New York: Vintage Books, 1973).

9 Paul Rabinow, "Introduction," in *The Foucault Reader*, ed. Paul Rabinow (New York: Pantheon Books, 1984), 3–29.

10 Ibid., 10.

11 Edward Said, *Orientalism* (New York: Pantheon Books, 1978).

12 Joan Brumberg, *The Body Project: An Intimate History of American Girls* (New York: Vintage Books, 1997).

13 Anne Fausto-Sterling, "The Five Sexes, Revisited," *Sciences* 40 (2000): 18–23.

14 Joel Frader, Priscilla Alderson, Adrienne Asch, Cassandra Aspinall, Dena Davis, Alice Dreger, James Edwards, Ellen Feder, Arthur Frank, Lisa Hedley, Eva Kittay, Jeffrey Marsh, Paul Miller, Wendy Mouradian, Hilde Nelson, and Erik Parens, "Health Care Professionals and Intersex Conditions," *JAMA Pediatrics* 158 (2004): 426–428.

15 See the Intersex Society of North America's website: http://www.isna.org/faq/what_is_intersex.

16 The summary of this case is taken from Susannah Cornwall, *Sex and Uncertainty in the Body of Christ: Insersex Conditions and Christian Theology* (London: Equinox, 2010), 35–41.

17 Margalit Fox, "Mary Daly, a Leader in Feminist Theology, Dies at 81," *The New York Times*, January 6, 2010, accessed June 25, 2013: http://www.nytimes.com/2010/01/07/education/07daly.html?hpw.

18 Mary Daly, *Gyn/Ecology: The Metaethics of Radical Feminism*, with a New Intergalactic Introduction by the Author (Boston: Beacon Press, 1990).

19 See Loretta Kopelman, "Medicine's Challenge to Relativism: The Case of Female Genital Mutilation," in *Philosophy of Medicine and Bioethics*, ed. Ronald Carson and Chester Burns (Dordrecht, NL: Kluwer Academic Publishers, 1997), 221–237.

20 Daly, *Gyn/Ecology*, 224.

21 Ibid.

22 Ibid.

23 Ibid., 244.

24 Ibid.

25 H. Gilbert Welch, "Screening Mammography – A Long Run for a Short Slide?" *NEJM* 363 (2010): 1276–1278.

26 See, for example, Harrison Pope Jr., Katharine Phillips, and Roberto Olivardia, *The Adonis Complex: The Secret Crisis of Male Body Obsession* (New York: The Free Press, 2000).

27 Daly, *Gyn/Ecology*, 233.

28 See, for example, Sabina Vaught and Angelina Castagno, "'I don't think I'm a racist': Critical Race Theory, Teacher Attitudes, and Structural Racism," *Race Ethnicity and Education* 11 (2008): 95–113.

29 U.S. Census Bureau, "Statistical Abstract of the United States: 2012," 131st Edition, Table 695: 455, Table 698: 457, Table 711: 465. Washington, DC, 2011, http://www.census.gov/compendia/statab/.

30 Quoted in Harriet Washington, *Medical Apartheid: The Dark History of Medical Experimentation on Black Americans from Colonial Times to the Present* (New York: Anchor Books, 2006), 347.

31 James Jones, *Bad Blood: The Tuskegee Syphilis Experiment* (New York: Free Press, 1981).

32 Eileen Welsome, *The Plutonium Files: America's Secret Medical Experiments in the Cold War* (New York: Dial Press, 1999).

33 Todd Savitt, *Medicine and Slavery: The Diseases of Health Care of Blacks in Antebellum Virginia* (Urbana: University of Illinois Press, 1978).

34 Allen Hornblum, *Acers of Skin: Human Experiments at Holmesburg Prison* (New York: Routledge, 1998).

35 Susan Reverby, *Examining Tuskegee: The Infamous Syphilis Study and Its Legacy* (Chapel Hill: University of North Carolina Press, 2009).

36 John Hoberman, *Black and Blue: The Origins and Consequences of Medical Racism* (Berkeley: University of California Press, 2012).

37 Ezekiel Emanuel, "Unequal Treatment," *The New York Times*, February 18, 2007: http://www.nytimes.com/2007/02/18/books/review/Emanuel.t.html.

38 Allan Brandt, "Racism and Research: The Case of the Tuskegee Syphilis Study," in *Ethical and Regulatory Aspects of Clinical Research: Readings and Commentary*, ed. Ezekiel Emanuel, Robert Crouch, John Arras, Jonathan Moreno, and Christine Grady (Baltimore, MD: The Johns Hopkins University Press, 2003), 20–21.

39 Ibid., 20.

40 Washington, *Medical Apartheid*, 157–185.

41 Brandt, "Racism and Research," 23.

42 On this point, see Kelly Brown Douglas, *Sexuality and the Black Church: A Womanist Perspective* (Maryknoll, NY: Orbis Books, 1999).

43 Washington, *Medical Apartheid*, 352–353.

44 See, for example, Emily Largent, David Wendler, Ezekiel Emanuel, and Franklin Miller, "Is Emergency Research without Initial Consent Justified?" *Archives of Internal Medicine* 170 (2010): 668–674.

45 S. Kay Toombs, *The Meaning of Illness: A Phenomenological Account of the Different Perspectives of Physician and Patient* (Dordrecht, NL: Kluwer Academic Publishers, 1992).

46 Havi Carel, *Illness: The Cry of the Flesh* (Stocksfield, UK: Acumen, 2008).

47 Fredrik Svenaeus, *The Hermeneutics of Medicine and the Phenomenology of Health: Steps Toward a Philosophy of Medical Practice* (Dordrecht, NL: Kluwer Academic Publishers, 2000).

18 JUST HEALTH CARE

1 Rashi Fein, "What's Wrong with the Language of Medicine," *New England Journal of Medicine* 306, no. 14 (1982): 864.

2 "Health Programme for the USA," *The Lancet* 253, no. 6557 (1949): 747–748.

3 Paul Starr, *Remedy and Reaction: The Peculiar American Struggle over Health Care Reform* (New Haven, CT: Yale University Press, 2011), 37–38.

4 Ibid., 39.

5 Among private organizations opposing the idea, the American Medical Association stands out. After Truman's surprise victory in the 1949 presidential contest, "the AMA thought Armageddon had come. It assessed each of its members an additional $25 just to resist health insurance and hired Whitaker and Baxter [a public relations firm] to mount a public campaign that cost $1.5 million in 1949, at that time the most expensive lobbying effort in American history." See Paul Starr, *The Social Transformation of American Medicine: The Rise of a Sovereign Profession and the Making of a Vast Industry* (New York: Basic Books, 1982), 284–285.

6 Ibid., 394.

7 Richard Nixon, "Statement on the Signing of the Health Maintenance Organization Act of 1973," December 29, 1973.

8 Starr, *Remedy and Reaction*, 63.

9 Starr, *Social Transformation*, 419.

10 Starr, *Remedy and Reaction*, 89. For a concise and accessible discussion of the theoretical underpinnings of the Clinton health plan, see Paul Starr, *The Logic of Health Care Reform*, rev. ed. (New York: Penguin Books, 1994).

11 Starr, *Remedy and Reaction*, 100.

12 What would reveal itself in retrospect as the one bright spot in Clinton's reform efforts was passage in 1997 of bipartisan legislation sponsored by Senators Edward Kennedy and Orrin Hatch establishing the State Children's Health Insurance Program (S-CHIP, later, simply CHIP)

that would later be reauthorized and expanded by Congress and signed into law by President Obama in 2009, following two vetoes by President George W. Bush.

13 Starr, *Remedy and Reaction*, 122–12.

14 Stephen M. Davidson, *A New Era in U.S. Health Care: Critical Next Steps Under the Affordable Care Act* (Stanford, CA: Stanford University Press, 2013).

15 For evidence of serious quality problems, see *State of Health Care Quality 2011*, National Committee for Health Care Quality, Washington, D.C., 2011.

16 David J. Rothman, "A Century of Failure: Health Care Reform in America," *Journal of Health Politics, Policy and Law* 18, no. 2 (1993): 273–274.

17 Deborah Stone, *The Samaritan's Dilemma: Should Government Help Your Neighbor?* (New York: Nation Books, 2008), 28.

18 Michael J. Sandel, *What Money Can't Buy: The Moral Limits of Markets* (New York: Farrar, Straus and Giroux, 2012), 6.

19 Ibid., 10–12.

20 Benjamin R. Barber, "Imperial Emporium," *Raritan: A Quarterly Review* 26, no. 3 (2007): 44–45. For an assessment of market influence on health care systems in both developed and developing countries, see Daniel Callahan and Angela A. Wasunna, *Medicine and the Market: Equity and Choice* (Baltimore, MD: Johns Hopkins University Press, 2006).

21 This idea is developed by Charles Taylor in *Philosophical Arguments* (Cambridge, MA: Harvard University Press, 1995), 127–145.

22 Michael Walzer, *Spheres of Justice: A Defense of Pluralism and Equality* (New York: Basic Books, 1983), 75. Also pertinent are Michael Walzer's book, *What It Means to Be an American* (New York: Marsilio Publishing Corp., 1992), a collection of thoughtful essays on citizenship in the American vein; and, on the concept of distributive justice, Michael Walzer, "Justice Here and Now," in *Justice and Equality Here and Now*, ed. Frank S. Lucash (New York: Cornell University Press, 1986), 136–150. For an insightful essay on the notion of needs, see Michael Ignatieff, *The Needs of Strangers: An Essay on Privacy, Solidarity, and the Politics of Being Human* (New York: Viking Penguin, 1985).

23 Howard H. Hiatt, "Protecting the Medical Commons: Who Is Responsible?" *New England Journal of Medicine* 293, no. 5 (1975): 235–241.

24 President's Commission for the Study of Ethical Problems in Medicine and Biomedical and Behavioral Research, *Securing Access to Health Care: The Ethical Implications of Differences in the Availability of Health Services* (Washington, D.C., 1983), 4. See also Richard Smith, Howard Hiatt, and Donald Berwick, "A Shared Statement of Ethical Principles for Those Who Shape and Give Health Care: A Working Draft from the Tavistock Group," *Annals of Internal Medicine* 130 (1999): 143–147.

25 For a concise overview of theoretically grounded arguments for a right to health care, see Allen Buchanan, "Justice: A Philosophical Overview," in *Justice and Health Care*, ed. Earl E. Shelp (Dordrecht: D. Reidel, 1981); a Roman Catholic perspective is discussed by B. Andrew Lustig in "The Common Good in 'Secular Society,'" *Journal of Medicine and Philosophy* 18 (1993): 569–583; on health equity and the social determinants of health, consult Norman Daniels, *Just Health: Meeting Health Needs Fairly* (Cambridge: Cambridge University Press, 2008); and Gopal Sreenivasan, "Health Care and Equality of Opportunity," with a commentary by Norman Daniels, *Hastings Center Report* 37, no. 2 (2007): 21–31 and 3, respectively. In a previous book, *Just Health Care*, Norman Daniels extended John Rawls's influential theory of justice to health care. See John Rawls, *Justice as Fairness* (Cambridge, MA: Harvard University Press, 1971).

26 See David Hume, *A Treatise of Human Nature* (1740), ed. L. A. Selby-Bigge and P. H. Nidditch (Oxford: Clarendon Press, 1978); and Annette Baier, *A Progress of Human Sentiments: Reflections on Hume's* Treatise (Cambridge, MA: Harvard University Press, 1991).

27 Larry R. Churchill, *Self-interest and Universal Health Care: Why Well-Insured Americans Should Support Coverage for Everyone* (Cambridge, MA: Harvard University Press, 1994), 51.

28 See Adam Smith, *The Theory of Moral Sentiments* (1759), eds., A. L. Macfie and D. D. Raphael (Indianapolis, IN: Liberty Press, 1982); Charles L. Griswold, Jr., *Adam Smith and the Virtues of the Enlightenment* (Cambridge: Cambridge University Press, 1999); and D. D. Raphael, *The Impartial Spectator: Adam Smith's Moral Philosophy* (New York: Oxford University Press, 2007).

29 See Larry R. Churchill, *Rationing Health Care in America: Perceptions and Principles of Justice* (Notre Dame, IN: Notre Dame University Press, 1987), especially ch. 4, "Principles of Justice: Rights and Needs," 70–103.

30 Churchill, *Self-Interest and Universal Health Care*, 15.

PART IV RELIGION AND MEDICINE

1 Stephen Pattison, "Absent Friends in Medical Humanities," *Medical Humanities* 33 (2007): 65–66.

2 See, e.g., Bonnie Miller-McLemore, "Thinking Theologically about Modern Medicine," *Journal of Religion and Health* 30 (1991): 287–298. Also see Nathan Carlin, "Bioethics and Pastoral Concern: Some Possible New Directions in Pastoral Theology," *Pastoral Psychology* 62 (2013): 129–138.

3 Daniel Callahan, "Religion and the Secularization of Bioethics," *The Hastings Center Report* 20 (1990): 2–4.

4 See, for example, Mark Cobb, Christinia Pulchaliski, and Bruce Rumbold, eds., *The Oxford Textbook of Spirituality in Healthcare* (Oxford: Oxford University Press, 2012).

5 Larry Churchill, "The Amoral Character of Our Attitudes about Death: Some Implications," *Journal of Religion and Health* 17 (1978): 169–176. Also see Larry Churchill, "The Human Experience of Dying: The Moral Primacy of Stories over Stages," *Soundings* 62 (1979): 24–37.

6 Leigh Turner, "Bioethics in Pluralistic Societies," *Medicine, Health Care and Philosophy* 7 (2004): 201–208.

7 Courtney Campbell, "Religion and Moral Meanings in Bioethics," *The Hastings Center Report*, 20 (1990): 4–10.

8 Gilbert Meilaender, "On Removing Food and Water: Against the Stream," *The Hastings Center Report* 14 (1984): 11–13.

9 Laurie Zoloth, "Yearning for the Long Lost Home: The Lemba and the Jewish Narrative of Genetic Return," *Developing World Bioethics* 3 (2003): 127–132.

10 B. Andrew Lustig, "Suffering, Sovereignty, and the Purposes of God: Christian Convictions and Medical Killing," *Christian Bioethics* 1 (1995): 249–255.

11 Daniel Sulmasy, "A Biopsychosocial-Spiritual Model for the Care of Patients at the End of Life," *The Gerontologist* 42 (2002): 24–33.

12 Paul Ramsey, *The Patient as Person: Explorations in Medical Ethics* (New Haven, CT: Yale University Press, 1970).

13 Richard McCormick, "Theology and Bioethics," in *On Moral Medicine: Theological Perspectives in Medical Ethics*, 2nd ed., eds. Stephen Lammers and Allen Verhey (Grand Rapids, MI: William B. Eerdmans Publishing Company), 63–71.

14 William May, "The Virtues in a Professional Setting," *Soundings* 67 (1984): 245–266.

15 David Smith, *Partnership with the Dying: Where Medicine and Ministry Should Meet* (New York: Rowman and Littlefield Publishers, Inc., 2005).

16 Albert Jonsen, "Beating Up Bioethics," *The Hastings Center Report* 31 (2001): 40–45.

17 Verlyn Barker, *Health and Human Values: A Ministry of Theological Inquiry and Moral Discourse* (United Ministries in Education, 1987).

18 Thomas McElhinney and Edmund Pellegrino, "The Institute on Human Values in Medicine: Its Role and Influence in the Conception and Evolution of Bioethics," *Theoretical Medicine* 22 (2001): 291–317.

19 Ronald Carson, "Focusing on the Human Scene: Thoughts on Problematic Theology," in *Notes from a Narrow Ridge: Religion and Bioethics*, eds. Dena Davis and Laurie Zoloth (Hagerstown, MD: University Publishing Group, 1999), 50.

20 Consider the following essay: Tod Chambers, "The Virtue of Incongruity in the Medical Humanities," *The Journal of Medical Humanities* 30 (2009): 151–154.

19 WORLD RELIGIONS FOR MEDICAL HUMANITIES

1 David Smith, "Introduction," in *Caring Well: Religion, Narrative, and Health Care Ethics*, ed. David Smith (Louisville, KY: Westminster John Knox Press, 2000), 13.

2 Daniel Sulmasy, *The Rebirth of the Clinic: An Introduction to Spirituality in Health Care* (Washington, DC: Georgetown University Press, 2006), 238.

3 See, for example, Nancy Waxler-Morrison, Joan Anderson, Elizabeth Richardson, and Natalie Cambers, eds., *Cross-Cultural Caring: A Handbook for Health Professionals*, 2nd ed. (Vancouver, BC: UBC Press, 2005); Larry Purnell, *Guide to Culturally Competent Health Care*, 2nd ed. (Philadelphia: F. A. Davis Company, 2009); Rachel Spector, *Cultural Diversity in Health and Illness*, 7th ed. (Upper Saddle River, NJ: Pearson/Prentice Hall, 2009).

4 Mark Furlong and James Wight, "Promoting 'Critical Awareness' and Critiquing 'Cultural Competence,': Towards Disrupting Received Professional Knowledges," *Australian Social Work* 64 (2011): 38–54.

5 For related issues in clinical ethics, see Jeffrey Spike, "When Ethics Consultation and Courts Collide: A Case of Compelled Treatment of a Mature Minor," *Narrative Inquiry in Bioethics* 1 (2011): 123–131.

6 See John Hoberman, *Black and Blue: The Origins and Consequences of Medical Racism* (Berkeley: University of California Press, 2012), 198–233.

7 Arthur Kleinman and Peter Benson, "Anthropology in the Clinic: The Problem of Cultural Competency and How to Fix It," *PLoS Medicine* 3 (2006): e294: doi:10.1371/journal.pmed.0030294.

8 See this blog by a medical student: Marianne DiNapoli, "When a Patient Just Won't Listen to You," timesunion.com, August 4, 2011: http://blog.timesunion.com/mdtobe/when-a-patient-just-wont-listen-to-you/1470/.

9 Patricia Marshall, "'Cultural Competence' and Informed Consent in International Health Research," *Cambridge Quarterly of Health Care Ethics* 17 (2008), 207.

10 Clifford Geertz, "Religion as a Cultural System," in *The Interpretation of Cultures: Selected Essays* (New York: Basic Books, 1973), 89.

11 Clifford Geertz, "Thick Description: Toward an Interpretive Theory of Culture," in *The Interpretation of Cultures: Selected Essays* (New York: Basic Books, 1973), 9.

12 Arthur Kleinman, *Writing at the Margins: Discourse between Anthropology and Medicine* (Berkeley: University of California Press, 1997), 8.

13 Harold Koenig, *Spiritualty and Patient Care: Why, How, When, and What*, 2nd ed. (Philadelphia: Templeton Foundation Press, 2007), 15–36.

14 Christina Puchalski and Anna Romer, "Taking a Spiritual History Allows Clinicians to Understand Patients More Fully," *Journal of Palliative Medicine* 3 (2000): 129–137.

15 On the definitional problem of religion and on defining the study of religion, see Diana Eck, "Dialogue and Method: Reconstructing the Study of Religion," in *A Magic Still Dwells: Comparative Religion in the Postmodern Age*, eds. Kimberley Patton and Benjamin Ray (Berkeley: University of California Press, 2000), 131–149. Also see Willi Braun and Russell McCutcheon, eds., *Guide to the Study of Religion* (London: Cassell, 2000).

16 Harold Koenig, *Faith and Mental Health: Religious Resources for Healing* (Philadelphia: Templeton Foundation Press, 2005), 44.

17 See Kenneth Pargament, *The Psychology of Religion and Coping: Theory, Research, Practice* (New York: The Guilford Press, 1997), 21–33.

18 See Gavin Flood, *An Introduction to Hinduism* (Cambridge: Cambridge University Press, 2004).

19 Manoj Shah and Siroj Sorajjakool, "Hinduism," in *World Religions for Health Care Professionals*, eds. Siroj Sorajjakool, Mark Carr, and Julius Nam (New York: Routledge, 2010), 39.

20 For these basic facts on Hinduism and more, see Huston Smith, *The Illustrated World's Religions: A Guide to Our Wisdom Traditions* (New York: HarperSanFrancisco, 1994), 17–57.

21 Manoj Shah and Siroj Sorajjakool, "Hinduism," 40–45.

22 Ibid., 40.

23 Prakash Desai, "Indian Religion and the Ayurvedic Tradtion," in *Oxford Textbook of Spirituality in Health Care*, eds. Mark Cobb, Christina Puchalski, and Bruce Rumbold (Oxford: Oxford University Press, 2012), 37.

24 Sudhir Kakar, *Shamans, Mystics, Doctors: A Psychological Inquiry into India and Its Healing Traditions* (Chicago: University of Chicago Press, 1982), 219.

25 See Desai, "Indian Religion and the Ayurvedic Tradtion," 40; as well as Manoj Shah and Siroj Sorajjakool, "Hinduism," 41–43.

26 Manoj Shah and Siroj Sorajjakool, "Hinduism," 41.

27 Ibid., 42.

28 Ibid., 44–45.

29 Koenig, *Spiritualty and Patient Care*, 215–218.

30 Purnell, *Guide to Culturally Competent Health Care*, 198–199.

31 For these basic facts on Buddhism and more, see Huston Smith, *The Illustrated World's Religions*, 58–97.

32 Kathleen Gregory, "Buddhism: Perspectives for the Contemporary World," in *Oxford Textbook of Spirituality in Health Care*, eds. Mark Cobb, Christina Puchalski, and Bruce Rumbold (Oxford: Oxford University Press, 2012), 11.

33 For more on the four noble truths, see Peter Harvey, *An Introduction to Buddhism: Teachings, History and Practices* (Cambridge: Cambridge University Press, 1990), 47–72.

34 Siroj Sorajjakool and Supaporn Naewbood, "Buddhism," in *World Religions for Health Care Professionals*, eds., Siroj Sorajjakool, Mark Carr, and Julius Nam (New York: Routledge, 2010), 55.

35 Ibid.

36 Harvey, *An Introduction to Buddhism*, 202.

37 Sorajjakool and Naewbood, "Buddhism," 58.

38 Ibid., 55–60.

39 Koenig, *Spiritualty and Patient Care*, 219.

40 For an introduction to Judaism, see Nicholas de Lange, *An Introduction to Judaism* (Cambridge: Cambridge University Press, 2000).

41 Douglas Kohn, "Judaism," in *World Religions for Health Care Professionals*, eds. Siroj Sorajjakool, Mark Carr, and Julius Nam (New York: Routledge, 2010), 114.

42 Ibid., 123.

43 Ibid., 120–128.

44 Ibid.,120.

45 Dawn Smith et al., "Male Circumcision in the United States for the Prevention of HIV Infection and Other Adverse Health Outcomes: Report from a CDC Consultation," *Public Health Reports* 125 (2010): 72–82.

46 Kohn, "Judaism," 120–128.

47 Koenig, *Spiritualty and Patient Care*, 206–210.

48 Dan Cohn-Sherbok, "Judaism," in *Oxford Textbook of Spirituality in Health Care*, eds. Mark Cobb, Christina Puchalski, and Bruce Rumbold (Oxford: Oxford University Press, 2012), 67.

49 For these basic facts on Christianity and more, see Huston Smith, *The Illustrated World's Religions*, 204–229.

50 For more on Christian history, see Alister McGrath, *Christian History: An Introduction* (Malden, MA: Wiley-Blackwell, 2013).

51 Alister McGrath, "Christianity," in *Oxford Textbook of Spirituality in Health Care*, eds. Mark Cobb, Christina Puchalski, and Bruce Rumbold (Oxford: Oxford University Press, 2012), 26.

52 David Larson, "Christianity," in *World Religions for Health Care Professionals*, eds. Siroj Sorajjakool, Mark Carr, and Julius Nam (New York: Routledge, 2010), 137–144.

53 Consider the cases of Karen Ann Quinlan and Terri Schiavo; see Gregory Pence, *Classic Cases in Medical Ethics: Accounts of the Cases that Have Shaped and Define Medical Ethics* (Boston: McGraw-Hill, 2008).

54 Timothy Quill, *Caring for Patients at the End of Life: Facing an Uncertain Future Together* (Oxford: Oxford University Press, 2001), 165–174.

55 David Larson, "Christianity," 139–140. Also see Robert Gagnon, *The Bible and Homosexual Practice: Texts and Hermeneutics* (Nashville, TN: Abingdon Press, 2001).

56 David Larson, "Christianity," 140.

57 See Donald Capps and Nathan Carlin, *Living in Limbo: Life in the Midst of Uncertainty* (Eugene, OR: Cascade Books, 2010).

58 Koenig, *Spiritualty and Patient Care*, 189–206.

59 For an introduction to Islam, see David Waines, *An Introduction to Islam* (Cambridge: Cambridge University Press, 1995).

60 For a brief overview of Islam, see Huston Smith, *The Illustrated World's Religions*, 144–177.

61 Ibid., 160–163.

62 Aasim Padela, "Islamic Medical Ethics: A Primer," *Bioethics* 21 (2007): 169–178.

63 Hamid Mavani, "Islam," in *World Religions for Health Care Professionals*, eds. Siroj Sorajjakool, Mark Carr, and Julius Nam (New York: Routledge, 2010), 103.

64 See Peter Brown, *The Body and Society: Men, Women, and Sexual Renunciation in Early Christianity* (New York: Columbia University Press, 1988).

65 Mavani, "Islam," 106.

66 Ibid., 104–110.

67 Ibid., 110.

68 Koenig, *Spiritualty and Patient Care*, 210–214.

69 Abdulaziz Sachedina, "Islam," in *Oxford Textbook of Spirituality in Health Care*, eds. Mark Cobb, Christina Puchalski, and Bruce Rumbold (Oxford: Oxford University Press, 2012), 62.

70 Quoted in Joan Anderson, Sheryl Reimer Kirkham, Nancy Waxler-Morrison, Carol Herbert, Maureen Murphy, and Elizabeth Richardson, "Conclusion," in *Cross-Cultural Caring: A Handbook for Health Professionals*, 2nd ed., Nancy Waxler-Morrison, Joan Anderson, Elizabeth Richardson, and Natalie Cambers, eds. (Vancouver: UBC Press, 2005), 343.

71 Ibid., 343–344.

72 Christina Puchalski and Anna Romer, "Taking a Spiritual History."

73 Eric Cassell, *The Nature of Suffering and the Goals of Medicine*, 2nd ed. (Oxford: Oxford University Press, 2204), xii.

74 Nancy Waxler-Morrison and Joan Anderson, "Introduction: The Need for Culturally Sensitive Health Care," in *Cross-Cultural Caring: A Handbook for Health Professionals*, 2nd ed., eds. Nancy Waxler-Morrison, Joan Anderson, Elizabeth Richardson, and Natalie Cambers (Vancouver: UBC Press, 2005), 1.

20 RELIGION AND HEALTH

1 William James, *The Varieties of Religious Experience* (New York: Simon & Schuster, 1997), 194–195.

2 Ibid., 109.

3 David M. Wulff, *Psychology of Religion: Classic and Contemporary*, 2nd ed. (New York: John Wiley and Sons, 1997), 205–206.

4 Harold G. Koenig, *Spirituality in Patient Care: Why, How, When, and What*, 2nd ed. (Philadelphia: Templeton Foundation Press, 2007), back cover. Our emphasis.

5 Robert Park, "Fraud in Science," *Social Research* 75 (2008): 1149. Also see Herbert Benson, et al., "Study of Therapeutic Effects of Intercessory Prayer (STEP) in Cardiac Bypass Patients: A Multicenter Randomized Trial of Uncertainty and Certainty of Receiving Intercessory Prayer," *American Heart Journal* 151 (2006): 934–942.

6 See, for example, Harold G. Koenig, Michael E. McCullough, and David B. Larson, eds., *Handbook of Religion and Health* (New York: Oxford University Press, 2001). Also see Harold G. Koenig, Dana King, and Verna Carson, eds., *Handbook of Religion and Health*, 2nd ed. (New York: Oxford University Press, 2012).

7 Hisham Abu-Raiya and Kenneth Pargament, "On the Links between Religion and Health: What Has the Empirical Research Taught Us?" in *The Oxford Textbook of Spirituality in Healthcare*, eds. Mark Cobb, Christina Puchalski, and Bruce Rumbold (Oxford: Oxford University Press, 2012), 335–337.

8 William B. Parsons, "Psychology of Religion," in *The Encyclopedia of Religion*, ed. Lindsay Jones, 2nd ed. (New York: Macmillan, 2005).

9 Ralph W. Hood Jr., et al., *The Psychology of Religion: An Empirical Approach*, 2nd ed. (New York: The Guilford Press, 1996), vii. The field of religion and health can also be seen as growing out of epidemiology. Unlike psychology of religion, epidemiology of religion has not been recognized as a field in its own right. Indeed, the term "epidemiology of religion" was not coined until the 1980s. See Jeffrey S. Levin and Harold Y. Vanderpool, "Is Frequent Religious Attendance Really Conducive to Better Health? Toward an Epidemiology of Religion," *Social Science & Medicine* 24 (1987): 589–600. Also, an important essay in establishing epidemiology of religion was published in 1987 by Jeffrey Levin and Preston Schiller. They note some of the growing interest in the potential associations between religion and health but point out that, at the time of writing, "next to nothing has been accomplished in terms of the refinement of concepts or measures" [see Jeffrey S. Levin and Preston L. Schiller, "Is There a Religious Factor in Health?" *Journal of Religion and Health* 26 (1987): 10]. They also note that a synthesis of findings had not yet been compiled. And so in their article they review theoretical and methodological issues and empirical findings in more than 200 research studies on the association between religion and health, covering such topics as cardiovascular disease, hypertension and stroke, and various types of cancer.

10 George C. Anderson, "Editorial," *Journal of Religion and Health* 1 (1961): 10.

11 Jeffrey S. Levin, "Foreword," in *Handbook of Religion and Health*, eds. Harold G. Koenig, Michael E. McCullough, and David B. Larson (New York: Oxford University Press, 2001), vii.

12 Larry Dossey, "Foreword," in *God, Faith, and Health: Exploring the Spirituality-Healing Connection*, Jeffrey Levin (New York: John Wiley and Sons, 2001), vii.

13 Jeffrey Levin, *God, Faith, and Health: Exploring the Spirituality-Healing Connection* (New York: John Wiley and Sons, 2001), 1–2.

14 Ibid., 7.

15 Ibid., 3, 23–29.

16 Koenig, *Spirituality in Patient Care*, 55.

17 Daniel E. Hall, Keith G. Meador, and Harold G. Koenig, "Measuring Religiousness in Health Research: Review and Critique," *Journal of Religion and Health* 47 (2008): 134–163.

18 Hall, Meador, and Koenig, "Measuring Religiousness in Health Research," 141. The authors reference an example of a study that tried to control for social connections: William J. Strawbridge, et al., "Frequent Attendance at Religious Services and Mortality Over 28 Years," *American Journal of Public Health* 87 (1997): 957–961.

19 Hall, Meador, and Koenig, "Measuring Religiousness in Health Research," 141. The authors reference Levin and Vanderpool, "Is Frequent Religious Attendance Really Conducive to Better Health?"

20 Hall, Meador, and Koenig, "Measuring Religiousness in Health Research," 140. The authors reference Alvan R. Feinstein, "Appraising the Success of Caring," in *The Lost Art of Caring: A*

Challenge to Health Professionals, Families, Communities, and Society, eds. Leighton E. Cluff and Robert H. Binstock (Baltimore, MD: Johns Hopkins University Press, 2001), 201–218.

21 Robert C. Fuller, *Spiritual, But Not Religious: Understanding Unchurched America* (New York: Oxford University Press, 2001).

22 Hall, Meador, and Koenig, "Measuring Religiousness in Health Research," 142.

23 Gordon W. Allport, *The Nature of Prejudice* (Cambridge, MA: Addison-Wesley Publishing, 1954).

24 Hall, Meador, and Koenig, "Measuring Religiousness in Health Research," 144.

25 Hall, Meador, and Koenig, "Measuring Religiousness in Health Research," 143. The authors reference Lee A. Kirkpatrick and Ralph W. Hood, Jr., "Intrinsic-Extrinsic Religious Orientation: The Boon or Bane of Contemporary Psychology of Religion," *Journal for the Scientific Study of Religion* 29 (1990): 442–462; and Lee A. Kirkpatrick and Ralph W. Hood, Jr., "Rub-A-Dub-dub: Who's in the Tub? Reply to Masters," *Journal for the Scientific Study of Religion* 30 (1991): 318–321.

26 Hall, Meador, and Koenig, "Measuring Religiousness in Health Research," 145. The authors reference Thomas G. Plante and Marcus T. Boccaccini, "Reliability and Validity of the Santa Clara Strength of Religious Faith Questionnaire," *Pastoral Psychology* 45 (1997): 429–437; and Thomas G. Plante and Marcus T. Boccaccini, "The Santa Clara Strength of Religious Faith Questionnaire," *Pastoral Psychology* 45 (1997) 375–387.

27 Hall, Meador, and Koenig, "Measuring Religiousness in Health Research," 146. The authors reference Harold G. Koenig, George R. Parkerson Jr., and Keith G. Meador, "Religion Index for Psychiatric Research," *American Journal of Psychiatry* 154 (1997): 885–886.

28 Hall, Meador, and Koenig, "Measuring Religiousness in Health Research," 146. The authors reference Fetzer/NIA Working Group, *Supplemental Appendix to the Multidimensional Measurement of Religiousness/Spirituality for Use in Health Research* (Kalamazoo, MI: John E. Fetzer Institute, 1999); and Ellen L. Idler, et al., "Measuring Multiple Dimensions of Religion and Spirituality for Health Research: Conceptual Background and Findings from the 1998 General Social Survey," *Research on Aging* 25 (2003): 327–265.

29 Hall, Meador, and Koenig, "Measuring Religiousness in Health Research," 146. The authors reference Jimmie C. Holland, et al., "A Brief Spiritual Beliefs Inventory for Use in Quality of Life Research in Life-Threatening Illness," *Psycho-Oncology* 7 (1998): 460–469.

30 Hall, Meador, and Koenig, "Measuring Religiousness in Health Research," 150. The authors reference Kenneth I. Pargament, et al., "Patterns of Positive and Negative Religious Coping with Major Life Stressors," *Journal for the Scientific Study of Religion* 37 (1998): 710–724. Also see Kenneth Pargament, *The Psychology of Religion and Coping* (New York: The Guilford Press, 1997).

31 Hall, Meador, and Koenig, "Measuring Religiousness in Health Research," 148.

32 C. Daniel Batson, "Religion as Prosocial: Agent or Double-Agent?" *Journal for the Scientific Psychosomatik, Medizinische Psychologie* 52 (1976): 306–313.

33 James W. Fowler, *Stages of Faith* (San Francisco: Harper and Row, 1981).

34 See Ralph W. Hood, Jr., "The Construction and Preliminary Validation of a Measure of Reported Mystical Experience," *Journal for the Scientific Study of Religion* 14 (1975): 29–41.

35 Hall, Meador, and Koenig, "Measuring Religiousness in Health Research," 153. The authors reference Lynn G. Underwood and Jeanne A. Teresi, "The Daily Spiritual Experience Scale: Development, Theoretical Description, Reliability, Exploratory Factor Analysis, and Preliminary Construct Validity Using Health-Related Data," *Annals of Behavioral Medicine* 24 (2002): 22–23.

36 For these various critiques, see Larry Dossey, "Foreword," viii.

37 Daniel Sulmasy, *The Rebirth of the Clinic: An Introduction to Spirituality in Health Care* (Washington, DC: Georgetown University Press, 2006), 115–120. Also see Joel Shuman and Keith Meador, *Heal Thyself: Spirituality, Medicine, and the Distortion of Christianity* (Oxford: Oxford University Press, 2003).

38 See Richard Sloan, et al., "Religion, Spirituality, and Medicine," *The Lancet* 353 (1999): 664–667; Richard Sloan, *Blind Faith: The Unholy Alliance of Religion and Medicine* (New York: St. Martin's Press, 2006).

39 See Harold Koenig, et al., "Religion, Spirituality, and Medicine: A Rebuttal to Skeptics," *International Journal of Psychiatry in Medicine* 29 (1999): 123–131; Harold Koenig, "Commentary: Why Do Research on Spirituality and Health, and What Do the Results Mean?" *Journal of Religion and Health* 51 (2012): 460–467.

40 See Harold Koenig, "Religion, Spirituality, and Medicine: Research Findings and Implications for Clinical Practice," *Southern Medical Journal* 97 (2004): 1194–1200.

21 RELIGION AND REALITY

1 William Blake, *William Blake: Selected Poetry*, ed. W. H. Stevenson (London: Penguin, 1988), 73.

2 Nancy Kehoe, *Wrestling with Our Inner Angels: Faith, Mental Illness, and the Journey to Wholeness* (San Francisco: Jossey-Bass, 2009), xvii–xviii.

3 Ibid., xvi.

4 One striking study involved putting three men who believed they were Jesus in a room together with the hope that these men could see through their delusion. See Milton Rokeach, *The Three Christs of Ypsilanti: A Psychological Study* (New York: Knopf, 1964).

5 Kehoe, *Wrestling with Our Inner Angels*, xix.

6 Some have called such an approach "biopsychosocial-spiritual." See Daniel Sulmasy, "A Biopsychosocial-Spiritual Model for the Care of Patients at the End of Life," *The Gerontologist* 42 (2002): 24–33.

7 See, e.g., Kenneth Pargament, *Spiritually Integrated Psychotherapy: Understanding and Addressing the Sacred* (New York: Guilford Press, 2007).

8 See Bernard Spilka, "Psychology of Religion: Empirical Approaches," in *Religion and Psychology: Mapping the Terrain*, eds. Diane E. Jonte-Pace and William B. Parson (New York: Routledge, 2001), 30.

9 Sigmund Freud, "A Religious Experience," in *The Standard Edition of the Complete Psychological Works of Sigmund Freud*, ed. and trans. James Strachey, vol. 21 (London: Vintage, 2001), 167–172 (first published 1928). All quotations in this section are from this essay. Also see Nathan Carlin, "A Religious Experience: A Psychological Interpretation of Kevin Kelly's Conversion to Christianity," *Pastoral Psychology* 62 (2013): 587–605. In this article, I provide a similar summary of Freud's essay.

10 Sigmund Freud, *The Future of an Illusion*, in *The Standard Edition of the Complete Psychological Works of Sigmund Freud*, ed. and trans. James Strachey, vol. 21 (London: Vintage, 2001), 1–56 (first published 1927).

11 Andrew Sullivan, *Love Undetectable: Notes on Friendship, Sex, and Survival* (New York: Vintage, 1999), 25–32. The material and quotations from this section come from these pages.

12 Fred Frohock, *Lives of the Psychics: The Shared Worlds of Science and Mysticism* (Chicago: University of Chicago Press, 2000), 145.

13 Ibid., 146–148.

14 Frederic Myers, *Human Personality and Its Survival of Bodily Death* (London: Longmans, 1903).

15 Sam Parnia, D. G. Waller, R. Yeates, and P. Fenwick, "A Qualitative and Quantitative Study of the Incidence, Features and Aetiology of Near Death Experiences in Cardiac Arrest Survivors," *Resuscitation* 48 (2001): 149–156.

16 David Derbyshire, "Scientists to Uncover the Truth of Out-of-Body Experiences," *Daily Mail*, September 19, 2008, accessed on April 2, 2013, http://www.dailymail.co.uk/sciencetech/article-1057506/Scientists-uncover-truth-body-experiences.html.

17 Rachel Stevenson, "Postcards from Heaven: Scientists to Study Near-Death Experiences," *The Guardian*, News Blog, September 18, 2008, accessed April 2, 2013, http://www.guardian.co.uk/news/blog/2008/sep/18/research.

18 William Styron, *Darkness Visible: A Memoir of Madness* (New York: Vintage, 1992). Unless otherwise noted, the quotations in this section come from the final section of the book (see pages 81–83).

19 Ibid., 1.

20 See, for example, Robert Segal, "In Defense of Reductionism," *Journal of the American Academy of Religion* 51 (1983): 97–124.

21 On this point, see William Parsons, *The Enigma of the Oceanic Feeling: Revisioning the Psychoanalytic Theory of Mysticism* (New York: Oxford University Press, 1999).

22 Rudolf Otto, *The Idea of the Holy*, trans. John Harvey (New York: Oxford University Press, 1923).

23 Styron, *Darkness Visible*, 7.

24 See Steven Miles, "A Challenge to Licensing Boards: The Stigma of Mental Illness," *JAMA* 280 (1998): 865; also see Kay Jamison, *An Unquiet Mind: A Memoir of Moods and Madness* (New York: Vintage, 1996).

25 Clifford Geertz, *Interpretation of Cultures* (New York: Basic Books, 1973).

26 See David Roe and Larry Davidson, "Self and Narrative in Schizophrenia: Time to Author a New Story," *Medical Humanities* 31 (2005): 89–94. Also see Albert Rothenberg, "Creativity, Self Creation, and the Treatment of Mental Illness," *Medical Humanities* 32 (2006): 14–19.

27 Paul Crawford and Charley Baker, "Literature and Madness: Fiction for Students and Professionals," *Journal of Medical Humanities* 30 (2009): 237–251.

28 Paula Gardner, "Distorted Packaging: Marketing Depression as Illness, Drugs as Cure," *Journal of Medical Humanities* 24 (2003): 105–130.

29 Michel Foucault, *Madness and Civilization: A History of Insanity in the Age of Reason*, trans. Richard Howard (New York: Pantheon Books, 1965).

30 For example, see Richard Tithecott, *Of Men and Monsters: Jeffrey Dahmer and the Construction of the Serial Killer* (Madison: University of Wisconsin Press, 1997) for a Foucauldian perspective on the construction of the serial killer and the construction of mental illness.

31 Geoff Hamilton, "Mythos and Mental Illness," *Journal of Medical Humanities* 29 (2008): 231–242.

32 See, for example, Rosemary Radford Ruether, *Many Forms of Madness: A Family's Struggle with Mental Illness and the Mental Health System* (Minneapolis: Fortress, 2010); Nick Flynn, *Another Bullshit Night in Suck City* (New York: W. W. Norton, 2005); Susanna Kaysen, *Girl, Interrupted* (New York: Vintage, 1994).

33 Anne Hawkins, "Pathography: Patient Narratives of Illness," *Western Journal of Medicine* 171 (1999): 127–129; Anne Jones, "Literature and Medicine: Narratives of Mental Illness," *The Lancet* 350 (1997): 359–361.

34 Jonathan Metzl, *The Protest Psychosis: How Schizophrenia became a Black Disease* (Boston: Beacon Press, 2009).

22 RELIGION AND BIOETHICS

1 Laurie Zoloth, "Faith and Reasoning(s): Bioethics, Religion, and Prophetic Necessity," in *Notes from a Narrow Ridge: Religion and Bioethics*, eds. Dena Davis and Laurie Zoloth (Hagerstown, MD: University Publishing Group, 1999), 247.

2 Albert Jonsen, "A History of Religion and Bioethics," in *Handbook of Bioethics and Religion*, ed. David Guinn (Oxford: Oxford University Press, 2006), 23.

3 See http://www.asbh.org/about/history/index.html. Also see Jonsen, "A History of Religion and Bioethics," 32.

4 Albert Jonsen, *The Birth of Bioethics* (New York: Oxford University Press, 2003).

5 Albert Jonsen and Stephen Toulmin, *The Abuse of Casuistry: A History of Moral Reasoning* (Berkeley: University of California Press, 1988).

6 Jonsen, "A History of Religion and Bioethics," 23–36.

7 Ibid., 25.

8 Ibid., 27.

9 Ibid.

10 Joseph Fletcher, *Morals and Medicine* (Princeton, NJ: Princeton University Press, 1954).

11 Joseph Fletcher, *Situation Ethics: The New Morality* (Philadelphia: Westminster Press, 1966).

12 Paul Ramsey, *Basic Christian Ethics* (New York: Scribner, 1950).

13 Jonsen, "A History of Religion and Bioethics," 28.

14 Paul Ramsey, *The Patient as Person: Explorations in Medical Ethics* (New Haven, CT: Yale University Press, 1970).

15 Jonsen, "A History of Religion and Bioethics," 29.

16 Ibid., 30–32.

17 Daniel Callahan, "Religion and the Secularization of Bioethics," *The Hastings Center Report* 20 (1990): 2–4.

18 Jonsen, "A History of Religion and Bioethics," 33.

19 Immanuel Jacobovits, *Jewish Medical Ethics: A Comparative and Historical Study of the Jewish Religious Attitude to Medicine and Its Practice* (New York: Philosophical Library, 1959).

20 J. David Bleich, *Judaism and Healing: Halakhic Perspectives* (New York: Ktav Publishing House, 1981).

21 Baruch Brody, *Life and Death Decision Making* (New York: Oxford University Press, 1988).

22 Jonsen, "A History of Religion and Bioethics," 32–33.

23 John Evans, "The Tension Between Progressive Bioethics and Religion," in *Progress in Bioethics: Sciences, Policy, and Politics*, eds. Jonathan Moreno and Sam Berger (Cambridge, MA: MIT Press, 2010), 119–141.

24 Tom Beauchamp and James Childress, *Principles of Biomedical Ethics*, 7th ed. (New York: Oxford University Press, 2013).

25 James Gustafson, quoted in John Evans, "The Tension between Progressive Bioethics and Religion," 123.

26 Kevin Wildes, "Religion in Bioethics: A Rebirth," *Christian Bioethics* 8 (2002): 163–174.

27 It will become more difficult as ASBH develops and refines credentialing standards for clinical ethics.

28 James Gustafson, *The Contributions of Theology to Medical Ethics* (Milwaukee, WI: Marquette University Press, 2006).

29 Ibid., 16.

30 Ibid., 18–19, 22.

31 Ibid., 93–94.

32 Ibid., p. 95.

33 Paul Ramsey, "On (Only) Caring for the Dying," in *The Essential Paul Ramsey: A Collection*, eds. William Werpehowski and Stephen Crocco (New Haven, CT: Yale University Press, 1994), 195–222.

34 Ibid., 222.

35 Bernard Lo, *Resolving Ethical Dilemmas*, 4th ed. (Philadelphia: Wolters Kluwer, 2009), 119–128.

36 Paul Ramsey, "The Indignity of 'Death with Dignity,'" in *The Essential Paul Ramsey: A Collection*, eds. William Werpehowski and Stephen Crocco (New Haven, CT: Yale University Press, 1994), 223–246.

37 Joseph Fletcher, "Four Indicators of Humanhood – The Enquiry Matures," in *On Moral Medicine: Theological Perspectives in Medical Ethics*, 2nd ed., eds. Stephen Lammers and Allen Verhey (Grand Rapids, MI: William B. Eerdmans Publishing Company, 1998), 377.

38 The National Commission for the Protection of Human Subjects of Biomedical and Behavioral Research, "The Belmont Report," *Department of Health, Education, and Welfare*, April 18, 1979, http://www.hhs.gov/ohrp/humansubjects/guidance/belmont.html.

39 R. Gillon, "Ethics Needs Principles – Four Can Encompass the Rest – and Respect for Autonomy Should Be 'First among Equals,'" *Journal of Medical Ethics* 29 (2003): 307–31.

40 Karen Lebacqz, "Philosophy, Theology, and the Claims of Justice," in *Handbook of Bioethics and Religion*, ed. David Guinn (Oxford: Oxford University Press, 2006), 253–263.

41 See Nathan Carlin, Thomas Cole, and Henry Strobel, "Guidance from the Humanities for Professional Formation," in *Oxford Textbook of Spirituality in Healthcare*, eds. Mark Cobb, Christina Puchalski, and Bruce Rumbold (Oxford: Oxford University Press, 2012), 443–450.

42 Lebacqz, "Philosophy, Theology, and the Claims of Justice," 257.

43 Ibid., 260.

44 William May, "Code and Covenant or Philanthropy and Contract?" in *On Moral Medicine: Theological Perspectives in Medical Ethics*, 2nd ed., eds. Stephen Lammers and Allen Verhey (Grand Rapids, MI: William B. Eerdmans Publishing Company, 1998), 121–137.

45 Ibid., 128.

46 H. Tristram Engelhardt Jr., *The Foundations of Bioethics*, 2nd ed. (New York: Oxford University Press, 1996).

47 H. Tristram Engelhardt Jr., "Bioethics in Pluralistic Societies," *Perspectives in Biology and Medicine* 26 (1982): 64–78.

48 Ibid., 66.

49 Ibid., 70.

50 Ibid., 66.

51 Bernard Lo, *Resolving Ethical Dilemmas*, 5–6, 182–189. Also see Jeffrey Spike, Thomas Cole, and Richard Buday, *The Brewsters: An Interactive Adventure in Ethics for the Health Professions* (Houston: Archimage, Inc., 2012), 161–162.

52 Engelhardt, Jr., "Bioethics in Pluralistic Societies," 76–77.

53 In contrast to Engelhardt's position, Laurence McCullough and Frank Chervenak offer a beneficence-based clinical ethics in *Ethics in Obstetrics and Gynecology*. Their model, while perhaps positivistic, offers one way that bioethics can offer content-full recommendations for specific circumstances. See Laurence McCullough and Frank Chervenak, *Ethics in Obstetrics and Gynecology* (New York: Oxford University Press, 1994).

54 Daniel Callahan, "Religion and the Secularization of Bioethics," 2.

55 Courtney Campbell, "Bioethics and the Spirit of Secularism," in *Secular Bioethics in Theological Perspective*, ed. Earl Shelp (Dordrecht, NL: Kluwer Academic Publishers, 1996), 4.

56 One of the authors of this textbook (Nathan Carlin) organized a conference on "Social Justice and the Health Professions," held at the University of Texas Health Science Center at Houston in 2011, and the papers from this conference became a special issue of *Pastoral Psychology*. In the special issue, Carlin outlined a vision for how pastoral theologians can contribute to bioethics, with the key point being that pastoral theologians ought to focus on both macro and micro issues in bioethics by building on established areas of intersections between bioethics and theology (e.g., justice), by drawing on the traditional resources of pastoral theology (e.g., psychology), and by following new directions in the field (e.g., by employing social scientific disciplines beyond psychology). See Nathan Carlin, "Bioethics and Pastoral Concern: Some Possible New Direction in Pastoral Theology," *Pastoral Psychology* 62 (2013): 129–138. Also, for a concrete example of how pastoral theology can contribute to bioethics, see the discussion of pastoral theologian Robert Dykstra in Chapter 23. Some material noted above is taken in a slightly revised form from this article. Also see David Smith, ed., *Caring Well: Religion, Narrative, and Health Care Ethics* (Louisville, KY: Westminster John Knox Press, 2000).

57 David Guinn, ed., *Handbook of Bioethics and Religion* (Oxford: Oxford University Press, 2006).

58 David Guinn, "Introduction: Laying Some Ground Work," in *Handbook of Bioethics and Religion*, ed. David Guinn (Oxford: Oxford University Press, 2006), 3.

59 Ibid., 6.

60 Ibid.

61 Ibid., 11–15.

62 Consider this book: Barrington Moore, *Moral Purity and Persecution in History* (Princeton, NJ: Princeton University Press, 2000).

63 Guinn, "Introduction," 8.

64 Ibid.

65 Ibid., our emphasis.

66 Relatedly, see Diogenes Allen, *Christian Belief in a Postmodern World: The Full Wealth of Conviction* (Louisville, KY: Westminster/John Knox Press, 1989).

67 Guinn, "Introduction," 10.

68 Ibid.

69 Arthur Caplan, James McCartney, and Dominic Sisti, eds., *The Case of Terri Schiavo: Ethics at the End of Life* (Amherst, NY: Prometheus Books, 2006).

70 H. Tristram Engelhardt, Jr., "Towards a Christian Bioethics," *Christian Bioethics* 1 (1995): 1.

71 Jonsen, "A History of Religion and Bioethics," 33.

23 SUFFERING AND HOPE

1 Quoted in Jerome Groupman, *The Anatomy of Hope: How People Prevail in the Face of Illness* (New York: Random House, 2004), ix.

2 Paul Tillich, *The Shaking of the Foundations* (New York: Charles Scribner's Sons, 1948), 106.

3 Arthur Kleinman and Joan Kleinman, "The Appeal of Experience; The Dismay of Images: Cultural Appropriations of Suffering in Our Times," in *Social Suffering*, eds. Arthur Kleinman, Veena Das, and Margaret Lock (Berkeley: University of California Press, 1997), 4. The following discussion is based on pages 1–9.

4 See the PEW Forum on Religion and Public Life, "The Global Religious Landscape," December 18, 2012: http://www.pewforum.org/global-religious-landscape-exec.aspx.

5 Kenneth Pargament, *The Psychology of Religion and Coping: Theory, Research, Practice* (New York: The Guilford Press, 1997).

6 Eric Cassell, *The Nature of Suffering and the Goals of Medicine*, 2nd ed. (Oxford: Oxford University Press, 2004).

7 Ibid., xii.

8 Ibid., 36–41.

9 Ibid., xii.

10 Eric Cassell, "Diagnosing Suffering," *Annals of Internal Medicine* 131 (1999): 532.

11 We would add that Simone Weil has coined the term "affliction" for such suffering. See Simone Weil, "Human Personality," in *Simone Weil: An Anthology*, ed. Siân Miles (New York: Grove Press, 1986), 70.

12 Bernard Lo, et al., "Discussing Religious and Spiritual Issues at the End of Life: A Practical Guide for Physicians," *JAMA* 287 (2002): 749–754.

13 C. S. Lewis, *The Problem of Pain* (New York: Simon & Schuster, 1996), 23.

14 Jeffry Zurheide, *When Faith Is Tested: Pastoral Responses to Suffering and Tragic Death* (Minneapolis: Fortress Press, 1997), 19–25.

15 Gavin Flood, *An Introduction to Hinduism* (Cambridge: Cambridge University Press, 2004), 75–76.

16 Houston Smith, *The Illustrated World's Religions: A Guide to Our Wisdom Traditions* (New York: HarperSanFrancisco, 1994), 43–44.

17 Bernard Faure, *The Power of Denial: Buddhism, Purity, and Gender* (Princeton, NJ: Princeton University Press, 2003), 99–103.

18 Peter Harvey, *Introduction to Buddhism: Teachings, History and Practices* (Cambridge: Cambridge University Press, 1990), 39.

19 Chokyi Nyima Rinpoche (with David Shlim), *Medicine and Compassion: A Tibetan Lama's Guidance for Caregivers* (Boston: Wisdom Publications, 2006), 26.

20 David Smith, *Partnership with the Dying: Where Medicine and Ministry Should Meet* (New York: Rowman & Littlefield, 2005), 1–13, 39–62.

21 Robert Dykstra, "The Intimate Stanger," in *Images of Pastoral Care*, ed. Robert Dykstra (St. Louis, MO: Chalice Press, 2005), 123–136.

22 Ibid., 124.

23 Donald Capps, "The Agent of Hope," in *Images of Pastoral Care*, ed. Robert Dykstra (St. Louis, MO: Chalice Press, 2005), 189.

24 Ibid., 191.

25 Ibid., 193–194.

26 Sherwin Nuland, *How We Die: Reflections on Life's Final Chapter* (New York: Vintage Books, 1995), 222.

27 Ibid., 225.

28 Ibid., 229.

29 Ibid., 236.

30 Ibid.

31 Ibid., 241.

32 Ibid.

EPILOGUE

1 Quoted in Isaiah Berlin, *The Crooked Timber of Humanity: Chapters in the History of Ideas*, ed. Henry Hardy (New York: Alfred A. Knopf, 1991), vii.

2 John Stephens, *The Italian Renaissance: The Origins of Intellectual and Artistic Change before the Reformation* (London: Longman, 1990), chs. 3–5; Robert Proctor, *Education's Great Amnesia: Reconsidering the Humanities from Petrarch to Freud* (Bloomington: Indiana University Press, 1988), part one. See also Douglas Biow, *Doctors, Ambassadors, Secretaries: Humanism and the Professions in Renaissance Italy* (Chicago: University of Chicago Press, 2002).

3 Bruce Kimball, *Orators and Philosophers: A History of the Idea of Liberal Education* (New York: The College Board, 1995), chs. 2, 4, and 5.

4 See Jean Lyotard, *The Postmodern Condition: A Report on Knowledge*, trans. Geoff Bennington (Minneapolis: University of Minnesota Press, 1984).

5 Martha Nussbaum, *Cultivating Humanity: A History of Reform in Liberal Education* (Cambridge, MA: Harvard University Press, 1998); *Not for Profit: Why Democracy Needs the Humanities* (Princeton, NJ: Princeton University Press, 2010).

INDEX

religion and health and, 330–331
religion and mental illness and, 333–336
suffering in, 362–364
Bicêtre, 49
Bichat, Xavier, 49, 50
Billings, John Shaw, 4, 21–22, 65
bimaristans (Islamic hospitals), 91–93
bioethics
access to health care and, 286–287
conservative turn in religion and, 353–355
contemporary discussions in religion and, 352–355
emergence of, 1–2
emergency room research, 273–274
gender malleability theory and, 266–268
healthcare reform and, 285–286
Hinduism and, 297–299
historical evolution of, 252–255
history of religion and, 340–343
House, M.D. television show and, 164–165
moral philosophy and, 251–261
non-Christian perspectives in, 355
philosophy and, 255–257
pluralism and, 350–351
proceduralism and, 257–259
professional ethics and, 348–350
public policy and religion, 352
religion and, 259, 340–355
secularization in, 291–293
theological founders of, 343–351
Tuskegee Syphilis Study and, 272–273
world religions and, 296–308
Bioethics at the Movies, 154
"Bioethics in Pluralistic Societies" (Engelhardt), 350–351
biomedical reductionism
dehumanization in health care and, 1–2, 36–38
in medical education, 4–6
physicians' experiences with religion and, 329–330
biomedical science, medical education and prominence of, 4–6
biomedicine
birth of, 49–51
disease model of, 242–245
biopolitics, medical humanities and, 11–12
biopsychosocial model of medicine, 9–10
bioscience
knowledge theory and, 214–216
limits of education in, 199–201
biostatistical theory, normative model of disease and, 242–243
biotechnology, current and future trends in, 85–87
birth. *See* pregnancy and childbirth
birth control, in Christianity, 304–306
The Birth of Bioethics (Jonsen), 340–343
The Birth of the Clinic (Foucault), 264
Bise, Michael, 83–84, 84f4
Black and Blue (Hoberman), 270–272
Black Death, 45–46, 91–93, 107
Blake, William, 131, 327
Blanton-Peale Institute, 317–318
Bleich, J. David, 342–343

blood transfusions, artificial blood substitutes and, 273–274
bloodletting
as early medical practice, 48
early technology for, 75–76
Boccaccio, Giovanni, 91–93
body. *See also* autopsy; dissection
in Buddhism, 300–301
in Christianity, 304–306
death and dying and, 105, 109–110
disease and, 8–9, 77–78, 247–249
feminist theory concerning, 264–266, 268–270
gender and, 266–268
genetic revolution and knowledge of, 53–55
health in antiquity and, 27–29, 41–44
health in Middle Ages and, 44–46
in Hinduism, 297–299
holistic concepts of, 238–242
illness and awareness of, 127–128
in Islam, 306–308
in Judaism, 301–304
in medical education, 63–64
medical preoccupation with, 225–226
medical technology and research on, 81–84
mind and, 245–247
nanotechnology and, 85–87
near-death experiences and, 331–333
normative model of disease and, 242–245
in pain, 9–10
in poetry, 170–171
Renaissance medicine and, 30–31, 46–47
scientific study of, 47–48, 213–214
x-ray images of, 80–81
Body Trauma TV, 154, 163
The Body Project (Brumberg), 264–266
Bok, Sissela, 342
Bologna, University of, early medical education at, 59–60
Bonner, Thomas, 24
Book of Job, suffering in, 362–364
Boorse, Christopher, 237, 242–245, 249
Boston Doctors (Southworth), 271f17
bottom-up reasoning, bioethics and, 259
Bowditch, H. I., 65
Brahma (Hindu Creator), 297–299
Brahms, Johannes, 130
brain death concept, 114–115
brain function
mental illness and, 245–247
personhood and, 347
Brâncusi, Constantin, 303
Brandt, Allen, 272–273
BRCA 1 and 2, breast cancer and, 53–54
Breaking Bad (television show), 156
Britain. *See* Great Britain
Brody, Baruch, 342–343
Brody, Howard, 239
Broyard, Anatole, 168, 195
Brumberg, Joan, 264–266
Buber, Martin, 220

bubonic plague and, 45–46
challenges to, 64–68
Renaissance examination of, 46–47
syphilis and, 46–47
"Humpty Dumpty" theory of medicalization, 54–55
Hunsberger, Bruce, 317

"iatrine" (woman physician), 58–59
The Idea of the Holy (Otto), 333–336
identity formation, in medical humanities, 14–15
idiographic inquiry, medical humanities and, 328
The Idiot (Dostoevsky), 246–247
Ikiru (film), 140–143
illness. *See also* mental health and illness
disease vs., 9–10, 247–249
mental illness as, 245–247
narratives of, 117, 123–124, 125–136, 219–221
public health and, 89–90
impaired newborns, bioethics of caring for, 252–255
Incan Empire, epidemic disease and destruction
of, 93–94
*Incidental Findings: Lessons from My Patients in the Art
of Medicine* (Ofri), 190–192
income disparities, structural racism and, 270–272
India
early medical education in, 58
early medical technology in, 75
Indiana Jones and the Kingdom of the Crystal Skull
(film), 149–150
indigenous Americans, colonialism and disease among,
46–47, 93–94
"The Indignity of 'Death with Dignity'" (Ramsey),
345–346
infectious disease
in antiquity, 90–91
colonialism and, 93–94
epidemiologic transition and, 98–99
global health and, 99–102
mortality from, 52
prevention, vaccination and antibiotics for, 52
public health and, 89–90
influenza epidemic of 1918, 51–53
informed consent principle
artificial blood substitutes and, 273–274
bioethics and, 252–255, 350–351
end of life care and, 226
Inniss, Leslie, 162
Innocent II (Pope), 75–76
insanity. *See* mental illness
Institute of Medicine, 233–234
Institute on Human Values in Medicine, 5–6, 291–293
Institutional Review Boards, 252–255
integrated care systems, medical education and, 68–72
intellect, emotion vs., 175
intensive care units
death and dying and, 113
evolution of, 83
interdisciplinary humanities
bioethics and, 255–257
emergence of, 2–4
medical humanities as, 7

intergeneration, aging and, 143–145
intermittent positive pressure ventilation (IPPV)
technique, 82–83, 112–113
internships
in doctor show formula, 156–157
experiential learning and, 201–206
medical education and evolution of, 68–72
students' accounts of, 201
The Interns (television show), 156–157
intersex conditions, 266–268
Intersex Society of North America, 266–268
"The Intimate Stranger" (Dykstra), 366–367
IPPV (intermittent positive pressure ventilation)
technique, 82–83, 112–113
Iris (film), 146
"iron lung," 82–83
The Iron Lady (film), 147
Islam
early medical education and, 59–60
Judaism and, 301
medicine and, 306–308
public health and, 91–93

Jackson, Mark, 24
Jacobovitz, Immanuel, 342–343
Jacobs, Jason, 154, 163
James, William, 314–316, 317, 324–325
Jamison, Kay, 246–247, 333–336
Jefferson, Thomas, 94, 352
Jehovah's Witnesses, 294–296
Jenner, Edward, 51
Jews, barriers to medical education for, 68–72
Jhally, Sut, 162
Jimenez, Luis, 118f6
John Money controversy, 266–268
Johns Hopkins baby case, 252–255
Johns Hopkins Hospital Historical Club, 21–22
Johns Hopkins University Medical School, 66
history of medicine at, 22
medical education theory and, 4, 21–22
women students at, 67–68
Johnson, Lyndon Baines, 279
Joint Commission on Accreditation of Health Care
Organizations, hospice care coverage
and, 233–234
Jonas, Hans, 255–257, 342
Jones, Anne, 8, 336–337
Jones, James, 270–272
Jones, Therese, 7–8, 154
Jones, Tommy Lee, 149–151
Jonsen, Albert R., 226, 252–255, 291–293, 340–343
Jotterand, Fabrice, 211–212
Journal of Religion and Health, 317–318
The Journal of Medical Humanities, 164–165
Judaism
bioethics and, 342–343
early medical education and, 58–59
health and medicine in, 301–304
suffering in, 362–364
Juengst, Eric, 230
Jung, C. G., 317

justice and, 347–348
  pastoral theology, 366–367
  suffering and, 365–366
theorizing stories, illness narratives and, 133
Theravada Buddhism, 300–301
thermometer, 78
Thessalius, 58–59
"They Decide Who Lives, Who Dies" (Alexander), 252–255
thick description, cultural competency and, 294–296
third-party payers, corporate transformation of American medicine and, 36–38
Thomas Aquinas (St.), 304–306
Thomasma, David, 8–9
Thornton, Helen, 331–333
Thurneisser zun Thurn, Leonhart, 41–44, 43f2
Tillich, Paul, 358
The Time of Their Dying, 125–127
Tolstoy, Leo, 110–111, 375–376
Tomes, Nancy, 154
Tooley, Michael, 347
Toombs, S. Kay, 274
top-down reasoning, bioethics and, 259
Topol, Eric, 85–87
Toulmin, Stephen, 213, 259–261, 340–343
Trachtman, Howard, 156
transplants. *See* organ transplantation
Trautmann, Joanne, 185
Treichler, Paule, 154
Treno, Joan M., 233–234
trepanation, history of, 75
Treponema pallidum, syphilis and, 47
Trilling, Lionel, 2–4, 398n7
triple contract theory, bioethics and, 257–259
The Trip to Bountiful (film), 143–145, 149
Truman, Harry, 279
tuberculosis
  ancient Greek study of, 41–44
  childbirth and, 79–80
  global health and, 99–102
  streptomycin and, 52
  in twentieth century, 51–53
Tuesdays with Morrie (film), 117
Türck, Ludwig, 78
Turner, Leigh, 291–293
Turow, Joseph, 153, 157, 161–162, 163–164
Tuskeegee Syphilis Study, 52, 252–255, 272–273
12 Angry Men (film), 142–143
Typa A/H1N1 virus, 51–53
typhus
  in antiquity, 90–91
  in Renaissance, 46–47
typography, art of, 175–176, 175f10

UDDA (Uniform Determination of Death Act), 114–115
The Uncertainty of the Signs of Death and the Dangers of Precipitate Interments and Dissections, 109
Unforgiven (film), 149–151

Uniform Determination of Death Act (UDDA), 114–115
United Kingdom. *See* Great Britain
United States
  death and dying in, 111–117
  early medical education in, 63–64
  epidemics in, 93–94
  eugenics in, 96–97
  public health in, 94–96, 98–99
  reform of medical education in, 65–68
  technological development in, 80–81
  twentieth-century technological advances in, 81–84
universities. *See specific universities, e.g.* Michigan, University of
university-based medical education, emergence of, 63–64
urban medicine, emergence in modern era of, 36–38
urbanization
  disease and, 90
  public health and, 94–96
"Use of Force" (Williams), 184–185

vaccines, historical development of, 50–51
valetudianarias (Roman infirmaries), 90–91
value-laden disease models, 242–245
Van Calcar, Jan, 60–63
The Varieties of Religious Experience (James), 314–316
vata (Hindu elements), 297–299
Vaux, Kenneth, 341–342
Veatch, Robert, 257–259, 341–342
Vedas (Hindu sacred writings), 297–299
vegetative state, death and dying and, 114–115
Verstehen, knowledge theory and, 215
Vesalius, Andreas, 30–31, 48, 60–63, 62f3, 83–84, 117–119, 318–321
Vico, Giambattista, 214
Viljanen, Anna Maria, 8–9
Virchow, Rudolf, 50, 53
virtue ethics, bioethics and, 259
viruses, twentieth-century theories concerning, 51–53
Vishnu (Hindu Preserver), 297–299
visual diagnosis, opthalmoscopy and, 78
Von Helmholtz, Hermann, 78
vulnerability and aging, 145–147

Wakley, Thomas, 95
Walters, LeRoy, 341–342
Warner, John Harley, 22, 24
Warnock, Mary, 175
Washington, Harriet, 270–272, 273–274
water supply and public health, 90–91, 94–96
Watkins, Melanie, 202
Watson, James, 53
Wear, Delese, 7–8
Webb, Sidney, 96
Weber, Max, 215
Weinberg, Richard, 221–223
Welch, William, 22, 66
Wells, John, 163
Welsome, Eileen, 270–272
Wertenbaker, Lael Tucker, 125–127